The Founders of Operative Surgery

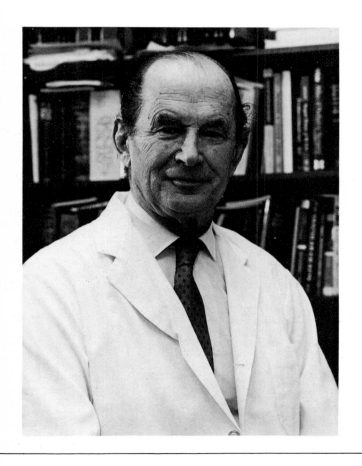

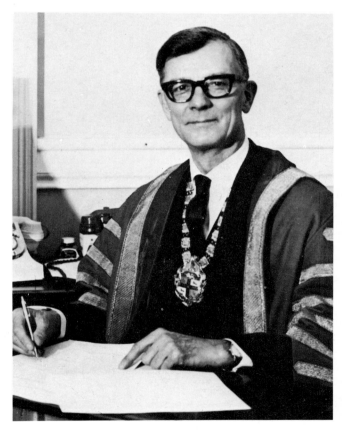

Charles Granville Rob MC, MChir, MD, FRCS, FACS
Professor of Surgery, Department of Surgery, Uniformed
Services University of the Health Sciences, F. Edward Hébert
School of Medicine, Bethesda, Maryland
Quondam: Professor of Surgery, St Mary's Hospital Medical
School, London 1950–1960;
Professor and Chairman, Department of Surgery, University of
Rochester, New York, 1960–1978;
Professor of Surgery, East Carolina University, 1978–1983

Lord Smith of Marlow KBE, MS, FRCS, Hon DSc
(Exeter and Leeds), Hon MD (Zurich), Hon FRACS,
Hon FRCS(Ed.), Hon FACS, Hon FRCS(Can.), Hon FRCSI,
Hon FRCS(SA), Hon FDS
Honorary Consulting Surgeon, St George's Hospital, London
Quondam: Surgeon, St George's Hospital, London,
1946–1978;
President of the Royal College of Surgeons of England,
1973–1977

Rob & Smith's
Operative Surgery

Vascular Surgery
Fourth Edition

Rob & Smith's
Operative Surgery

General Editors

Hugh Dudley ChM, FRCS(Ed.), FRACS, FRCS
Professor of Surgery, St Mary's Hospital, London, UK

David C. Carter MD, FRCS(Ed.), FRCS(Glas.)
St Mungo Professor of Surgery, University of Glasgow;
Honorary Consultant Surgeon, Royal Infirmary, Glasgow, UK

Rob & Smith's
Operative Surgery

Vascular Surgery

Fourth Edition

Edited by

James A. DeWeese MD, FACS
Professor and Chairman, Division of Cardiothoracic Surgery,
University of Rochester Medical Center, Rochester, New York, USA

Butterworths
London Boston Durban Singapore Sydney Toronto Wellington

© Butterworths 1985

First edition published in eight volumes 1956–1958
Second edition published in fourteen volumes 1968–1971
Third edition published in nineteen volumes 1976–1981
Fourth edition published 1983–1985

British Library Cataloguing in Publication Data
Rob, Charles
   Rob & Smith's operative surgery. – 4th ed.
   Vascular surgery.
   1. Surgery
   I. Title   II. Smith, Rodney Smith, *Baron*
   III. DeWeese, James A.   IV. Rob, Charles.
   Operative surgery
   617   RD31

   ISBN 0-407-00659-1

Library of Congress Cataloging in Publication Data
(Revised for pt. 3)
Main entry under title:

Rob & Smith's operative surgery

   Rev. ed. of: Operative surgery. 3rd. 1976–
   Includes bibliographies and index
   Contents: [1] Alimentary tract and abdominal wall.
1. General principles, oesophagus, stomach, duodenum, small intestine, abdominal wall, hernia / edited by Hugh Dudley – –[3] Vascular surgery / edited by James A. DeWeese.
   1. Surgery, Operative.   I. Rob, Charles.   II. Smith of Marlow, Rodney Smith, Baron, 1914– .   III. Dudley, Hugh Arnold Freeman.   IV. Pories, Walter J.
V. Carter, David C. (David Craig)   VI. Operative surgery. [DNLM: 1. Surgery, Operative.
WO 500 061 1982]
RD32.06   1983   617'.91   83-14465
ISBN 0-407-00651-6 (v. 1)

Volumes and Editors

Alimentary Tract and Abdominal Wall

1 **General Principles · Oesophagus · Stomach · Duodenum · Small Intestine · Abdominal Wall · Hernia**

Hugh Dudley ChM, FRCS(Ed.), FRACS, FRCS
Professor of Surgery, St Mary's Hospital, London, UK

2 **Liver · Portal Hypertension · Spleen · Biliary Tract · Pancreas**

Hugh Dudley ChM, FRCS(Ed.), FRACS, FRCS
Professor of Surgery, St Mary's Hospital, London, UK

3 **Colon, Rectum and Anus**

Ian P. Todd MS, MD(Tor), FRCS, DCH
Consulting Surgeon, St Bartholomew's Hospital, London;
Consultant Surgeon, St Mark's Hospital and
King Edward VII Hospital for Officers, London, UK

L. P. Fielding MB, FRCS
Chief of Surgery, St Mary's Hospital, Waterbury, Connecticut, USA;
Associate Professor of Surgery, Yale University, Connecticut, USA

Cardiac Surgery

Stuart W. Jamieson MB, BS, FRCS
Assistant Professor of Cardiovascular Surgery,
Stanford University School of Medicine, California, USA

Norman E. Shumway MD, PhD, FRCS
Professor and Chairman, Department of Cardiovascular Surgery,
Stanford University School of Medicine, California, USA

The Ear

John C. Ballantyne FRCS, HonFRCSI, DLO
Consultant Ear, Nose and Throat Surgeon,
Royal Free and King Edward VII Hospital for Officers, London, UK;
Honorary Consultant in Otolaryngology to the Army

Andrew Morrison FRCS, DLO
Senior Consultant Otolaryngologist, The London Hospital, UK

General Principles, Breast and Extracranial Endocrines

Hugh Dudley ChM, FRCS(Ed.), FRACS, FRCS
Professor of Surgery, St Mary's Hospital, London, UK

Walter J. Pories MD, FACS
Professor and Chairman, Department of Surgery, School of Medicine,
East Carolina University, Greenville, North Carolina, USA

Gynaecology and Obstetrics

J. M. Monaghan MB, FRCS(Ed.), MRCOG
Consultant Surgeon, Regional Department of Gynaecological Oncology,
Queen Elizabeth Hospital, Gateshead, UK

The Hand

Rolfe Birch FRCS
Consultant Orthopaedic Surgeon, PNI Unit and Hand Clinic,
Royal National Orthopaedic Hospital, London and
St Mary's Hospital, London, UK

Donal Brooks MA, MB, FRCS, FRSCI
Consulting Orthopaedic Surgeon, University College Hospital
and Royal National Orthopaedic Hospital, London, UK;
Civilian Consultant in Hand Surgery to the Royal Navy and
Royal Air Force

Neurosurgery

Lindsay Symon TD, FRCS, FRCS(Ed.)
Professor of Neurological Surgery, Institute of Neurology,
The National Hospital, Queen Square, London, UK

David G. T. Thomas MRCP, FRCSE
Senior lecturer and Consultant Neurosurgeon,
Institute of Neurology, The National Hospital,
Queen Square, London, UK

Kemp Clarke MD
Professor and Chairman, Division of Neurological Surgery,
Southwestern Medical School, Dallas, Texas, USA

Nose and Throat

John C. Ballantyne FRCS, HonFRCSI, DLO
Consultant Ear, Nose and Throat Surgeon,
Royal Free and King Edward VII Hospital for Officers, London, UK;
Honorary Consultant in Otolaryngology to the Army

D. F. N. Harrison MD, MS, FRCS, FRACS
Professor of Laryngology and Otology,
Royal National Throat, Nose and Ear Hospital, London, UK

Ophthalmic Surgery

Thomas A. Rice MD
Assistant Clinical Professor of Ophthalmology,
Case Western Reserve University School of Medicine,
Cleveland, Ohio, USA;
formerly of the Wilmer Ophthalmological Institute

Ronald G. Michels MD
Professor of Ophthalmology, The Wilmer Ophthalmological Institute,
The Johns Hopkins University School of Medicine,
Maryland, USA

Walter W. J. Stark MD
Professor of Ophthalmology, The Wilmer Ophthalmological Institute,
The Johns Hopkins University School of Medicine,
Maryland, USA

Orthopaedics (in 2 volumes)

George Bentley ChM, FRCS
Professor of Orthopaedic Surgery, Institute of Orthopaedics,
Royal National Orthopaedic Hospital, London, UK

Paediatric Surgery

L. Spitz PhD, FRCS
Nuffield Professor of Paediatric Surgery and Honorary
Consultant Paediatric Surgeon, The Hospital for Sick Children,
Great Ormond Street, London, UK

H. Homewood Nixon MA, MB, BChir, FRCS, HonFAAP
Consultant Paediatric Surgeon, The Hospital for Sick Children,
Great Ormond Street, London and Paddington Green Children's
Hospital, St Mary's Hospital Group, London, UK

Plastic Surgery

T. L. Barclay ChM, FRCS
Consultant Plastic Surgeon, St Luke's Hospital,
Bradford, West Yorkshire, UK

Desmond A. Kernahan, MD
Chief, Division of Plastic Surgery,
The Children's Memorial Hospital, Chicago, Illinois, USA

Thoracic Surgery

J. W. Jackson MCh, FRCS
Formerly Consultant Thoracic Surgeon, Harefield Hospital, Middlesex, UK

D. K. C. Cooper MD, PhD, FRCS
Department of Cardiac Surgery, University of Cape Town
Medical School, Cape Town, South Africa

Trauma

John V. Robbs FRCS
Associate Professor of Surgery,
Department of Surgery, University of Natal, South Africa

Howard R. Champion FRCS
Chief, Trauma Service;
Director, Surgery Critical Care Services,
The Washington Hospital Center, Washington, DC, USA

Donald Trunkey MD
San Francisco General Hospital, San Francisco, California, USA

Urology

W. Scott McDougal MD
Professor and Chairman, Department of Urology, Vanderbilt
University, Nashville, Tennessee, USA

Vascular Surgery

James A. DeWeese MD
Professor and Chairman, Division of Cardiothoracic Surgery,
University of Rochester Medical Center, Rochester, New York, USA

Contributors

James T. Adams MD
Professor of Surgery, University of Rochester Medical Center, Rochester, New York, USA

Carl H. Andrus MD
Clinical Associate Professor of Surgery, University of Rochester Medical Center, Rochester, New York, USA

Elethea H. Caldwell MD
Associate Professor of Plastic Surgery, University of Rochester School of Medicine and Dentistry, Rochester, New York, USA

F. B. Cockett MS(Lond.), FRCS
Teacher and Examiner in Surgery, The University of London; Consulting Surgeon, St Thomas's Hospital, London; Consultant Surgeon to King Edward VII Hospital for Officers, London, UK

James A. DeWeese MD, FACS
Professor and Chairman, Division of Cardiothoracic Surgery, University of Rochester Medical Center, Rochester, New York, USA

H. H. G. Eastcott MS, FRCS
Honorary Consultant Surgeon, St Mary's Hospital, London, UK

W. G. Fegan MCh, FRCSI
Formerly Research Professor of Surgery, University College of Dublin, Trinity College at Sir Patrick Dun's Hospital, Dublin, Irish Republic

John Franklin MD
Plastic Surgery Associates of Chattanooga, Tennessee, USA

Alastair J. Gillies MB, ChB
Professor, Department of Anesthesiology, and Professor of Pharmacology, University of Rochester School of Medicine and Dentistry, Rochester, New York, USA

Richard M. Green MD, FACS
Clinical Assistant Professor of Surgery, University of Rochester Medical Center, New York, USA

John T. Hobbs MD, FRCS
Senior Lecturer in Surgery, University of London; Consultant Surgeon, St Mary's Hospital, London, UK

Robert W. Hobson II MD
Professor of Surgery and Chief, Section of Vascular Surgery, University of Medicine and Dentistry of New Jersey, New Jersey Medical School, Newark, New Jersey, USA

E. A. Husni MD
Associate Director, Department of Surgery, Huron Road Hospital, Cleveland, Ohio, USA

Anthony M. Imparato MD
Professor of Surgery and Director, Division of Vascular Surgery, New York University Medical Center, New York, USA

Barry T. Katzen MD, FACR
The Alexandria Hospital, Alexandria, Virginia; Clinical Professor of Radiology, George Washington University Medical Center, Washington, DC, USA

Elliot O. Lipchik MD
Associate Chief, Department of Radiology, Mount Sinai Medical Center, Milwaukee, Wisconsin; Clinical Professor of Radiology, the Medical College of Wisconsin, Milwaukee, Wisconsin, USA

Thomas G. Lynch MD
Assistant Professor of Surgery, Section of Vascular Surgery, University of Medicine and Dentistry of New Jersey, New Jersey Medical School, Newark, New Jersey, USA; Chief, Vascular Surgical Section, VA Medical Center, East Orange, New Jersey, USA

Allyn G. May MD, FACS
Professor of Surgery, University of Rochester Medical Center, Rochester, New York, USA

David Negus DM, MCh, FRCS
Teacher in Surgery, the University of London, United Medical Schools of Guy's and St Thomas's; Consultant Surgeon, Lewisham and Hither Green Hospitals, London, UK

Joseph A. O'Donnell MCh, FRCSI
Consultant Surgeon, Department of Surgery, UCC, Regional Hospital, Cork, Ireland

Nicholas Ogburn MD
Instructor in Surgery, East Carolina University School of Medicine, Greenville, North Carolina, USA

Malcolm O. Perry MD
Professor of Surgery, Cornell University Medical College, New York, USA

Walter J. Pories MD, FACS
Professor and Chairman, Department of Surgery, East Carolina
University School of Medicine, Greenville, North Carolina, USA

John J. Ricotta MD
Assistant Professor of Surgery, University of Rochester School of
Medicine and Dentistry, Rochester, New York, USA

Charles G. Rob MC, MChir, MD, FRCS, FACS
Professor of Surgery, Department of Surgery, Uniformed Services
University of the Health Sciences, F. Edward Hébert School of
Medicine, Bethesda, Maryland, USA

Seymour I. Schwartz MD
Professor of Surgery, University of Rochester School of Medicine and
Dentistry, Rochester, New York, USA

Michael E. Snell MChir, FRCS
Consultant Urologist, St Mary's Hospital, London, UK

A. E. Thompson MS, FRCS
Consultant Surgeon, St Thomas's Hospital, London, UK

Harold C. Urschel, Jr MD
Clinical Professor of Thoracic and Cardiovascular Surgery, University
of Texas Health Science Center, Baylor University Medical Center,
Dallas, Texas, USA

J. Leonel Villavicencio MD, FACS
Professor of Surgery, Uniformed Services University of the Health
Sciences, F. Edward Hébert School of Medicine, Bethesda, Maryland;
Director, Vein and Lymphatic Clinic, Water Reed Army Medical
Center, Washington, DC, USA

Thomas J. Whelan, Jr MD
Professor and Chairman, Department of Surgery, University of Hawaii,
Honolulu, Hawaii, USA

John H. N. Wolfe MS, FRCS
Consultant Surgeon, St Mary's Hospital, London, UK

Contributing Medical Artists

Susan Y. Anderson
Director and Medical Illustrator, Health Instructional Resources Unit,
University of Hawaii, John A. Burns School of Medicine, Honolulu,
Hawaii 96813, USA

Robert M. Bride
Operations Coordinator, Art Section, University of Medicine and
Dentistry of New Jersey Educational Communications Center, 100
Bergen Street, Newark, New Jersey 07103, USA

Angela Christie
14 West End Avenue, Pinner, Middlesex, HA5 1JB, UK

Fernando Diez-Zamora MA
Vice-Chairman and Staff, Medical Illustrations Department, Hospital
General de Mexico, Mexico City, Mexico

Diane Elliott
Medical Illustrator, Photography and Illustration Service, University of
Rochester School of Medicine and Dentistry, Rochester, New York,
USA

Jane Hurd
Medical Illustration Studio, 4002 Virginia Place, Brookmont,
Maryland 20016, USA

Kathleen Jung MS, BS, AMI
The Cleveland Clinic Foundation, Cleveland, Ohio, USA

Robert N. Lane MMAA
Medical Artist, Studio 19a, Edith Grove, Chelsea, London, SW10, UK

Gillian Lee FMAA
Medical Illustrator, Burnham, 15 Little Plucketts Way, Buckhurst Hill,
Essex, IG9 5QU, UK

Kevin Marks
3 Hilltop Court, Grange Road, Upper Norwood, London, SE19 3BQ,
UK

Anita Matthews BFA, AMI
Medical Illustrator, Photography and Illustration Service, University of
Rochester School of Medicine and Dentistry, Rochester, New York,
USA

Gillian Oliver AIMBI
Medical Illustrator, 71 Crawford Road, Hatfield, Herts AL10 0PF, UK

Carol J. Pienta
Medical Illustrator, Audio-Visual Services Center, School of Medicine,
East Carolina University, Greenville, North Carolina, USA

Lou Sadler
Assistant Professor in Biomedical Illustrations, University of Texas
Science Center, Texas, USA

Jorge Perez-Vela
Professor of Medical Art, University of Toronto, Canada

Robert Wabnitz AMI
Medical Illustrator, Photography and Illustration Service, University of
Rochester School of Medicine and Dentistry, Rochester, New York,
USA

Contents

Preface to the 4th Edition
James A. DeWeese

xvii

Preface to the 3rd Edition
Charles G. Rob

xviii

Arterial Surgery

Vascular laboratory examinations for arterial disease
John J. Ricotta

1

Arteriography
Elliot O. Lipchik

15

Percutaneous transluminal angioplasty in the treatment of peripheral vascular disease
Barry T. Katzen

24

Exposure of major blood vessels
H. H. G. Eastcott
A. E. Thompson

36

Arterial suture and anastomoses
H. H. G. Eastcott
A. E. Thompson

63

Operative angiography
John J. Ricotta

70

Carotid endarterectomy
James A. DeWeese

73

Operations for occlusive disease of the vertebral artery
Anthony M. Imparato

82

Treatment of occlusion of branches of the aortic arch and subclavian arteries
James A. DeWeese

92

Treatment of dissecting thoracic aortic aneurysms
James A. DeWeese

104

Treatment of intrathoracic aneurysms and thoracoabdominal aneurysms
James A. DeWeese

111

Treatment of abdominal aortic aneurysms   123
James A. DeWeese

Aortoiliac reconstruction: thromboendarterectomy, bypass graft   136
John J. Ricotta
James A. DeWeese

Reconstruction of the mesenteric and coeliac arteries   152
Nicholas Ogburn
Walter J. Pories

Renal artery reconstruction   166
Michael E. Snell

Axillofemoral and femorofemoral bypass grafts   179
Allyn G. May
James A. DeWeese

Arterial reconstruction below the inguinal ligament   183
Richard M. Green
James A. DeWeese

Arterial embolectomy   201
James A. DeWeese

Management of peripheral arterial aneurysms   207
John J. Ricotta

Popliteal artery entrapment syndrome   214
Thomas J. Whelan, Jr

Management of vascular injuries   219
Malcolm O. Perry

Treatment of iatrogenic vascular injuries   229
Richard M. Green
Charles G. Rob

Treatment of acquired arteriovenous fistulae   239
H. H. G. Eastcott
A. E. Thompson

Treatment of congenital arteriovenous fistulae   246
J. Leonel Villavicencio

Venous Surgery

Role of the vascular laboratory in the diagnosis of venous disease   253
Robert W. Hobson II
Thomas G. Lynch
Joseph A. O'Donnell

Phlebography   263
James A. DeWeese

Operations for varicose veins 271
John T. Hobbs

Injection treatment of varicose veins 291
W. G. Fegan

Venous ulcers 301
John T. Hobbs

Ligation of the ankle-perforating veins 310
F. B. Cockett
David Negus

Venous thrombectomy 318
James A. DeWeese

Interruptions of the inferior vena cava and femoral veins 325
James T. Adams

Venous reconstructive procedures 334
E. A. Husni

Portal hypertension 342
Seymour I. Schwartz

Lymphography 356
John H. N. Wolfe

Direct operations on the lymphatics 365
J. Leonel Villavicencio

Operative management of lymphoedema 377
Elethea H. Caldwell

Sympathetic ganglion block 382
Alastair J. Gillies

Sympathectomy of the upper extremity 386
Richard M. Green
Charles G. Rob

Lumbar sympathectomy 394
John J. Ricotta

Amputations 398
Richard M. Green
Charles G. Rob

Fasciotomy 415
Richard M. Green
James A. DeWeese

Meralgia paraesthetica 422
Charles G. Rob
James A. DeWeese

Thoracic outlet syndrome   **424**
Harold C. Urschel, Jr

Excision of carotid body tumours   **430**
John J. Ricotta

Vascular access   **435**
Allyn G. May
Carl H. Andrus

Index   **449**

Preface to the 4th Edition

It is most fitting that Charles Rob's preface to the 3rd edition of *Vascular Surgery* should be included in this volume. Many of the chapters in the current edition are written by contemporaries of Charles Rob or his students in London, England or Rochester, New York. Most of the chapters describing the standard operations contain certain techniques that evolved from a close association with Charles Rob in the same operating room, in nearby operating rooms, on vascular rounds, in conferences, or in the clinics. Some of the chapters from previous editions are unchanged, others contain only minor changes attesting to the soundness of the techniques. They were able to withstand the test of both time and the natural fierce desire of the independent young surgeon to reinvent the wheel.

I did choose guest authors with special expertise for new chapters on operations for more unusual conditions such as vertebral artery stenosis, popliteal artery entrapment syndromes, vascular injuries, congenital arteriovenous fistulae, chronic venous occlusions and thoracic outlet syndromes.

The most dramatic change that has occurred in the management of patients with vascular disease since publication of the last edition has been the widespread development of non-invasive vascular laboratories. Most of the newer tests are based on technological improvements in the older Doppler and ultrasound equipment, allowing more accurate estimations of blood flow, and the imaging of vessel walls. These are applicable to the study of patients with both arterial and venous disease and are important enough to be covered in separate chapters.

Although Dotter made pioneering efforts in the balloon dilatation of stenotic arterial lesions in the 1960s, it was the technological development of improved equipment by Gruentzig in 1974 that stimulated the rapid growth of balloon angioplasty in the management of renal, iliac, femoral and coronary arterial lesions. These procedures are performed by both radiologists and surgeons and therefore a chapter is included on this subject.

As diseases of the lymphatics remain a challenge, it was felt important to present the current status of attempts to manage lymphatic lesions more effectively, and new chapters on lymphography and direct operations on the lymphatics have therefore been included.

James A. DeWeese

Preface to the 3rd Edition

Vascular surgery may be defined as the surgery of the arteries, the veins and the lymphatics, together with certain related procedures such as amputations for ischaemia and fasciotomy for acute vascular occlusion. For convenience most cardiac operations have been placed in the Cardiothoracic Surgery volume. There is also a close association between vascular surgery and organ transplantation, because the success or failure of an organ transplant procedure depends in no small measure upon the vascular anastomoses between the host and the transplanted organ.

A brief history of the development of vascular surgery is now given because a note of this type is a useful introduction to any subject.

The first permanent union of two blood vessels either in the laboratory or clinical practice appears to have been accomplished in 1897 by Eck, a Russian surgeon. Before this there were occasional reports of lateral suture of blood vessels, but in 1900 Dörfler reviewed this subject and he concluded that the literature contained reports of only nine patients with a successful arterial repair by direct suture. In 1906 Carrel and Guthrie began experimenting with the anastomosis of blood vessels in the Hull Physiological Laboratory of the University of Chicago, and the techniques they developed have, except for minor variations, remained unchanged to the present time.

In the field of operative surgery some events stand out as milestones where a genuinely new clinical procedure was performed for the first time. Murphy in 1897 reported the first successful end-to-end arterial anastomosis using an invagination technique of the proximal into the distal artery. In 1906 Jose Goyanes used an autogenous vein graft for the first time to replace a peripheral aneurysm; this procedure was repeated in 1907 by Lexer, and in 1913 Pringle was the first English-speaking surgeon to report the insertion of a vein graft into the human arterial system. In 1947 Dos Santos was the first to perform the procedure of thromboendarterectomy in the way we use this technique today. In 1949 Kunlin introduced the procedure of femoropopliteal bypass grafting using an autogenous vein, and in 1951 Dubost, Allery and Oeconomos reported for the first time the successful resection of an aneurysm of the abdominal aorta and its replacement by an arterial homograft. In 1952 Voorhees, Jaretzki and Blakemore were the first to report the use of porous plastic cloth tubes to bridge arterial defects, a procedure which DeBakey and others have developed and improved. In 1963 Fogarty introduced the balloon embolectomy catheter which bears his name.

We must not forget sympathectomy and the surgery of the venous system. In 1890 Trendelenburg reported ligature of the long saphenous vein for lower limb varices and admitted a recurrence rate of 22 per cent after a four-year follow-up. This led to the improved techniques used today. Sympathectomy was performed as a periarterial procedure by Jaboulay in 1899 and it appears that Jonnesco in 1923 was the first to resect the sympathetic ganglia.

Finally, we should remember the debt that vascular surgeons owe to those who developed arteriography and phlebography. In 1923 Berberich and Hirsch performed phlebograms in humans and in 1924 Brooks injected sodium iodide into a patient's femoral artery, producing the first arteriogram. These techniques were improved and developed by Moniz and Dos Santos in Portugal together with many of our Swedish colleagues.

Charles G. Rob

Vascular laboratory examinations for arterial disease

John J. Ricotta MD
Assistant Professor of Surgery, University of Rochester
School of Medicine and Dentistry, Rochester, New York, USA

Introduction

Application of laboratory techniques to the evaluation of the patient with vascular disease has been one of the most significant contributions to vascular surgery in the last decade. The technology of the vascular laboratory has increased exponentially to the point where confusion often exists over the various techniques available. In this chapter, general comments about the various types of instrumentation and their applications will be made. For more detailed descriptions of specific techniques, references are provided at the end of this chapter[1,2,3]. It must be remembered that even the best vascular laboratory examination, often performed by a technician and interpreted by a physician who may not have examined the patient, is not meant to replace a thoughtful history and careful physical examination.

The vascular laboratory serves several purposes: (1) to screen patients at high risk for certain types of vascular disease (e.g. carotid stenosis); (2) to quantify objectively the degree of disease present; (3) to provide quantitative reproducible physiological information. This information is most useful in patient follow-up, especially after arterial reconstruction, and for objective comparison of different patient groups. There are some techniques (e.g. B-mode Doppler ultrasound) which provide anatomical rather than physiological data. The anatomical accuracy of these methods has yet to be proven and their role is uncertain at present. In contrast, the physiological, or 'functional', studies have become widely accepted, and these techniques will be the focus of this chapter.

For the purposes of this discussion, the chapter will be divided into evaluation of the peripheral arterial and cerebrovascular circulation.

Evaluation of the peripheral arterial circulation

Two general methods are used to evaluate the peripheral arterial circulation: doppler ultrasound and plethysmography. Within these broad categories there are various applications of each technology. The two methods may provide different and often complementary information in the individual patient.

The techniques

DOPPLER

1

Doppler principle

Sound beams are emitted from a transducer and reflected at the interface of two surfaces. The reflected waves can be sensed by a receiver. As the Doppler signal strikes red cells in the bloodstream, it is reflected back to the transducer. A shift in the frequency of the reflected signal occurs which is proportional to the velocity of the red cells in the blood: the faster the cells are travelling, the higher the frequency shift. Using different technology, the magnitude and direction of the frequency shift can be expressed as a wave on a strip chart recorder, converted to an audible signal, or frequency shifts can be analysed using techniques such as Fast Fourier Transform. If the angle θ is known, quantitation of blood flow is possible. Interested readers are referred to the monograph by Dean and Yao[1] for a more detailed description. Each of these techniques gives information about the blood flow at that point in the artery sampled. Additional information can be gained by placing a blood pressure cuff over the arterial segment of interest and determining the systolic pressure in that segment by monitoring a distal artery with a Doppler probe. This technique – determination of segmental limb pressures – is one of the simplest, most useful and most widely practised methods of non-invasive vascular evaluation.

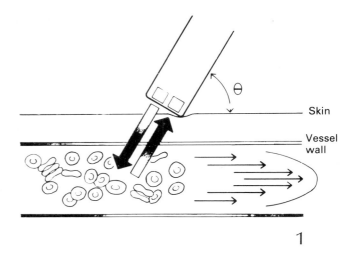

1

Doppler wave forms

2

The Doppler wave form is characteristic for a normal and a stenotic artery: as the stenosis increases, the wave form is altered in a characteristic fashion. An unobstructed artery has a brisk upstroke, sharp peak, definite reversal of flow and then a return to baseline. This is heard as a crisp biphasic signal. As the artery becomes diseased, its compliance is lost and so is the reversal of flow; the signal becomes monophasic. As stenosis progresses, the upstroke is blunted and the signal becomes more attenuated. Finally, as the artery occludes, the wave form and Doppler signal disappear or are replaced by a flat line or monotonous hum indicating collateral flow.

Doppler interrogation can be used to identify sites of major arterial occlusion. Doppler wave forms are combined with determination of segmental limb pressure to localize areas of arterial stenosis or occlusion. Doppler analysis allows interrogation of major arteries and provides direct information on their status. It is particularly useful in objectively evaluating the common femoral artery which cannot be specifically examined by plethysmographic techniques. Doppler techniques do not evaluate total limb flow and in certain patients with extensive small vessel disease (e.g. diabetes) do not reliably reflect the severity of disease. In patients with Monckeberg's calcinosis, Doppler signals, although abnormal in quality, are often present and cannot be obliterated even by pressures far exceeding systolic pressure. In such circumstances, Doppler spectral analysis or plethysmographic techniques become important.

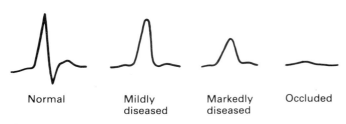

Normal   Mildly diseased   Markedly diseased   Occluded

3

Doppler spectral analysis

This technique analyses the spectral frequencies of the Doppler signal. The Doppler shift signals reflect the velocities found in the bloodstream. Distal to a stenosis there will be turbulent flow which will be manifest by a broadening of the Doppler spectrum. Analysis of 'spectral broadening' and amplitude of frequency shift are used to quantitate the severity of stenosis. At present, these techniques are being applied both clinically and experimentally in a number of centres. Quantification of blood flow requires expensive and elaborate technology which is currently under evolution. The interested reader is referred to the discussion by Johnson[4].

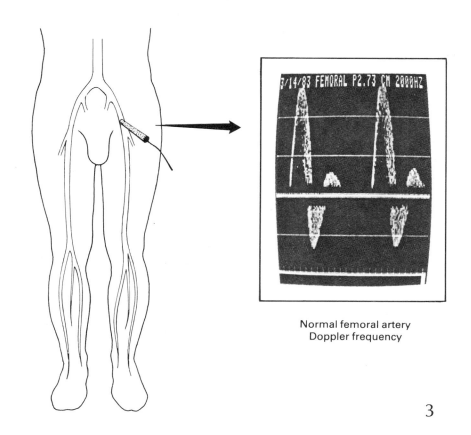

Normal femoral artery
Doppler frequency

3

4

PLETHYSMOGRAPHY

Common plethysmographic techniques include a mercury strain gauge, plethysmography and air plethysmography (pulse volume recorder)[3]. In the former, changes in leg volume that accompany arterial pulsation are sensed by the strain gauge and translated as a wave form on a strip chart recorder. In the latter, changes in leg volume produce changes in the volume of an inflated air bladder which are expressed on a strip chart recorder. In each case, changes in the volume of the examined part are measured rather than changes in blood velocity of a particular artery. Thus while plethysmographic tracings and Doppler wave forms may appear similar, they are measuring two related but separate parameters and provide different information. Although plethysmographic tracings measure total flow quite well, they do not give information about individual arteries. In fact, short segmental occlusions with abundant collateral circulation often give near-normal plethysmographic tracings. However, plethysmography is particularly useful in patients with diffuse small vessel arterial disease, especially diabetics. Plethysmography can be combined with segmental compression to give a topographical evaluation of the extremity[3], but we find it only rarely adds any information.

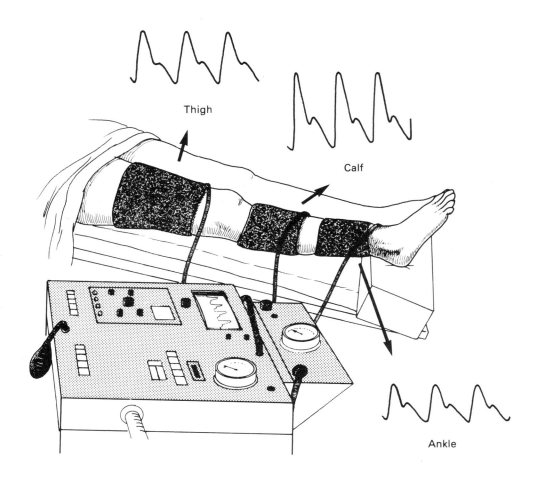

Thigh

Calf

Ankle

4

Arterial pulse volume recordings

The examination

The patient is examined in a comfortable room equipped with an examining table and treadmill for exercising. Some authors have questioned the value of treadmill testing; however, we feel that it continues to be valuable, especially in evaluating patients with claudication. During exercise, the patient may be monitored with an ECG although this is not routinely our practice. Reports from several centres suggest that the incidence of cardiac complications with treadmill exercise in a vascular laboratory is extremely small. Nevertheless, when treadmill testing is indicated, it should be performed by someone trained in cardiopulmonary resuscitation and appropriate equipment for resuscitation should be readily available.

The history

A pertinent history is taken with special emphasis on the severity, duration and distribution of symptoms, their relationship to exercise and their progression over time. Special attention should be paid to medications the patient takes including analgesics and cardioactive drugs as well as any history of coronary or cerebral insufficiency. Additional demographic data such as presence or absence of diabetes, family history of atherosclerosis and amount of cigarette consumption is important. Following the interview, blood pressure is auscultated in each arm. The highest systolic pressure is used to calculate the ankle/brachial indices described below.

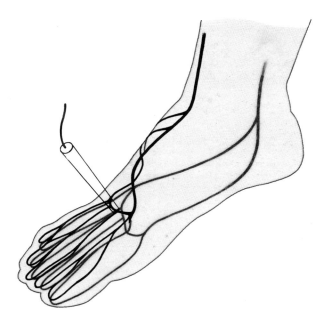

5

Evaluation of distal vessels

Attention is next turned to palpation of the distal pulses. Femoral, popliteal, posterior tibial, and dorsalis pedis arteries are palpated. Pulses are classified as present, diminished or absent. Each artery is then interrogated using the Doppler instrument. The audible quality of the signal is assessed and, if possible, the wave form is recorded on a strip chart recorder. this is particularly important in the common femoral artery. The anatomy of the pedal arch can be assessed by evaluating the dorsalis pedis artery while sequentially compressing the posterior tibial, lateral malleolar or lateral tarsal arteries[5]. In this way, the most significant arterial supply to the plantar arch can be determined. It should be noted, however, that with severe multisegmental disease, pedal arch signals may not be heard despite patency of the vessel on angiography. Conversely, Doppler signals may be present indicating a patent artery when this is not demonstrated by angiography.

5

6

Segmental limb pressures

Following direct vessel interrogation, segmental limb pressures are recorded again using the Doppler probe. The popliteal and pedal arteries are isolated with the probe, and an appropriately sized cuff is placed on the segment (calf or thigh) immediately proximal to the probe. Several authors still employ a 'high thigh' cuff to identify aortoiliac disease. We have not found this useful and rely instead on palpation and Doppler interrogation of the common femoral artery. The leg cuff is then inflated until the signal disappears; this is the segmental systolic pressure and is used in calculating the ankle-brachial index (see below). Finally, plethysmographic tracings are made over the thigh, calf, ankle and forefoot. Tracings and Doppler pressure can be carried out on the digits as well. These procedures are identical when the upper extremity requires evaluation.

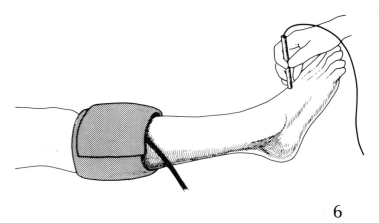

6

Exercise testing

Exercise testing is done on all patients with a history of claudication who do not have significant medical contraindication to treadmill testing. Continuous ECG monitoring has been suggested for all patients during exercise testing but in our opinion is not essential. The patient is exercised on a treadmill placed on a 10 per cent gradient at either a slow (1½ mph; 2.4 km/h) or fast (2¼ mph; 3.6 km/h) rate. Exercising continues for 5 min or until disabling symptoms appear. The onset of symptoms is noted as well as the pattern of their distribution (thigh, calf, hip and buttock). Other symptoms such as angina or shortness of breath are also recorded. Following exercise, ankle pressures and ankle plethysmographic tracings are repeated. If ankle pressures drop, they are followed every 1–2 min until they return to normal[1].

7

Interpretation of the tests

Interpretation depends on segmental Doppler pressures and plethysmographic tracings. Changes in wave forms or drop in pressure as one proceeds down the leg are important in localizing the site of stenosis or occlusion. In general, a drop in systolic pressure of 20 mmHg or greater from one segment to the next indicates a significant stenosis or occlusion in that segment. Similarly, a change in the quality of wave form from one segment to the next can indicate the level of disease. A major difficulty remains in differentiating iliac or common femoral stenosis from lesions in the high superficial femoral artery. Palpation of the femoral pulse and interrogation of the femoral artery with the Doppler are helpful, as is the distribution of symptoms, especially after exercise. Nevertheless, differentiation of aortoiliac and proximal femoral disease may remain difficult.

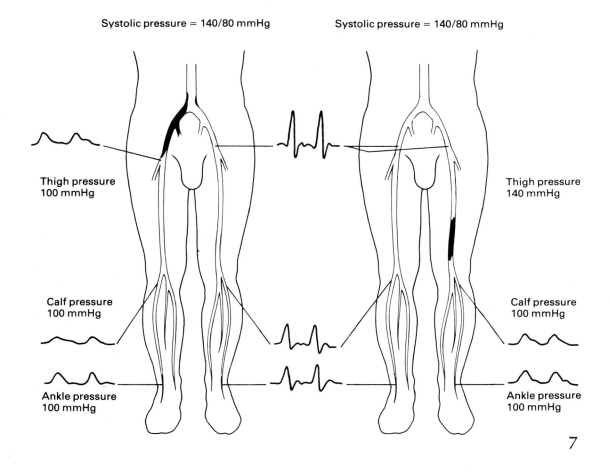

Systolic pressure = 140/80 mmHg   Systolic pressure = 140/80 mmHg

Thigh pressure 100 mmHg   Thigh pressure 140 mmHg

Calf pressure 100 mmHg   Calf pressure 100 mmHg

Ankle pressure 100 mmHg   Ankle pressure 100 mmHg

7

Calculation of an ankle/brachial ratio, using the highest ankle pressure, is helpful in evaluating severity of ischaemia. In general, a ratio ankle pressure:brachial pressure ≥0.9 is normal, 0.5–0.9 indicates ischaemia associated with claudication, <0.5 is usually associated with severe arterial ischaemia and rest pain, and <0.3 indicates impending tissue loss. These criteria have been helpful in categorizing patients with arterial disease.

Occasionally a patient with claudication will have a normal arterial examination at rest. Abnormalities can almost always be brought out by exercise on a treadmill. This phenomenon was noted by DeWeese in 1960[6] and is explained by vasodilation of the distal arterial bed causing a pressure drop distal to a critical stenosis. If the patient cannot be exercised, reactive hyperaemia can be achieved by inflating the thigh cuff over systolic pressure and maintaining ischaemia for 5 min. The vasodilation which follows release of the cuff will be followed by a distal pressure drop if a flow-limiting stenosis exists.

Special considerations

8

Vasculogenic impotence

Considerable interest has been focused on alterations in pelvic haemodynamics as a cause of impotence. Several papers discussing the laboratory criterion for vasculogenic impotence are listed in the references[7,8]. Doppler pressures and plethysmography have both been employed as well as a penile brachial index. In our experience, these data have been unreliable and we are currently not convinced of the value of these techniques. However, others have reported excellent results with these methods in identifying patients with 'vasculogenic impotence'. A special cuff is placed around the base of the penile shaft, the dorsal penile artery is found with a Doppler probe and the penile systolic pressure is determined.

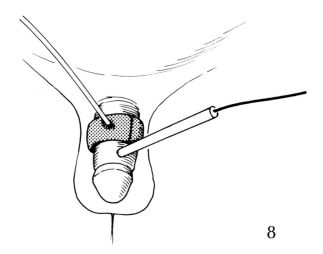

8

Thoracic outlet syndrome

The techniques described for the lower extremities can be applied to the upper extremities as well. We have studied a number of patients with thoracic outlet compression using Doppler and plethysmographic techniques. As might be expected, these techniques yielded little additional information not apparent on careful physical examination. In isolated instances, however, the tests have been helpful in identifying intrinsic disease in the forearm, alerting us to the possibility of a proximal arterial lesion.

Raynaud's phenomenon

Like thoracic outlet compression, this diagnosis is best made by thorough history and physical examination. We are currently evaluating patients with Raynaud's phenomenon using digital plethysmography at room temperature, after immersion in warm water and after immersion in cool (50°F; 10°C) water. This has been helpful in separating patients with intrinsic arterial disease from those with pure vasospasm. Serial measurements are helpful in patients with Raynaud's phenomenon as they often demonstrate a prolonged recovery time after cold induces vasospasm.

Cerebrovascular evaluation

Evaluation of the carotid circulation again involves two basic techniques: Doppler examination and plethysmography. In addition, however, there have been significant developments in carotid imaging using B-mode ultrasound. This technique has significant potential for providing anatomical information about the common carotid and carotid bifurcation.

DOPPLER TECHNIQUES

9

Supraorbital Doppler examination

The simplest Doppler examination is the supraorbital Doppler test as described by Barnes[9]. This test is based on monitoring the quality and direction of blood flow in either the supraorbital or frontal artery. This artery is supplied by branches of both the internal carotid (ophthalmic) and external carotid (superficial temporal, facial, mandibular) arteries. Under normal conditions, the majority of flow is from the internal carotid artery outward, toward the probe. After the supraorbital artery has been located, the flow signal is evaluated by a directional Doppler. Reversal of flow (toward the orbit, away from the probe) indicates dominance of the external

carotid system and suggests an internal carotid stenosis. Supraorbital flow is then monitored as the branches of the external carotid artery are serially compressed. Diminution or obliteration of the Doppler signal by arterial compression indicates an internal carotid lesion (unmasked by obliterating the major flow from one of the external carotid branches). Ipsilateral and contralateral compression are used on each side. Contralateral common carotid compression has been advocated by Barnes but is not routinely used in our laboratory and probably should be done only in the presence of a physician.

The advantage of this test is its relative simplicity. Chart recordings are rarely required; only the audible signal is used. The examination can be performed at the patient's bedside with a pocket Doppler. The overall accuracy of the test, however, is only in the 70–80 per cent range. It is able to detect only severe stenosis or occlusions and, while highly specific, is not very sensitive. Finally, the accuracy of the examination is directly related to the experience of the person performing it and considerable interpretive skill may be required. However, it remains a rapid method of evaluation in experienced hands.

Recently, the technique has been modified using photoplethysmography with arterial compression. In this examination, skin blood flow over the eyebrow is monitored. A one-third reduction in blood flow with compression indicates a significant internal carotid stenosis[10]. While this technique has the advantages of being easier to do and providing graphic information, it has the same problems with sensitivity as supraorbital Doppler and is not used in our laboratory.

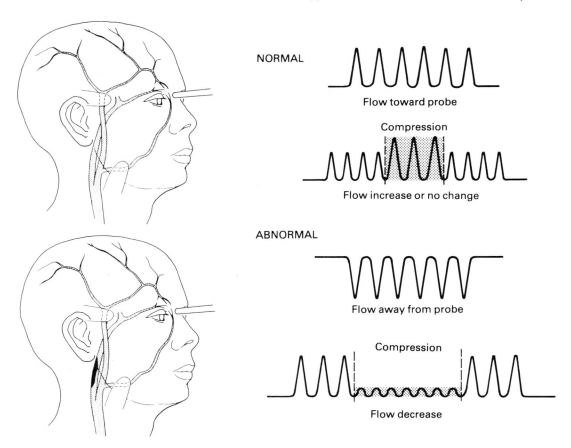

NORMAL

Flow toward probe

Compression

Flow increase or no change

ABNORMAL

Flow away from probe

Compression

Flow decrease

10

Direct Doppler examination frequency analysis

Direct Doppler examination of the carotid artery by pulsed and continuous wave Doppler instrumentation has become an important technique for evaluating the carotid bifurcation. The Doppler probe is placed directly on the carotid artery and the common carotid artery and its branches are investigated. Doppler signals can be stored on an oscilloscope to give a visual picture of the carotid bifurcation.

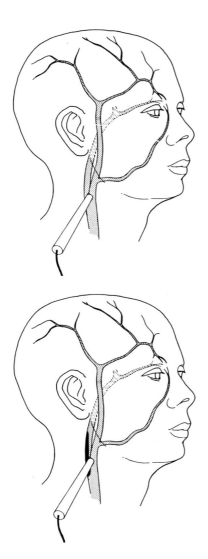

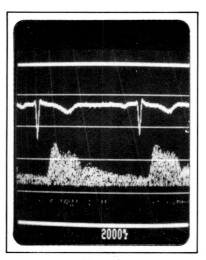

Normal

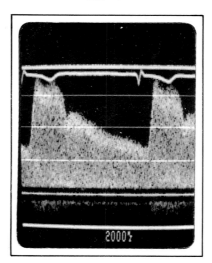

Internal carotid stenosis

11

Doppler carotid imaging

Doppler frequency shifts can also be analysed and either stored visually or displayed on a screen. Analysis of these frequency patterns permits categorization of stenoses as minimal, moderate and severe[12]. Frequency shifts can be colour coded: normal (0–2 kHz) – red; moderate (4–6 kHz) – yellow; and high (>6 kHz) – blue. Areas with abnormal frequency elevation can thus be visually represented. These techniques are quite satisfactory at present and continue to be improved. However, their performance requires a significant degree of time and technical skill. Even in experienced hands mistakes can be made, particularly in the identification of total occlusions of the internal carotid artery. This is because the diagnosis of an occlusion relies on negative information, and we have often found that a branch of the external carotid may be confused with the internal carotid when the latter is occluded.

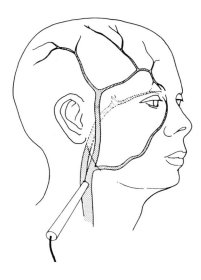

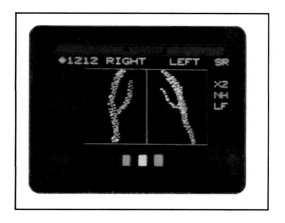

Normal   Internal carotid stenosis

11

PLETHYSMOGRAPHIC TECHNIQUES

These techniques involve measurement of eye pulsation and/or pressures as a reflection of internal carotid artery flow. As such, they are indirect evaluations of the internal carotid artery and cannot be used to distinguish between disease at the carotid bifurcation and siphon, or in the ophthalmic artery. There are two basic types of examination: ocularplethysmography (developed by Kartchner and MacRae[13]) and ocularpneumoplethysmography (developed by Gee[14]).

12

Ocularplethysmography (Kartchner)

Ocularplethysmography is based on measuring ocular pulse wave forms simultaneously in each eye. Suction cups are placed on the cornea of each eye and secured with low level suction (40–45 mmHg). Either air or water contact can be used. With arterial pulsations the volume of the globe is distorted and a pulse wave is produced. External carotid flow is monitored by a photosensor placed on the ear lobe. Tracings are made simultaneously of both eye pulses and ear pulses. A delay in eye pulse arrival time of >10 ms indicates a significant internal carotid stenosis on that side. Bilateral carotid disease results in a blunted ocular pulse and a delay in arrival of the eye pulse as compared to the ear pulse. The overall accuracy of this technique in detecting flow-limiting carotid stenoses is variously reported as 80–90 per cent. We have found this technique less accurate and more cumbersome than ocularpneumoplethysmography.

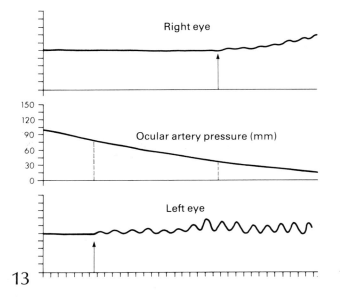

12

Ocularplethysmographic tracing (Kartchner) – left carotid stenosis

13

Ocularpneumoplethysmography (OPG – Gee)

In this technique, suction cups are applied to the sclera of each eye. High levels of suction are then applied to the eye (up to 500 mmHg) for a brief period to obliterate ocular artery pulsation. As the pressure is decreased, appearance of ocular pulsations are noted on a strip chart recorder indicating ocular systolic pressure. A difference of greater than 5 mmHg in ocular systolic pressure between eyes or an abnormally low ratio of ocular:brachial systolic pressure indicates a haemodynamically significant carotid stenosis. Accuracy of this technique is 92–97 per cent[15]. We have been impressed with the simplicity and reproducibility of this technique as well as the relative ease of interpretation. It also has the added advantage of providing absolute pressure information and can be used to determine carotid back pressure if desired. This technique remains our preferred method of non-invasive carotid evaluation.

13

Ocularpneumoplethysmographic tracing (Gee) – right carotid stenosis

14

CAROTID IMAGING – B-MODE ULTRASOUND SCANS

Recent advances in direct carotid imaging have been made using B-mode ultrasound. This technique allows visualization of the carotid artery and its branches in both longitudinal and transverse views. Anatomical rather than physiological information is obtained. It is hoped that this technique will detect non-haemodynamically significant lesions and ulcerative plaques not identified by other non-invasive tests. A number of studies have found the technique to be promising but some difficulty has been encountered in the diagnosis of high grade stenosis or total occlusion[16]. Our experience with over 400 patients confirms these observations. At present, we feel that anatomical information gained from B-scanning is helpful but not accurate enough to replace arteriography and that expectations to the contrary are unrealistic at present. However, combining anatomical information from B-scanning with functional information obtained by Doppler frequency analysis or ocularpneumoplethysmography can be valuable.

Uses of non-invasive testing in the diagnosis of cerebrovascular disease

Non-invasive tests are helpful in identifying haemodynamically significant internal carotid stenoses. Although B-mode ultrasound has the potential for identifying smaller lesions which might give rise to platelet emboli, at present it is not sensitive enough to substitute for arteriography. Arteriography should not be deferred in symptomatic patients on the basis of negative non-invasive tests.

Non-invasive tests are helpful in screening for significant stenosis in four groups of patients: (1) patients with asymptomatic carotid bruits; (2) patients with peripheral vascular or coronary artery disease; (3) patients with non-localizing symptoms of cerebrovascular insufficiency; and (4) follow-up patients after carotid endarterectomy.

It is generally accepted that patients with high grade carotid stenosis are at greater risk of stroke than patients with less severe lesions. Asymptomatic bruits associated with positive ocularpneumoplethysmography are more likely to give rise to symptoms of cerebrovascular insufficiency than those bruits not associated with a haemodynamically significant stenosis[17]. Many vascular surgeons currently perform prophylactic carotid endarterectomy on patients with asymptomatic high grade stenosis of the carotid artery. Functional tests (in our clinic, ocularpneumoplethysmography) are used to screen patients with asymptomatic neck bruits in order to select those candidates suitable for arteriography and surgery.

Recent studies have shown as high as 30 per cent incidence of significant carotid stenosis in asymptomatic patients with peripheral vascular or coronary artery disease. Many of these patients did not have a neck bruit and this group therefore constitutes a second group where vascular screening is helpful.

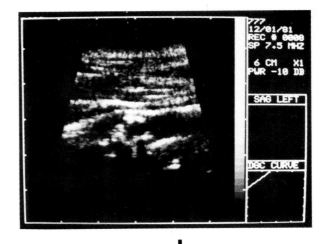

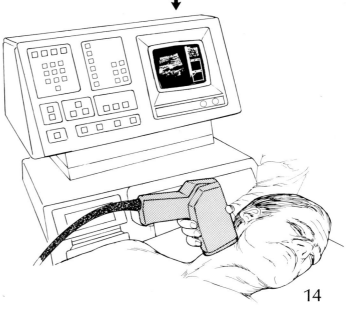

14

It is known that certain patients with non-focal symptoms or symptoms suggesting vertebrobasilar insufficiency can be improved by carotid endarterectomy. Patients who are best surgical candidates have haemodynamically significant lesions in their anterior circulation. Again, non-invasive studies have been helpful to us in identifying these patients.

Recent work has suggested an unexpectedly high incidence of restenosis following carotid endarterectomy, over 25 per cent in one series[18]. Many of these patients remain asymptomatic. Non-invasive studies may be helpful in identifying these patients as well as following progression of contralateral disease. Finally, non-invasive testing (OPG–Gee) has been used in the immediate postoperative period to check patency of the endarterectomy site[19]. We find this particularly helpful in the patient who develops a neurological deficit during or after surgery. A positive test suggests occlusion of the endarterectomized segment and the need for prompt surgical exploration. If the OPG is normal, however, re-exploration is not warranted, or should be performed only after angiographic study. Unnecessary and potentially dangerous re-exploration can be avoided.

References

1. Dean, R. H., Yao, J. S. Hemodynamic measurements in peripheral vascular disease. Current Problems in Surgery 1976; 13: 1–76

2. Barnes, R. W. Noninvasive diagnostic techniques in peripheral vascular disease. American Heart Journal 1979; 97: 241–258

3. Raines, J., Traad, E. Noninvasive evaluation of peripheral vascular disease. Medical Clinics of North America 1980; 64: 283–304

4. Johnston, K. W. Peripheral arterial doppler blood flow velocity wave form analysis. In: Kempczinski, R. F., Yao, J. S. T., eds. Practical noninvasive vascular diagnosis. Chicago, London: Yearbook Medical Publishers, 1982: 119–144

5. Roederscheimer, L. R., Feins, R., Green, R. M. Doppler evaluation of the pedal arch. American Journal of Surgery, 1981; 142: 601–604

6. DeWeese, J. A. Pedal pulses disappearing with exercise: A test for intermittent claudication. New England Journal of Medicine 1960; 262: 1214–1217

7. Kempczinski, R. F. Role of the vascular diagnostic laboratory in the evaluation of male impotence. American Journal of Surgery 1979; 138: 278–282

8. Queral, R. A., Whitehouse, W. M., Flinn, W. R., Zarins, C. K., Bergan, J. J., Yao, J. S. T. Pelvic hemodynamics after aortoiliac reconstruction. Surgery 1979; 86: 799–809

9. Barnes, R. W., Russel, H. E., Bone, G. E., Slaymaker, E. E. Doppler cerebrovascular examination: Improved results with refinements in technique. Stroke 1977; 8: 468–471

10. Lynch, T. G., Wright, C. B., Miller, E. V. Oculopneumoplethysmography, Doppler examination and supraorbital photoplethysmography. Annals of Surgery 1971; 194: 731–736

11. Mozersky, D. J., Hokanson, D. E., Sumner, D., Strandness, D. E. Ultrasonic visualization of the arterial lumen. Surgery 1972; 72: 253–259

12. White, D. N., Curry, G. R. A comparison of 424 carotid bifurcations examined by angiography and the doppler echoflow. In: White, D. N., Lyons, E. A., eds. Ultrasound in medicine. New York: Plenum, 1978: 363

13. Kartchner, M. M., McRae, L. P., Morrison, F. D. Noninvasive detection and evaluation of carotid occlusive disease. Archives of Surgery 1973; 106: 528–535

14. Gee, W., Oller, D. W., Homer, L. D., Bailey, C. R. Simultaneous bilateral determination of the systolic pressure of the ophthalmic arteries by ocular pneumo-plethysmography. Investigative in Ophthalmology and Visual Science 1977; 16: 86–89

15. McDonald, P. T., Rich, N. M., Collins, G. J., Anderson, C. A., Kozloff, L. Doppler cerebrovascular examination, oculoplethysmography and ocularpneumoplethysmography: use in detection of carotid disease: a prospective clinical study. Archives of Surgery 1978; 113: 1341–1349

16. Hobson, R. W., Berry, S. M., Katocs, A. S., O'Donnell, J. A., Jamil, Z., Savitsky, J. P. Comparison of pulsed Doppler and real time B-mode echo arteriography for noninvasive imaging of the extracranial carotid arteries. Surgery 1980; 87: 286–293

17. Busutil, R. W., Baker, J. D., Davidson, R. K., Machleder, H. I. Carotid artery stenosis – hemodynamic significance and clinical course. Journal of American Medical Association 1981; 245: 1438–1441

18. Zierler, R. E., Bandyk, D. F., Thiele, B. O., Strandness, D. E. Carotid artery stenosis following endarterectomy. Presented at 30th Meeting of the International Society for Cardiovascular Surgery, NA Chapter, Boston, Mass., 1982

19. Ortega, G., Gee, W., Kaupp, H. A., McDonald, K. M. Postendarterectomy carotid occlusion. Surgery 1981; 90: 1093–1098

Illustrations by Anita Matthews

Arteriography

Elliot O. Lipchik MD
Associate Chief, Department of Radiology, Mount Sinai Medical Center, Milwaukee, Wisconsin;
Clinical Professor of Radiology, the Medical College of Wisconsin, Milwaukee, Wisconsin, USA

Introduction

The Roentgen demonstration of the vascular system continues to be vital in the delineation of pathology. It has become routine in all departments of radiology. Arteriography is an interventional radiographic procedure, requiring training, experience and skill. It is not to be dealt with casually. Arteriography is the preliminary diagnostic technique necessary for accurate planning of many therapeutic procedures, such as endarterectomy, bypass grafting, angioplasties, and embolization of vessels and organs. The mechanics of the exam can easily be learned, but in order to obtain the maximum and proper information with the least risk and the least radiation dose to the patient, a thorough knowledge of the technique and the tools required is mandatory.

Essential equipment

X-ray unit and film changers

There are many X-ray units, tables, films, screens and film-changers of varying design and cost. Rapid serial film changers capable of at least two films per second are essential for areas of high-velocity bloodflow – for example, in the thoracic and abdominal aorta and their branches. A manually operated serial changer capable of 3–5 films, spanning any desired length of time, may be sufficient for peripheral limb arteriography or venography where the contrast or bloodflow has a decidedly slower course. However, apparatus of this sort is not considered optimal. Single plane units are sufficient for most arteriographic procedures, but biplane studies may be necessary more truly to evaluate the anatomy of a vessel, particularly the posterior walls. Since 70–85 kV give the best diagnostic quality films, high milliamperage generators of 1000 or more are recommended for arteriographic work.

The dynamics of bloodflow may best be evaluated by cineroentgenography, but at the risk of sacrificing anatomical detail and shrinking the field size recorded. Cine is recommended for cardiac studies but not for peripheral angiography. The shortest possible exposure times, proper coning, and the smallest practicable focal spot, all help to improve detail. Magnification radiography is a luxurious refinement, but not essential in a routine practice. A relatively long series of films may be necessary to encompass the complete circulation of contrast material from the arteries to the veins. For example, in visceral arteriography the veins may maximally opacify from 8 to 20 s after the start of the injection.

Pressure injectors

A pressure injector is universally used for catheter aortography and in most areas of non-selective arteriography where a large bolus of contrast material has to be injected in a relatively short period of time. The units of pressure indicated for the different makes of injectors do not correspond: the same 'dial' readings produce different effective pressure and therefore different flow rates. In any event, the radiologist is a specialist who should be fully conversant with the problems of apparatus and its use. He must know the capabilities and characteristics of the entire injection system, which includes the injector, connecting tubes, connectors, catheters and contrast material.

Contrast materials

The newer and safer contrast materials are all water-soluble organic molecules with bound iodine. There are many brand names, different in every country. Most contrast materials are hypertonic, viscid solutions, some with high sodium as well as iodine content; all are expensive. In proper dosage they are quite safe, but they are toxic in overdosage, and when stasis allows longer periods of tissue contact, particularly with dehydration and low cardiac output. The toxicity of contrast material varies depending on the region or organ perfused. No one contrast agent necessarily qualifies as best for all regional circulations. For example, pure methylglucamine salts of low or no sodium content are least toxic in the cerebral circulation, whereas methylglucamine-sodium diatrizoate mixtures are recommended for the heart, aorta and its branches. Non-ionic, water-soluble contrast materials, at present utilized primarily for myelograms, are available for peripheral arteriography and venography. They cause no discomfort during injection and should elicit no untoward cardiovascular responses (as do the usual hypertonic contrast media), but they are prohibitively expensive.

The trade names and numbers of the various agents are confusing. For example, the iodine content of Renografin 60 (meglumine diatrizoate) and Hypaque 50 (sodium diatrizoate) are almost identical. It is the iodine content which determines the radiodensity of the material. The exact concentration of iodine is listed on the label, not in the trademark.

In all aspects of arteriography, the examination has to be tailored and modified to suit the individual and the specific problem. Thus the amount and the site of injection of contrast cannot be rigidly applied to every patient. Non-selective aortography may require from 30–50 ml of the more concentrated materials at a rate of 10–25 ml/s. Selective arterial injections – for example, carotid studies – require 10–12 ml at 7–8 ml/s; 8–15 ml are recommended for selective renal arteriograms, and 30–60 ml for selective superior mesenteric or coeliac artery injections at a rate of 6–10 ml/s. Less concentrated opaque material is recommended for the selective studies. The volume and the flow rate of the contrast material into the vessel are the determining factors in the quality of the opacification of that vessel. Repeat injections may safely be made after several minute intervals.

In the demonstration of peripheral arteriosclerosis, relatively slow rates and larger volumes is the usual successful combination. With a slower injection of 8–10 ml/s, the distal aorta and iliac vessels are usually fully opacified by the first exposure just before the end of the injection (4–6 s). The popliteal and trifurcation vessels in the calf are usually opacified from within 6–12 s after the beginning of the injection. Vessels in the ankle and foot begin to fill after 12–18 s. For adequate opacification of the very distal vessels it may be necessary to prolong the time of filming up to 45 s. Reflex hyperaemia, by either having the patient actively exercise the symptomatic foot or by occluding the femoral pulse for 2 min just prior to the injection of contrast, helps to opacify the vessels of the ankle and feet. Two mg of 1 per cent lignocaine per ml of contrast material, well mixed, provides sufficient relief from pain in most patients. Lignocaine should only be used in the lower aorta and peripheral vessels.

1a–d

Catheter, needles and cannulae

New catheter materials are continually appearing on the market. Selective catheterization of vessels often requires specially designed preformed catheters. The smaller the radius of the catheter, the safer the procedure. Thin-wall catheters of sizes 5 Fr to 7 Fr are sufficient for almost every application. Catheters with multiple sideholes are recommended for non-selective aortograms (a). Selective catheterization of branch vessels, whether into the head (b), heart (c) or viscera (d), should be attempted only by experienced workers in the field. All catheters should be frequently or continuously flushed with normal saline with a small amount of heparin in the flush (2000 u/500 ml).

Many different needle-cannula assemblies are available. Most consist of an innermost obturator within a sharp, pointed needle and an external cannula with a blunt, tapered end. The most useful size is 18 Fr gauge. The guidewires also come in various diameters and lengths which have to correspond with the internal diameter and length of the catheter used. A very useful guidewire is one with a 'floppy' curve at the end which facilitates the negotiation of tortuous, arteriosclerotic vessels.

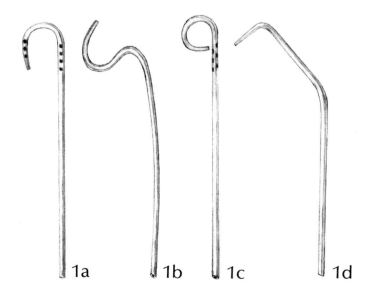

1a 1b 1c 1d

Percutaneous catheterization

The percutaneous catheter placement of Seldinger allows easy entrance into almost any vessel system in the body. The transfemoral route is the method of choice for most patients except those with obstruction due to advanced aortoiliac atherosclerosis. Via this route one may easily study the entire aorta and its branches, including the head as well as the lower limbs, depending on the position of the tip of the catheter. It is recommended that the intracranial circulation be studied by manoeuvring a properly shaped catheter into the desired brachiocephalic vessel. The catheter tip should rest in the common carotid at least several centimetres below the carotid bifurcation. For arch aortography a multihole pigtail loop catheter is recommended. The loop should be just proximal to the innominate artery. By either selective or arch technique, the anatomy of the brachiocephalic vessels has to be completely depicted, including their origins. Biplane studies are mandatory for the carotid bifurcation and for the intracranial circulation.

Preoperative preparation

The patient may feel pain only at the time of needle insertion for induction of local anaesthesia and during the injection of contrast, which may cause a feeling of intense heat, verging into pain, in the region of perfusion. Pain at any other time during the catheter manipulation is abnormal, and most often due to intramural placement of catheter or wire (or improper anaesthesia).

The patient should not eat solids, but should be allowed, and in most instances encouraged, to drink clear fluids, starting approximately 6–8 hours prior to the examination. For most selective abdominal angiography, including renal angiography, a mild laxative bowel preparation is highly recommended, if clinically feasible. Light sedation with tranquillizing agents, such as diazepam (Valium) 5–10 mg intravenously just prior to the examination, is used by the author. The author does not use barbiturates or antihistamines. Pethidine (Demerol) is contraindicated in all angiographic procedures as it may act as a vasoplegic with resultant hypotension. We are no longer using anticoagulants prior to insertion of the catheter. Routine sterile skin preparation is done with the patient on the X-ray table.

CATHETERIZATION OF FEMORAL ARTERY

2

Identification of femoral artery

The femoral artery pulsation is identified in either groin in the inguinal crease and well below the inguinal ligament. A needle puncture above this ligament makes haemostasis difficult during and after the examination. The surgeon also has easier access to a damaged or thrombosed artery below the inguinal ligament. The skin and subcutaneous tissues are infiltrated with locally acting anaesthetics, down to the arterial wall. For increased patient comfort, the subcutaneous layers of the skin should be infiltrated prior to the raising of the intracutaneous weal with a 25–26 gauge needle. Proper anaesthesia ensures a painless procedure. A tiny slit puncture is made through the skin by a No. 11 scalpel blade, followed by insertion of a small haemostat to spread the subcutaneous tissues. This allows free passage of catheter and guidewire through the skin layers into the artery.

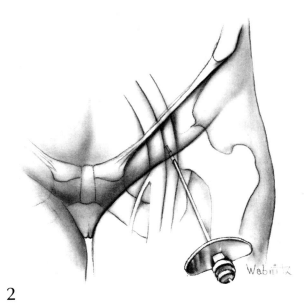

2

3

Insertion of needle-cannula

The needle-cannula is then inserted until the pulsations of the vessel are felt at its tip. The needle is inserted quickly at an approximate angle of 45–60°, with fixation of the tissues and vessel by the left index and middle fingers. At first it may be wise to transfix both walls of the vessel. With practice, puncture of only the anterior wall may be accomplished, but the added danger of subintimal placement of wire and catheter may offset the gain in haemostasis.

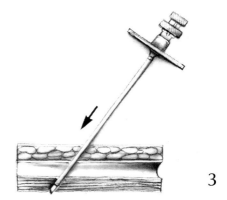

3

4

Withdrawal of cannula

After withdrawal of the inner needle and obturator, the cannula is gently and slowly withdrawn until blood spurts forcefully from the open end. The cannula should only then be lowered to almost 20° to the horizontal for guidewire passage.

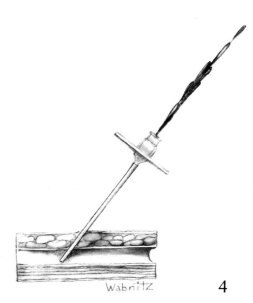

4

5

Removal of cannula

The guidewire is then inserted through the cannula 20–30 cm past the tip into the artery. It should pass through the needle into the vessel without any resistance.

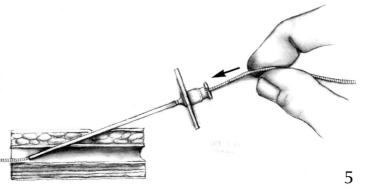

5

6

With the guidewire remaining in the vessel, the cannula is removed. Compression is applied over the puncture site, since the guidewire has a narrower diameter than the cannula. The catheter is threaded over the spring guidewire and advanced to the skin. Obviously, the guide has to be longer than the catheter so that it protrudes outside and can be grasped for removal. Wire guides have various shapes and flexible tip configurations.

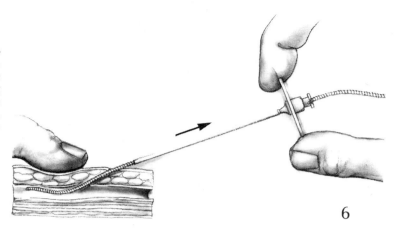

6

Insertion of guide and catheter

7

Both guide and catheter are inserted into the vessel by firm pressure and rotation. A curved tip catheter should be inserted with the curve opened – i.e., the tip pointed upwards. The compressing finger thereby straightens the catheter into the artery. The catheter is then positioned at its proper level under fluoroscopic control.

The guide is withdrawn and the catheter flushed with normal saline. A drip infusion provides reliable, continuous flushing of an endhole catheter, but catheters with multiple sideholes require frequent, continual, forceful manual flushes.

When the arteriogram is completed, the catheter is withdrawn from the vessel. Firm, but not occlusive manual, pressure must be maintained on, and slightly proximal to, the puncture site for at least 10 min. The patient is advised to remain on bedrest for at least 6 hours, or most often till the next morning. A pressure bandage is usually not necessary unless there is a heightened risk of bleeding or if a haematoma has already formed.

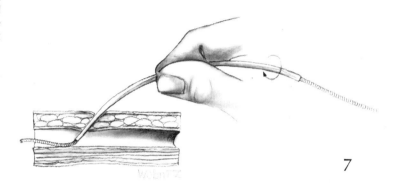

7

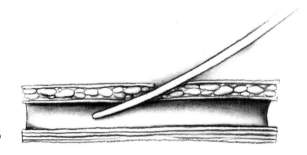

8

8

A closed-tip catheter or even a balloon-tipped catheter may be inserted into a vessel by the same technique. A wide-bore sheath is slipped into the vessel over a guidewire and tapered catheter.

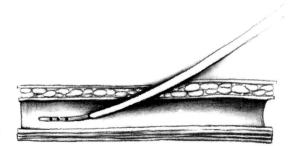

9

9

The catheter and wire are removed and the special catheter inserted through the short sheath. The balloon-tipped catheters may be used for pressure monitoring, removal of clots or purposeful occlusion of smaller branch vessels.

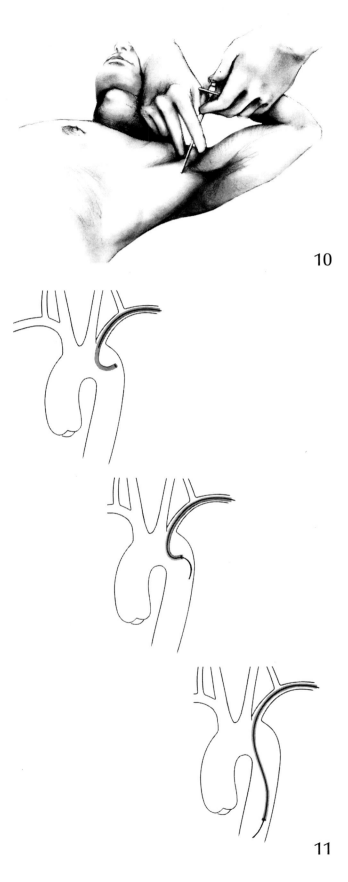

10

10 & 11

CATHETERIZATION OF AXILLARY ARTERY

Either axillary artery may be easily catheterized. The left axillary artery provides easy access (with some extra manipulation required in the elderly) to the aorta and vessels below the diaphragm. A curved-tip catheter with the tip directed laterally just within the arch is recommended. The patient should be supine with the appropriate arm abducted and the hand resting under his head. The artery may be palpated in the axilla, preferably just distal to the fold of the pectoralis muscle, but frequently the artery is more easily fixated and catheterized several centimetres distal to the axilla. The arterial puncture is the same as described above for the femoral artery, except that the needle has to be inserted almost at right-angles to the axillary artery. Extra care has to be taken to prevent brachial plexus injury. When using the left axillary artery approach, the catheter usually enters the descending aorta in patients under 40 years of age without need for manipulation.

OTHER VESSEL PUNCTURES

Other vessels which can be punctured percutaneously for catheterization are the carotid arteries; the subclavian arteries, by either intra or supraclavicular approaches; and the brachial arteries. Surgical arteriotomy is preferred for brachial artery catheterization since this vessel is highly prone to spasm and resultant thrombosis.

11

Translumbar aortography

If there is severe occlusive disease of the aortoiliac system and arteriograms of this system are needed, translumbar puncture of the aorta may be necessary. Throughout the years and despite its limitations, this method of angiography has been comparatively free of complications and certainly belongs in the armamentarium of angiographers.

This method makes it more difficult to inject the contrast selectively at a particular level. There is no control or possibility, short of major surgery, of applying haemostasis. Manipulation of the needle is impossible and excessive movement of the patient may be hazardous.

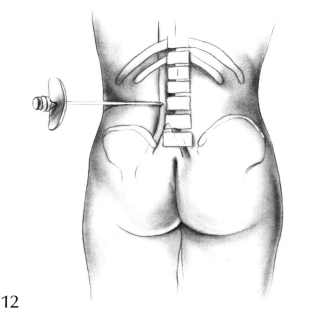

12

Insertion of needle

12

An 18 gauge, 20 cm aortographic needle or preferably a flexible Teflon sleeve needle, catheter may be used. After sterile preparation and local anaesthesia, the needle is inserted between the 12th rib and the iliac crest, 8–12 cm (5–6 fingerbreadths) to the left of the midline, with the patient prone. The author prefers to begin with a 'low' aortogram (below the renal arteries) by directing the tip of the needle medially towards L2 or L3. The needle may be directed medially and cranially towards the anterior portion of the 12th vertebral body if a 'higher' aortogram is desired. Fluoroscopic control of the site and direction of the needle can lead to a shortening of the procedure time and to a more accurate placement, but is not mandatory.

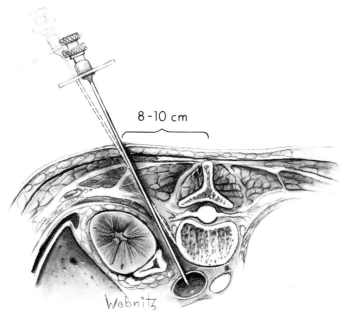

13

13

Direct puncture of the aorta may be accomplished most of the time. Occasionally it may be necessary to gently strike the anterior part of the vertebral body, withdraw somewhat and redirect the needle slightly more vertical. The pulsatile jet of blood from the needle when it enters the aorta is not as dramatic as from the femoral artery. A curved-tip guidewire is then advanced through the flexible catheter into the aorta to aid several more centimetres of intraluminal catheter placement. A film or fluoroscopic control of a test injection of 5–10 ml contrast material is highly recommended.

Following removal of the catheter, the patient is instructed to remain on bedrest till the next morning.

Carotid arteriography

Carotid arteriography should be accomplished by percutaneous transfemoral catheterization, as described. For direct carotid angiography, the author recommends a short bevel 19 or 20 gauge needle, 6–7 cm in length, fitting snugly inside a flexible Teflon or polyethylene sleeve or cannula of gauge 18 (*see* inset to *Illustration 14*). When the arterial puncture is made, the sharp needle may be withdrawn, leaving the blunt but flexible cannula in the lumen of the vessel. This flexible atraumatic cannula may easily be inserted further into the vessel with or without the use of a guidewire, without causing intimal damage. There is also less danger of vessel wall damage if the patient has to be moved or moves inadvertently.

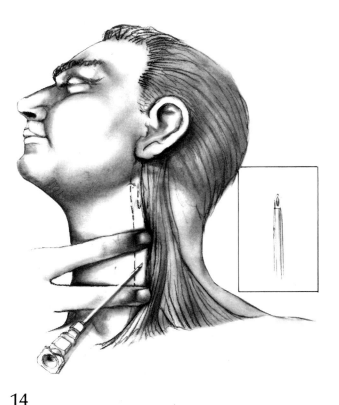

14

14

The head should be mildly extended (a soft support under the shoulder helps). Sterile preparation and local anaesthesia are carried out. The common carotid artery is fixed with the second and third fingers of the left hand. The sternocleidomastoid muscle is displaced posterolaterally by these fingers. The bifurcation of the common carotid artery is usually above the level of the superior margin of the thyroid cartilage, just below the angle of the jaw. A nearly right-angle approach of the needle, using exactly the technique of arterial puncture described above, should be employed. Both walls of the vessel may be transfixed. Slow, gentle withdrawal of the inner needle is advised so that as the posterior wall 'pops' away, the cannula tip remains within the vessel lumen. The cannula hub should then be lowered to a more horizontal position and eased inwards. Control of the intraluminal position is maintained and secured by the pulsatile jet of blood. Ten to 12 ml of lower concentration, low sodium, methylglucamine contrast material gives adequate detail of the intracranial vessel system. The normal intracranial circulation may be successfully mapped if rapid, serial films are exposed to span at least a 6 second period. The author recommends X-ray texts for a proper discussion of head positioning and programming for intracranial arteriography.

Complications of percutaneous catheterization

A relatively simple examination can lead to a catastrophe if measures are not instituted to prevent and treat emergencies. Total complication rates should be below 2 per cent.

Fatal allergic or idiosyncratic reactions to contrast material are unusually rare. Subcutaneous, conjunctival and intravenous tests of contrast material have proved unreliable in eliciting allergic reactions. The best safeguard against any serious reaction is its immediate recognition and treatment. A history of serious reaction to previous injections of contrast is only a relative contraindication to further studies; 24–48 hour pretreatment with steroids allows safe angiography in such patients. Antihistamines may be useful for minor allergic phenomena – for example, itching and urticaria. Adrenaline (1:1000) and steroids may be necessary to treat life-threatening allergic complications such as laryngeal oedema.

Contrast-materials are potent vasodilators. Most of the haemodynamic effects of contrast media injection, such as increased stroke volume, heart rate and cardiac output, as well as expansion of the circulatory blood volume, fall of the haematocrit, and hypotension, are due to the hypertonicity of the injectate and the introduction of large volumes of fluid. Adequate hydration of the patient and electrolyte balance should be assured before attempting arteriography. Cardiovascular collapse and shock are rarely seen with routine arteriographic procedures, but oxygen, airways, emergency drugs and a defibrillator have to be within easy reach.

Since renal failure is more frequent in the diabetic, extra precaution for adequate hydration is mandatory; 25–50 gm of mannitol may be used as an osmolar diuretic in diabetic patients and in those with poor renal function.

The majority of complications of percutaneous catheterization are local – that is, occurring at the site of arterial puncture. The incidence of serious complications should be less than 0.5 per cent. These are as follows:

Haemorrhage may occur during two phases of the procedure: just after the puncture of the artery with the guidewire *in situ*, as the catheter is being slipped on; or when the catheter is removed at the end of the examination. Digital pressure at both times prevents this complication. Hypertensive patients bleed more readily.

Thrombosis of the punctured artery should be recognized immediately. The typical signs are a cool, blanched, painful lower limb, with no peripheral pulse. This complication is usually due to excessive manipulation of the catheter, prolonged duration of the catheter in the vessel, low cardiac output, hypotension or a catheter which was too large for the blood vessel. Rapid intervention is recommended.

Spasm of the artery is more often seen in younger individuals and may lead to stasis and thrombus formation. Spasm may be caused by multiple traumatic punctures and excessive, prolonged catheterization time. The brachial artery is much more prone to spasm than the femoral or the axillary artery and ought not to be percutaneously catheterized.

Other complications False aneurysm, intravascular breakage of the guidewire tip, haematomas, arteriovenous fistulae and intramural injections have all been reported. These may usually be avoided by meticulous, correct technique. Non significant para-aortic bleeding is a constant finding after translumbar aortography. Embolic phenomena – air, cholesterol and foreign matter – have been reported.

Further reading

American College of Radiology. Prevention and management of adverse reactions to intravascular contrast media. Committee on Drugs Bulletin 1977, p. 2

Amplatz, K. Translumbar catheterization of the abdominal aorta. Radiology 1963; 81: 927–931

Hanafee, W. Axillary artery approach to carotid, vertebral, abdominal aorta, and coronary angiography. Radiology 1963; 81: 559–567

Haut, G., Amplatz, L. Complication rates of transfemoral and transaortic catheterization. Surgery 1968; 63: 594–596

Kahn, P. C., Boyer, D. N., Moran, J. M., Callow, A. D. Reactive hyperemia in lower extremity arteriography: an evaluation. Radiology 1968; 90: 975–980

Seldinger, S. I. Catheter replacement of the needle in percutaneous arteriography. Acta Radiologica 1953; 39: 368–376

Lipchik, E. O., Rogoff, S. M. In: Abrams, H. L., ed. Abdominal aortography: translumbar, femoral and axillary artery catheterization techniques and the normal lumbar aortogram in Angiography, 3rd ed. Boston: Little, Brown & Co., 1982

Stocks, L. O., Halpern, M., Turner, A. F. Complete translumbar aortography: the Teflon sleeve technique. American Journal of Roentgenology 1969; 107: 835–839

Widrich, W. D., Robbins, A. H., Goldstein, S. A., Singer, R. J. Adjuvant intra-arterial Lidocaine in aortofemoral arteriography. Radiology 1978; 129: 371–373

Fischer, H. W. Some factors in selection of intravascular and urographic contrast agents. In: Potchen, E. J., ed. Current concepts in radiology. Vol. I. St. Louis: Mosby Co., 1972: 210–224

Percutaneous transluminal angioplasty in the treatment of peripheral vascular disease

Barry T. Katzen MD, FACR
The Alexandria Hospital, Alexandria, Virginia;
Clinical Professor of Radiology, George Washington University Medical Center, Washington, DC, USA

Introduction

History

Percutaneous transluminal angioplasty (PTA) has recently become an accepted alternative method for therapy of stenotic and occlusive disease of the peripheral circulation, having been demonstrated to be effective in both initial reports and reports of long-term follow-up. The ability to increase blood flow through a stenotic area by catheter technique was first described by Dotter and Judkins in 1964[1,2]. Although relatively little further application and development occurred in the United States during the following 10 years, considerable interest and application occurred in European centres, where it remains the 'Dotter' procedure. Lack of further development was the result of many factors, including scepticism about efficacy, the considerable development of bypass surgery, and the technical difficulties presented by existing dilating instruments. Coaxial dilatation required the introduction of 12 Fr catheters, and which resulted in trauma at the puncture site. This led to multiple attempts to develop balloon catheters[3] which could produce dilatation of larger vessels with smaller catheters. The most successful of these, developed by Porstmann[4,5], allowed dilatation of iliac arteries using a caged balloon apparatus, but there were considerable technical limitations.

In 1974, a major technical advance was described by Gruntzig[6]: employing new plastics polymers, a 'rigid' balloon dilatation catheter was developed. The balloon had the unique ability to be inflated to relatively high pressures without significant change in outer diameter. This was followed by further improvements in balloon technology, as well as increasing experience by multiple investigators in Europe and the United States.

Pathophysiology of angioplasty

Initial theories of the mechanism of angioplasty advocated compression of plaque as the most significant factor[7,8]. More recent extensive evaluation in cadavers, animals and patients by Castaneda-Zuniga et al.[9,10,11] has demonstrated that plaque compression is a relatively insignificant part of the angioplasty process, with trauma or 'cracking' of the plaque being the predominant process. This accounts for the intimal defects noted at the angioplasty site by angiography. A subsequent healing process occurs, with neointima forming at the site of trauma, ultimately producing a smooth lumen at the site of angioplasty. Damage to the media has also been demonstrated microscopically. Adventitial injury can occur, but is generally not part of the angioplasty process.

Mechanics of dilatation and selection of balloon size

Balloon dilatation catheters currently manufactured inflate reliably to prescribed dimensions of outer diameter under high pressures, with stretching of the balloon. Effective angioplasty is the result of force applied to a lesion by a balloon under pressure[11,12]. One should remember, however, that the *inflation pressure* and *force* applied to the lesion are only indirectly related. The force applied is dependent on other factors, including the degree of stenosis and the outer diameter of the balloon relative to the vessel size. Balloon sizing and selection is therefore a critical element affecting successful angioplasty. Selection of a balloon with too small an outer diameter may result in underdilatation and early restenosis, and too large a diameter might increase the risk of vessel rupture. Most angiographers base their selection of the outer diameter upon direct measurement from conventional angiograms, allowing for magnification. This generally results in the use of a balloon 10–20 per cent larger than the actual internal diameter. Balloon length should be sufficient to extend 1–2 cm on each side of the lesion. It is axiomatic that the angiographer must understand the mechanics of dilatation as well as the potential hazards of inflating balloons under high pressure in the vascular tree.

General principles of technique

Many techniques and variations have been described for performing successful angioplasty, reflecting the varied backgrounds of angiographers. However, the following concepts are generally followed.

1. Safe and effective angioplasty demands cautious approach to and passage through the diseased area, and frequently requires a variety of catheters and guide-wires used in subselective catheterization. It should therefore be performed only by physicians with the skill and training in the techniques of selective percutaneous angiography.

2. Passage of a guide-wire through a lesion is the most critical part of the procedure and should be performed only once if possible.
3. Once the dilatation has been performed, further manipulation through the lesion by guide-wires should not be performed because of the known trauma at the angioplasty site and the risk of thrombosis.
4. Detailed angiographic evaluation or 'road mapping' should be performed to define the lesion optimally.
5. Antegrade puncture of the common femoral artery is the optimal approach for superficial femoral artery occlusions and most stenoses.
6. Aggressive steps to prevent and reverse spasm should be employed during procedures.
7. Close cooperation with vascular surgeons in patient selection and discussion of alternative methods of therapy is essential.

Iliac angioplasty

Patient selection

Morphologically, the ideal lesion is a focal stenosis of haemodynamic significance not directly involving a vessel orifice[14,15]. Longer stenoses (greater than 2 cm) and orifice lesions can be dilated but may require some technical variations and may have lesser initial and long-term success rates. Treatment of iliac artery occlusions has also been reported with some success[16], but in the United States, these are generally considered to be best treated surgically.

The angiographic approach, whether antegrade or retrograde, may vary depending on the anatomical location, the presence of concomitant lesions, the state of the aortic bifurcation and the preferences of the individual angiographer. Direct measurement of intra-arterial pressure across stenotic lesions is helpful in establishing the physiological significance of a given stenosis. It also provides baseline information for subsequent evaluation of the adequacy of the dilatation, with elimination of any pressure gradients and morphological improvement defining the end-point of the angioplasty. Ideally, evaluation of the patient before angioplasty using segmental Doppler pressure analysis, pulse volume recordings or other non-invasive techniques will have determined the physiological significance of lesions before angiography. These non-invasive studies are extremely helpful[17], both in patient selection and in confirming the significance of otherwise questionable stenoses. For instance, it is possible for an iliac stenosis of 40–50 per cent to have no change in intra-arterial pressure across the stenosis at rest. However, when the patient exercises, peripheral vasodilatation occurs, creating a drop in pressure across the stenosis and resultant symptoms. Preangioplasty non-invasive studies are also helpful in determining the significance of various lesions when they are positioned in tandem ipsilaterally (i.e. tandem iliac and femoral stenoses).

1a–g

Technique

The most common technical approach is from the ipsilateral side, but the contralateral approach is occasionally used[18]. Generally, a catheter is placed from the contralateral side to perform diagnostic angiography and facilitate contrast injections during the course of angioplasty.

Perhaps the most critical aspect of all types of angioplasty is in passing the guide-wire safely across the lesion. A variety of types of angiographic guide-wires may be necessary, including 'J' shaped and straight with long, tapered mandrils.

Once the lesion has been traversed, the guide-wire is passed into the abdominal aorta to provide secure access for catheter exchange. The angioplasty catheter is then introduced and positioned under fluoroscopic control. To facilitate anatomical localization, a metallic marker such as a haemostat may be placed on the skin surface, localizing the lesion. The guide-wire is generally left in place along with the balloon catheter to facilitate access. Dilatation is then performed while monitoring under fluoroscopy. Inflation to 5–6 atmospheres of pressure (505–606 kPa) is performed while a defect on the balloon is viewed on the video monitor. When the balloon is completely inflated, the defect should be obliterated and this may occur in rather sudden fashion. Duration of inflation is generally 10–15 seconds. A second inflation is performed during which residual defects are carefully looked for; if any are present, employment of a slightly larger balloon should be considered.

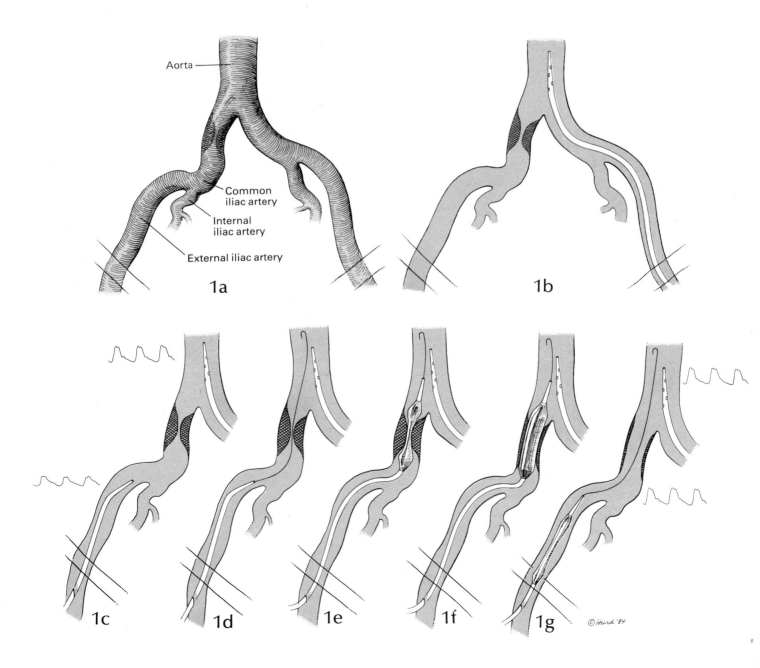

Aorta

Common iliac artery

Internal iliac artery

External iliac artery

1a

1b

1c   1d   1e   1f   1g

© Herd '84

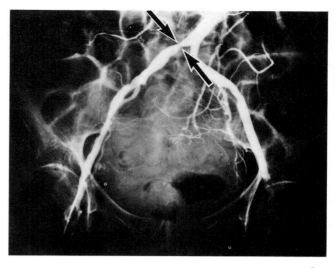

2a

2a & b

When the procedure is complete, the catheter may be withdrawn distal to the angioplasty site and intra-arterial pressure may be measured while the guide-wire is in place. Additionally, injection of contrast through the contralateral catheter will allow morphological evaluation. When completion of the angioplasty has been confirmed by fluoroscopic and physiological evaluation, conventional angiography is done via the catheter from the contralateral side to document the efficacy of the angioplasty and the degree of trauma caused.

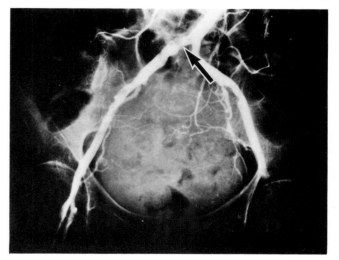

2b

(Opposite page) *Technique of iliac angioplasty. (a) An angiographic demonstration of a high-grade right common iliac stenosis. (b) A 5 Fr flush catheter is placed in the lower abdominal aorta. (c) A 5 Fr multipurpose catheter is placed in the ipsalateral external iliac artery and pressure gradient is established. (d) An angiographic guide-wire is carefully used to traverse the lesion. A multipurpose catheter curve is used to help direct the guide-wire towards the central portion of the stenosis. Contrast may be injected through the flush catheter to monitor the position of the wire. (e) An angioplasty balloon is then exchanged for the diagnostic catheter, being careful to maintain the guide-wire across the stenosis. (f) Dilatation to 5–6 atmospheres of pressure (505–606 kPa) is performed. (g) The angioplasty balloon is deflated and moved distally in the vessel, with the guide-wire remaining across the lesion.*

(Above) *Common iliac angioplasty – evaluation. (a) High-grade lesion involving the proximal portion of the right common iliac artery. (b) Following angioplasty, there is marked morphological improvement in the stenosis with a widely patent lumen demonstrated.*

Antegrade puncture of the common femoral artery

3a & b

Lesions of the superficial femoral artery, both stenoses and occlusions, are best approached following percutaneous antegrade puncture of the common femoral artery. Although the superficial femoral artery can be punctured directly, this approach has several disadvantages including the inability to obtain adequate compression post procedure and the possibility of inadvertently missing lesions at the orifice of the superficial femoral artery. The objective of antegrade puncture is to puncture the common femoral artery as it exits from the inguinal canal; this requires an approach originating at the inguinal ligament. Careful palpation and anatomical orientation should be made to avoid inadvertent puncture of the common femoral artery above the inguinal ligament. Using fluoroscopy to confirm final needle placement may be helpful.

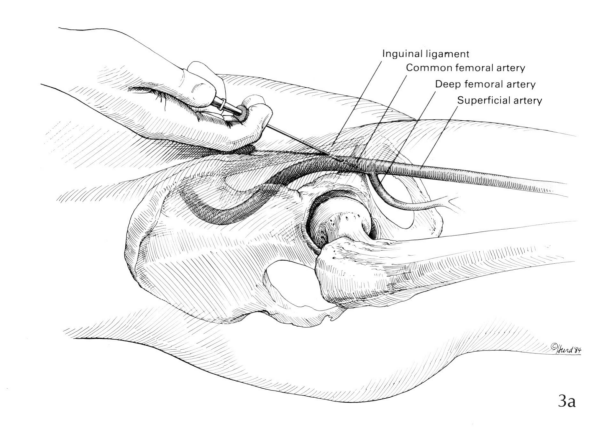

Inguinal ligament
Common femoral artery
Deep femoral artery
Superficial artery

3a

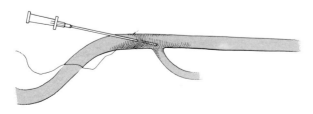

3b

Antegrade puncture of the common femoral artery. (a) Needle path is planned to achieve an oblique puncture coursing over to the inguinal ligament and puncturing the common femoral artery as it exits from the inguinal canal. This allows adequate room for compression post procedure and permits puncture proximal to the origin of the profunda femoral artery. (b) The puncture is made and good retrograde flow achieved.

Femoral angioplasty

4a–d

Following the antegrade puncture of the common femoral artery, a guide-wire is placed in the superficial femoral artery. If the guide-wire preferentially passes into the profunda femoral artery, small injections of contrast are made to evaluate the potential for catheterizing the superficial femoral artery. If needle placement has been made directly into the profunda femoral artery, or too low

in the common femoral artery, withdrawal of the needle, compression and attempt at repuncture at a slightly higher site is recommended.

Once the guide-wire has been placed in the superficial femoral artery, a 5 Fr multipurpose catheter is introduced for initial access, morphological evaluation and better delineation of the lesion.

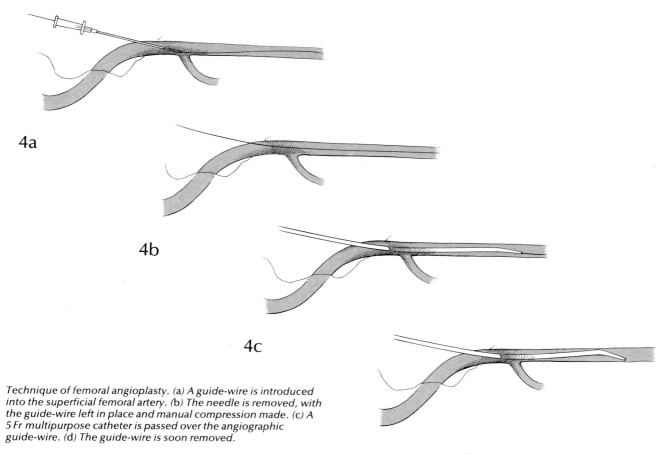

4a

4b

4c

Technique of femoral angioplasty. (a) A guide-wire is introduced into the superficial femoral artery. (b) The needle is removed, with the guide-wire left in place and manual compression made. (c) A 5 Fr multipurpose catheter is passed over the angiographic guide-wire. (d) The guide-wire is soon removed.

4d

Superficial femoral artery stenosis

5a–f

A guide-wire is first employed to traverse the lesion. Since lesions are frequently eccentric, a multipurpose catheter with a slight curve facilitates optimal passage of the guide-wire. Various straight wires are generally used to traverse the lesion since the overall vessel calibre and lumen size through the stenosis will not allow J-wire passage. Once the guide-wire has traversed the lesion and is positioned sufficiently distal to the lesion to allow safe catheter exchange, one should consider exchanging the straight guide-wire for a J-wire which will be positioned in the popliteal artery during the angioplasty. This can be done by passing the 5 Fr multipurpose catheter through the lesion and exchanging the straight guide-wire for a 1.5 mm 'J'. Maintaining the wire at the level of the tibial plateau will minimize development of popliteal spasm.

Prior to dilatation, all areas of significant disease should be inspected on the preliminary arteriogram.

Dilatation is performed in a manner similar to that described above for iliac angioplasty. Since an antegrade approach is employed, when dilatation is complete, the catheter may be withdrawn and a contrast injected over the guide-wire to allow inspection of the angioplasty site. Following completion of the angioplasty and dilatation of all segments, a follow-up arteriogram is performed for documentation purposes and evaluation of distal run-off.

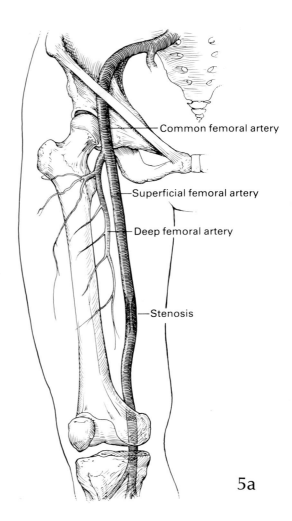

Common femoral artery

Superficial femoral artery

Deep femoral artery

Stenosis

5a

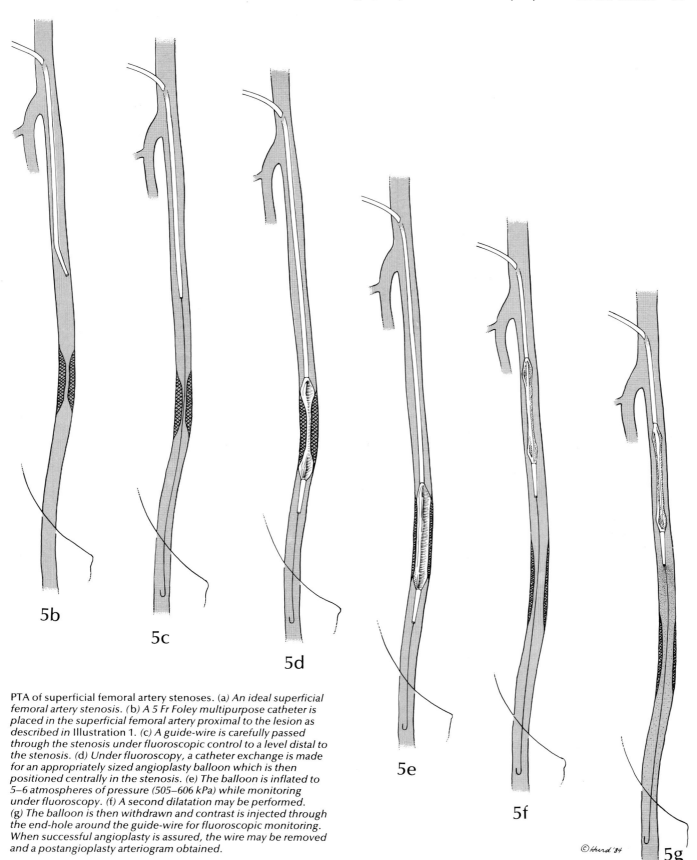

5b

5c

5d

5e

5f

5g

PTA of superficial femoral artery stenoses. (a) *An ideal superficial femoral artery stenosis. (b) A 5 Fr Foley multipurpose catheter is placed in the superficial femoral artery proximal to the lesion as described in* Illustration 1. *(c) A guide-wire is carefully passed through the stenosis under fluoroscopic control to a level distal to the stenosis. (d) Under fluoroscopy, a catheter exchange is made for an appropriately sized angioplasty balloon which is then positioned centrally in the stenosis. (e) The balloon is inflated to 5–6 atmospheres of pressure (505–606 kPa) while monitoring under fluoroscopy. (f) A second dilatation may be performed. (g) The balloon is then withdrawn and contrast is injected through the end-hole around the guide-wire for fluoroscopic monitoring. When successful angioplasty is assured, the wire may be removed and a postangioplasty arteriogram obtained.*

©Hurd '84

Superficial femoral artery occlusion

6a–f

Treatment of femoral artery occlusions involves recanalization as well as dilatation. Access to the artery is performed in the manner described above. The most common technique of recanalization employs a reducible core, a J-wire, which becomes a rigid straight wire when the mandrel is placed at the tip of the wire. This results in a straightening of the multipurpose catheter. The multipurpose catheter should be placed as close to the occlusion as possible, and the guide-wire is then passed through the occluded segment. Preprocedure marking of the occlusion using a radiopaque haemostat on both the proximal and distal ends of the occlusion is helpful. When the guide-wire has reached the terminal portion of the occlusion, the inner mandrel is moved approximately 1–2 cm, reconstituting the 'J' configuration. Once recanalization has been successfully achieved, the multipurpose catheter may be passed through the occlusion and intra-arterial vasodilators may be administered. Injection of contrast and visualization under fluoroscopy should be employed to exclude early distal embolization or distal arterial spasm. Exchange for a dilatation balloon is then performed as described above, and dilatation may be carried on as in treatment of stenotic lesions.

During the course of recanalization of any arterial occlusion, the patient should feel no pain. The sensation of pain during the passage of a guide-wire indicates the presence of subintimal dissection and passage of the guide-wire into the wrong space. The guide-wire should be withdrawn and a repeat attempt of recanalization performed by repositioning the 5 Fr multipurpose catheter proximal to the occlusion.

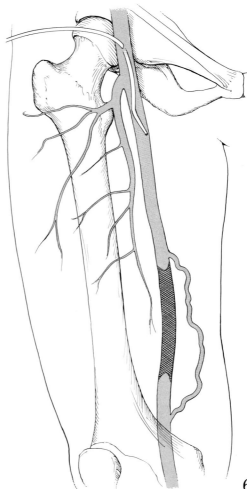

6a

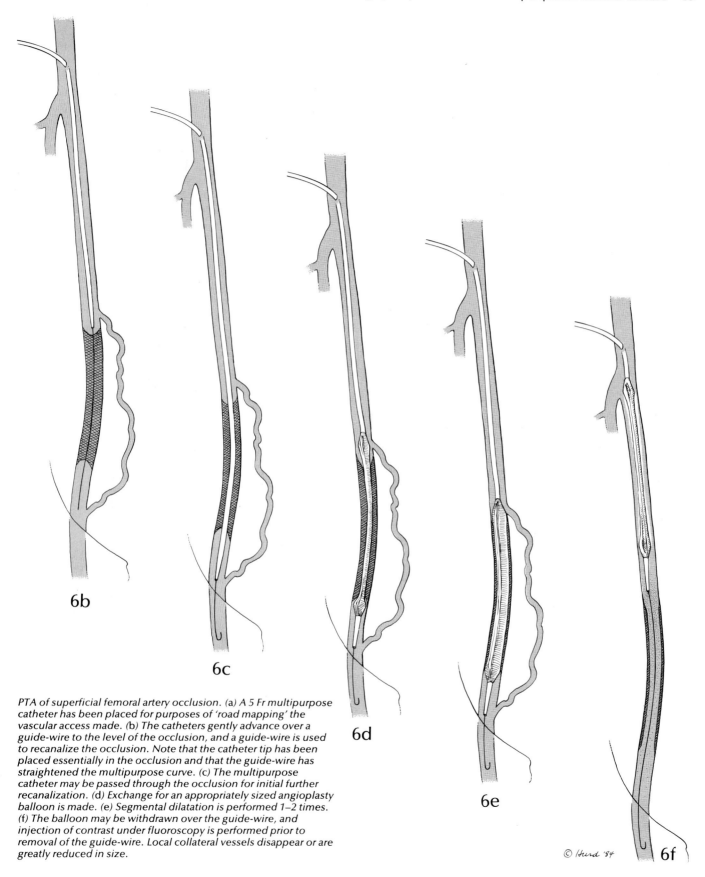

6b

6c

6d

6e

6f

PTA of superficial femoral artery occlusion. (a) A 5 Fr multipurpose catheter has been placed for purposes of 'road mapping' the vascular access made. (b) The catheters gently advance over a guide-wire to the level of the occlusion, and a guide-wire is used to recanalize the occlusion. Note that the catheter tip has been placed essentially in the occlusion and that the guide-wire has straightened the multipurpose curve. (c) The multipurpose catheter may be passed through the occlusion for initial further recanalization. (d) Exchange for an appropriately sized angioplasty balloon is made. (e) Segmental dilatation is performed 1–2 times. (f) The balloon may be withdrawn over the guide-wire, and injection of contrast under fluoroscopy is performed prior to removal of the guide-wire. Local collateral vessels disappear or are greatly reduced in size.

© Hurd '84

7a & b

Following angioplasty, angiographic evaluation should be performed to document the morphological success of the angioplasty as well as the degree of vascular trauma created, and to exclude the presence of distal emboli or other pathology.

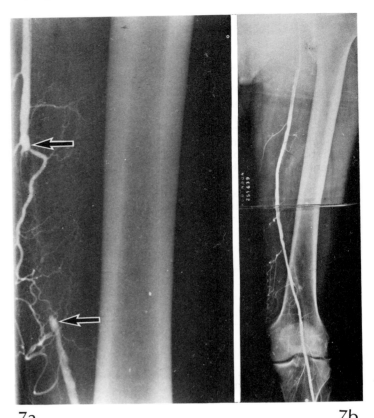

7a   7b

PTA of superficial femoral artery occlusion – evaluation. (a) 8 cm total occlusion of a superficial femoral artery. (b) Following recanalization and dilatation of a widely patent lumen; there is a small intimal defect.

Treatment of run-off vessels

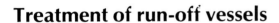

Attempts at percutaneous transluminal angioplasty of arteries below the popliteal vessels should be limited to patients in whom rest pain or frank ischaemia is present, and a limb salvage problem is present clinically. Small balloon catheters and coaxial dilatation catheters are occasionally used but the hazards of treatment of these lesions are considerably greater than with treatment of larger vessels. Technical considerations are beyond the scope of this discussion[19].

Results

In general, percutaneous transluminal angioplasty has success rates comparable to equivalent surgical procedures. Larger vessels are associated with higher initial and long-term success rates than smaller vessels, so that results are generally better in iliac arteries than in superficial femoral arteries and run-off vessels[20–23].

As reported in several long-term series[20, 22], one can expect the following results from angioplasty of non-occlusive iliac artery stenosis: initial success – 96 per cent; one year patency – 90–95 per cent; 3 year patency – 85–90 per cent; and 5 year patency – 85–90 per cent. As in all methods of interventional treatment of vascular disease, individual results will be affected by adverse variables including diabetes, the presence of diffuse disease and smoking. Average results from a variety of investigators[19, 22] allow one to anticipate an initial success rate of 75–80 per cent for superficial femoral artery stenosis and a 2 year success rate of 50–75 per cent. For superficial femoral artery occlusions (<15 cm), the initial success rate is 70–80 per cent and the 2 year success rate is 50–70 per cent. Certainly the most 'ideal' lesion is the focal (< 2 cm) stenosis, although these are probably the least commonly available lesions for dilatation. Occlusions of the superficial femoral artery can be recanalized and dilated and best results occur when obstructions are less than 15 cm.

Experience has shown that one can obtain an initial success rate of 80–90 per cent for popliteal stenosis and a 2 year patency rate of 70–80 per cent. For popliteal occlusion, the initial success rate is 70–75 per cent and the 2 year patency rate is 60–70 per cent. As in all therapeutic procedures, the specific patient, associated risk factors and the extent of disease must be carefully weighed before proceding. Dilatation of vessels below the popliteal artery is generally approached with great caution and primarily when limb salvage is the main consideration.

Complications

Complications of transluminal angioplasty may result from the arterial puncture and associated catheter manipulation, thrombosis at the site of angioplasty, distal embolization and contrast-related problems. In general, the complication rates in the literature are between and 1 and 4 per cent, with approximately 1–2 per cent occasionally requiring surgical intervention. Adequate patient selection based on appropriate clinical and morphological criteria will generally help to maintain low complication rates[24].

Recent experience has shown that vasospasm and its associated reduction in blood flow and platelet activation contribute significantly to complications and aggressive use of vasodilators has become frequently employed. Commonly used agents are listed in Table 1.

Table 1 Appropriate administration of vasodilators

Drug	Dose	Method of administration
Nitroglycerin	100–200 μg	Intra-arterial
Nitroglycerin	0.4 mg	Sublingual
Nifedipine	5–10 mg	Mucosal
Lignocaine (lidocaine)	100 mg	Intra-arterial
Tolazoline hydrochloride (Priscoline)	25 mg	Intra-arterial

Conclusion

Percutaneous transluminal angioplasty is an effective method of treatment of peripheral vascular disease in patients with appropriate lesions and symptomatology. Advantages of local anaesthesia, reduced hospital stay and repeatability make this technique frequently the procedure of choice in specific patients. Performance of the procedure by an experienced angiographer and careful attention to technique and control of the angioplasty environment will contribute significantly to high initial and long-term success rates, and will reduce morbidity.

References

1. Dotter, C. T., Judkins, M. P. Transluminal treatment of arteriosclerotic obstruction: description of a new technic and a preliminary report of its application. Circulation 1964; 30: 654–670

2. Dotter, C. T., Judkins, M. P. Percutaneous transluminal treatment of arteriosclerotic obstruction. Radiology 1965; 84: 631–643

3. Staple, T. W. Modified catheter for percutaneous transluminal treatment of arteriosclerotic obstructions. Radiology 1968; 91: 1041–1043

4. Portsmann, W. Ein neuer Korsett-Balloon Katheter zur transluminalen Rekanalisation nach Dotter unter besonderer Berucksichtigung von Obliterationend an den Beckenarterien. Radiologica Diagnostica (Berlin) 1973; 14: 239–244

5. Dotter, C. T., Rösch, J., Andersen, J. Transluminal iliac artery dilation. Circulation 1983; Suppl. 48: IV–119 (abstract 469)

6. Gruntzig, A., Hopff, H. Perkutane Rekanalisation chronischer arterieller Verschlusse mit einem neuen Dilatationskatheter: Modifikation der Dotter-Technik. Deutsches Medizinische Wochenschrift 1974; 99: 2502–2510

7. Dotter, C. T. Transluminal angioplasty; pathologic basis. In: Zeitler, E., Gruntzig, A., Schoop, W., eds. Percutaneous vascular recanalization. New York: Springer-Verlag, 1978: 3–12

8. Lue, H. J., Gruntzig, A. Histopathological aspects of transluminal recanalization. In: Zeitler, E., Gruntzig, A., Schoop, W., eds. Percutaneous vascular recanalization. New York: Springer-Verlag, 1978: 39–50

9. Castaneda-Zuniga, W. R., Formanek, A., Tradavarthy, M., et al. The mechanism of balloon angioplasty. Radiology 1980; 135: 565–571

10. Castaneda-Zuniga, W. R., Sibley, R. K., Laerum, F., et al. Mechanics of angioplasty: an experimental approach. Radiographics 1981; 1: 1–14

11. Amplatz, K. A. The method of transluminal angioplasty. In: Castaneda-Zuniga, W. R., ed. Transluminal angioplasty. New York: Thieme-Stratton, 1983: 3–10

12. Abele, J. E. Technical considerations: physical properties of balloon catheters, inflation devices, and pressure measurement devices. In: Casteneda-Zuniga, W. R., ed. Transluminal angioplasty. New York: Thieme-Stratton, 1983: 20–27

13. Abele, J. E. Balloon catheters and transluminal dilatation: technical considerations. American Journal of Roentgenology 1980; 135: 901–906

14. Motarjeme, A., Keifer, J. W., Zuska, A. J. Percutaneous transluminal angioplasty and case selection. Radiology 1980; 135: 573–581

15. Katzen, B. T., Chang, J., Knox, W. G. Percutaneous transluminal angioplasty with the Gruntzig balloon catheter: a review of 70 cases. Archives of Surgery 1979; 114: 1389–1399

16. Colapinto, R. F., Harries-Jones, E. P., Johnston, K. W. Percutaneous transluminal dilatation and recanalization in the treatment of peripheral vascular disease. Radiology 1980; 135: 583–587

17. Friedman, M. H., Katzen, B. T. Noninvasive evaluation procedures. In Castaneda-Zuniga, W. R., ed. Transluminal angioplasty. New York: Thieme-Stratton, 1983: 48–53

18. Bachman, D. M., Casarella, W. J., Sos, T. A. Percutaneous iliofemoral angioplasty via the contralateral femoral artery. Radiology 1979; 130: 617–621

19. Sniderman, K. W., Sos, T. A., The popliteal artery and its branches. In: Castaneda-Zuniga, W. R., ed. Transluminal angioplasty. New York: Thieme-Stratton, 1983: 118–127

20. van Andel, G. J. Transluminal iliac angioplasty: long-term results. Radiology 1980; 135: 607–611

21. Katzen, B. T. Transluminal angioplasty in ischemic peripheral vascular disease. Section A: transluminal angioplasty of the iliac arteries. In: Castaneda-Zuniga, W. R., ed. Transluminal angioplasty. New York: Thieme-Stratton, 1983: 93–102

22. Katzen, B. T. Percutaneous transluminal angioplasty for arterial disease of the lower extremities. American Journal of Roentgenology 1984; 142: 23–25

23. Wierny, L., Plass, R., Portsmann, W. Long-term results in 100 consecutive patients treated by transluminal angioplasty. Radiology 1974; 112:543–548

24. Laerum, F., Castaneda-Zuniga, W. R., Amplatz, K. A. Complications of transluminal angioplasty. In: Castaneda-Zuniga, W. R., ed. Transluminal angioplasty. New York: Thieme-Stratton, 1983: 41–44

Illustrations by Kevin Marks

Exposure of major blood vessels

H. H. G. Eastcott MS, FRCS
Honorary Consultant Surgeon, St Mary's Hospital, London, UK

A. E. Thompson MS, FRCS
Consultant Surgeon, St Thomas's Hospital, London, UK

Indications

The exposure of the blood vessels is necessary in both emergency and elective surgery. Access to the great vessels is most commonly required in major elective cardiovascular procedures.

Exposure of the peripheral vessels has become more complex as expertise in the surgery of smaller vessels becomes more successful. It is also routinely required for extracorporeal circulation, regional perfusion or rapid blood transfusion.

Contraindications

Surgery on blood vessels carries considerable risk and is best undertaken when adequate support is available: good operating facilities, adequate anaesthetic support and blood replacement. Control of blood loss may be more effectively obtained by exposure of vessels proximal to an infected or scarred area.

Exposure

The use of a wide approach for dealing thoroughly with nerves and vessels needs no defence[1]. When reconstructive surgery is necessary, flexures may be crossed, muscles and tendons divided and the abdomen opened to its fullest extent. Good illumination and effective self-retaining retractors are essential.

The operations

EXPOSURE OF THE ASCENDING AORTA

1

The incision

The incision is made in the midline, extending from the suprasternal notch to just beyond the xiphisternum. The extent is dictated by the need for extracorporeal circulation. A transverse component at the upper end may be added. However, if the upper end of the incision is kept below the level of the sternal notch the transverse component is not needed to achieve a good cosmetic result.

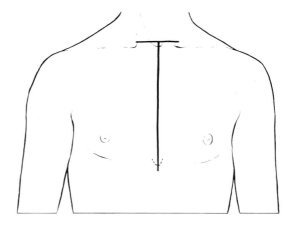

2

Entering the mediastinum

The sternum is divided with a power-driven saw. The line of division deviates slightly to the left in its lower half to avoid entering the right pleural cavity.

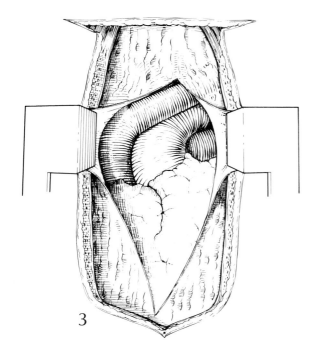

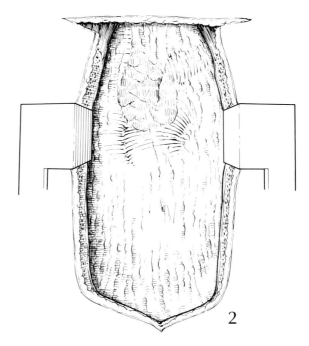

3

Deep dissection

The thymic remnant is divided and the innominate vein identified. Final access to the ascending aorta is obtained by opening the pericardium longitudinally.

EXPOSURE OF INNOMINATE ARTERY AND THORACIC PART OF RIGHT SUBCLAVIAN ARTERY

4

The incision

The shoulder girdle is displaced backwards by placing a sandbag between the patient's shoulders. The incision is centred over the right sternoclavicular joint, exposing the medial third of the clavicle, the manubrium and the first two intercostal spaces.

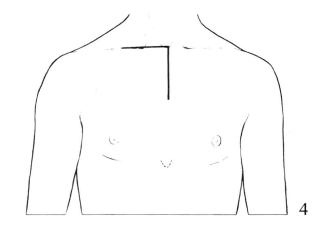

5

Splitting the manubrium

The manubrium is divided in the midline with a power-driven saw. The two halves are separated by a self-retaining retractor. Further exposure can then be obtained by transecting the sternum below the manubrium or by dividing the clavicle and anterior ends of the first and second ribs.

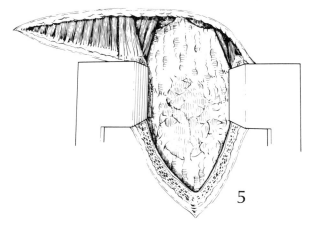

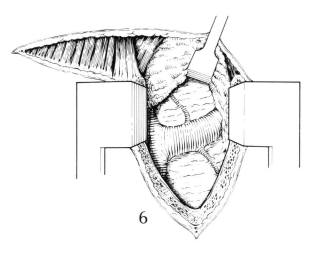

6

Deep dissection

The thymic remnant and anterior mediastinal fat are cleared to expose the innominate vein. The anterior borders of the pleural cavities are swept away laterally.

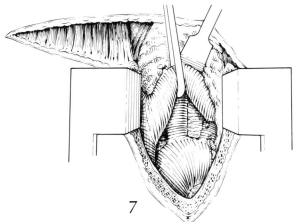

7

Exposure of the great vessels

Mobilization of the innominate vein permits it to be retracted upwards, revealing the origins of the great vessels.

EXPOSURE OF THORACIC PART OF LEFT SUBCLAVIAN ARTERY

This can be exposed by modifying the approach for the innominate and right subclavian arteries (above), or by the lateral approach through the 4th left intercostal space.

8

The incision

With the patient in the right lateral position a curved incision is made skirting the angle of the left scapula. Care must be taken to keep the incision inferior to breast tissue anteriorly and to carry it high posteriorly.

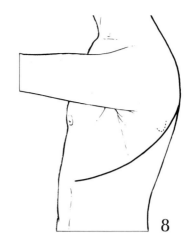

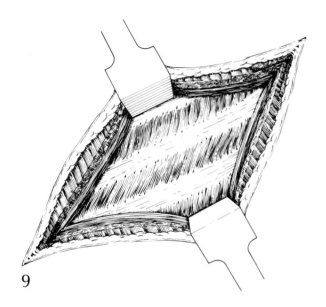

9

Deep dissection

The latissimus dorsi and serratus anterior muscles are divided and the chest is entered through an incision along the upper border of the fifth rib. Adequate exposure may require division of the fifth rib (and fourth if necessary) at the posterior end.

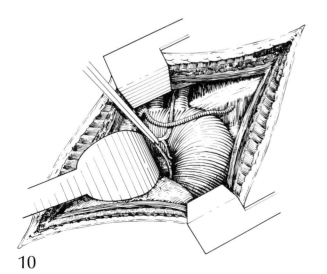

10

Intrathoracic exposure

The intrathoracic segment of the left subclavian artery can be exposed by incision of the overlying mediastinal pleura. The left superior intercostal vein is divided during incision of the mediastinal pleura. The vagus nerve is carefully preserved and the thoracic duct lying posterior to the subclavian artery is avoided.

EXPOSURE OF THE AORTIC ARCH

The aortic arch is approached as for the thoracic part of the subclavian artery. Access is improved if the anaesthetist uses a technique allowing deflation of the left lung. The left main bronchus and left pulmonary artery lie beneath the arch, with oesophagus and thoracic duct on the deep aspect.

11

EXPOSURE OF THE DESCENDING THORACIC AORTA

This vessel can be exposed in the same way as the aortic arch, entering the thorax through a lower rib space (see *Illustrations 8–10*).

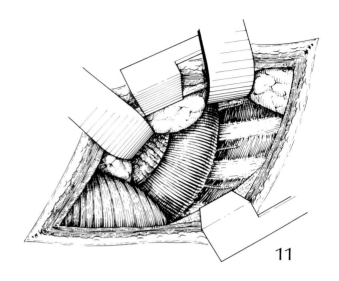

11

EXPOSURE OF CERVICAL PART OF SUBCLAVIAN ARTERY AND ORIGIN OF VERTEBRAL ARTERY

12

The incision

The patient's neck is extended and turned to the opposite side of the planned incision. A skin crease incision is made one fingerbreadth above the middle third of the clavicle. The platysma and the clavicular head of the sternomastoid are divided.

12

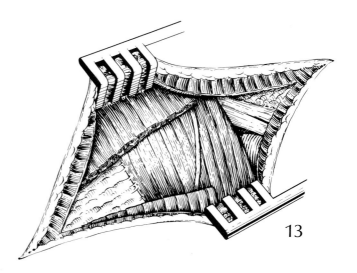

13

13 & 14

Deep dissection

The omohyoid fascia is incised and the scalenus anterior muscle exposed with the phrenic nerve on its surface. The internal jugular vein and the termination of the thoracic duct (on the left side) lie in the medial end of the field. The phrenic nerve is delicately mobilized and retracted medially, before the scalenus anterior muscle is divided piecemeal to avoid damage to the underlying vessel and its branches. The artery is finally exposed by incision of its sheath. The lower trunks of the brachial plexus lie above and lateral to the vessel.

More extensive exposure of the distal part of the vessel and the axillary artery is obtained by subperiosteal excision of the appropriate part of the clavicle.

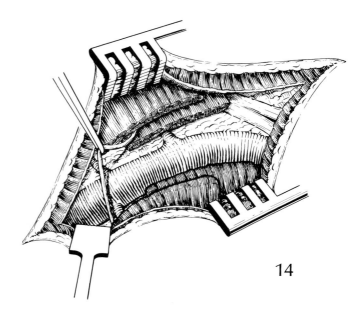

14

EXPOSURE OF AXILLARY ARTERY (FIRST PART)

15

The incision

With the arm abducted to a right angle, the incision is made just below and parallel to the clavicle.

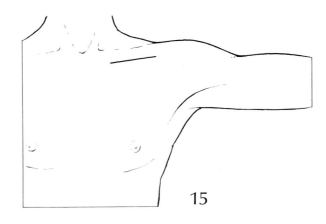

15

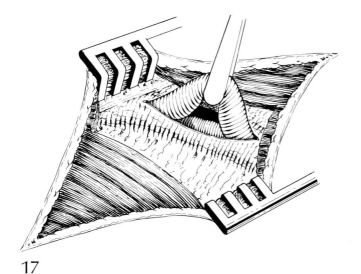

16

16

Dissection

The pectoral fascia is divided along the line of the muscle fibres of the clavicular head of the pectoralis major, which are then split to expose the vascular sheath. The pectoral branch of the acromiothoracic axis may require division.

17

17

Division of sheath

The pulsations of the artery are palpated and the vascular sheath is divided along the line thus indicated. Here the only other important structure is the axillary vein. This lies below and medial to the artery from which it is then carefully separated. This is the site for axillofemoral bypass.

EXPOSURE OF AXILLARY ARTERY (SECOND AND THIRD PARTS)

18

The incision

With the arm abducted to a right angle the incision is made along the line of the pulsating artery up to the lower border of the pectoralis major muscle. If the artery is pulseless the groove between the coracobrachialis and triceps is the guide.

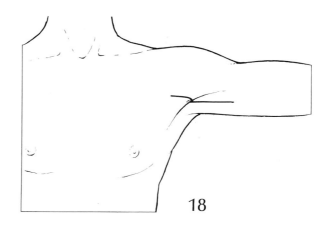

18

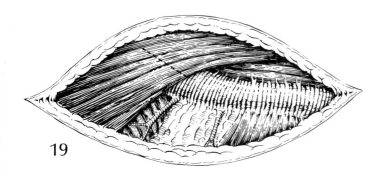

19

19

Dissection

The pectorals are retracted upwards and medially to expose the distal two-thirds of the axillary artery. If necessary, both muscles are divided and a portion of the clavicle resected to gain exposure of the whole length of the subclavian-axillary vessel. Sections of bone need not be replaced[2,3].

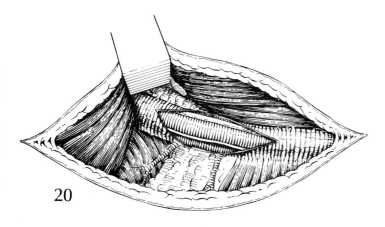

20

20

Exposure of artery

The axillary sheath is opened to reveal the vein medially and the brachial plexus laterally. The artery will be found between these two structures. It can also be identified by following the subscapular artery to its origin.

EXPOSURE OF BRACHIAL ARTERY

21

The incision

The incision is made along the line of the pulsating artery or in the line of the sulcus separating the biceps muscle from the triceps muscle. The length of the incision is governed by the procedure to be performed. In order to facilitate exposure, a sandbag is placed supporting the elbow extension.

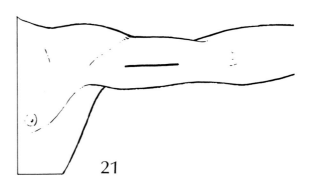

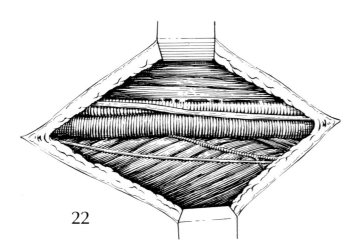

22

Dissection

The neurovascular sheath is opened. The veins and the median nerve, which crosses the artery from the lateral to the medial side, are separated from the artery. Care must be taken to recognize a high bifurcation of the vessel. The ulnar collateral artery and medial cutaneous nerve of the forearm lie close to the brachial artery and must not be included in clamps. The dissection is further complicated by the basilic vein which perforates the deep fascia and joins the brachial vein in this region.

EXPOSURE OF BRACHIAL ARTERY AT THE ELBOW

23

The incision

A skin crease incision is made at the elbow with longitudinal extensions along the line of the brachial artery medially and down the brachioradialis laterally. The skin should be marked to allow an accurate closure.

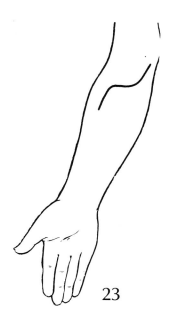

23

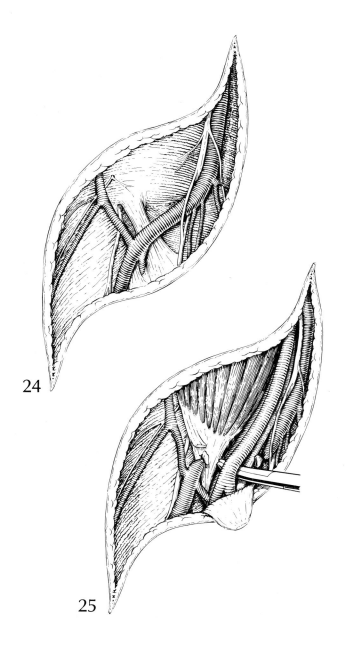

24

24

Superficial dissection

The artery is obscured by the cubital veins, the deep fascia and the bicipital aponeurosis. The two cutaneous nerves to the forearm lie deep to the veins at the medial and lateral ends of this plane of the incision and should be avoided.

25

Deep dissection

The overlying superficial veins and the bicipital aponeurosis are divided. This exposes the artery, with its accompanying deep veins, just above the bifurcation which is close to the medial side of the biceps tendon. Opening the sheath allows the vessel to be lifted away from its venae comitantes and from the median nerve, which lies on its medial side. This exposure is most commonly indicated when the brachial artery has been damaged in a supracondylar fracture. Spasm in the intact vessel can be overcome by the injection of saline into the lumen of the affected segment between arterial clamps[4].

25

EXPOSURE OF RADIAL ARTERY AT THE WRIST

26

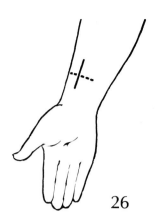

The incision

A longitudinal or transverse incision centred 3–4 cm above the radial styloid is used.

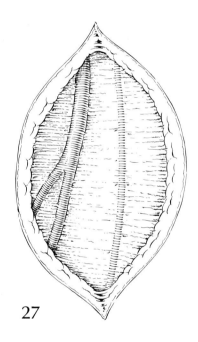

27

Dissection

The lower end of the cephalic vein lies in the superficial fascia at the radial side of the wrist. The radial artery lies at a deeper level beneath the deep fascia with its venae comitantes. Both vessels can be mobilized easily and approximated to allow a side-to-side anastomosis, creating an arteriovenous fistula for haemodialysis.

EXPOSURE OF COMMON CAROTID ARTERY

28

The incision

With neck slightly extended, and the head turned to the opposite side, a 6 cm incision is made along the anterior edge of the sternomastoid with its centre three finger-breadths above the clavicle.

For a wider exposure of the common carotid artery and internal jugular vein the incision is extended along the dotted lines, dividing the origin of the sternomastoid.

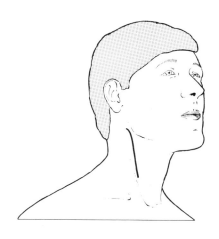

28

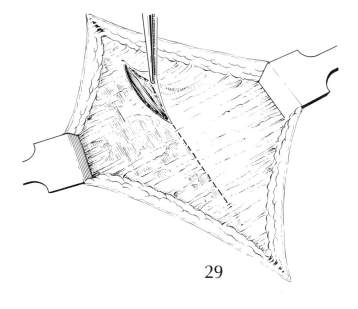

29

29

Dissection

The deep fascia is opened in the same line and the sternomastoid and infrahyoid muscles are separated from the underlying vascular sheath. This plane of dissection is bloodless except for a sternomastoid branch of the superior thyroid artery.

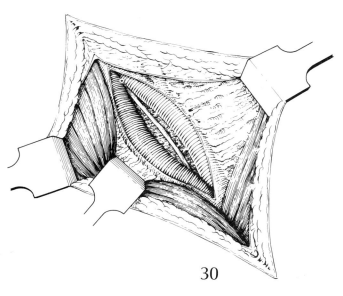

30

30

Exposure

The sheath is opened above the omohyoid. The jugular vein is dissected free and retracted laterally to isolate the artery. The vagus lies well back between the vessels, and the sympathetic trunk back further still and more medially. Lower in the neck the inferior thyroid artery crosses behind the carotid artery.

EXPOSURE OF INTERNAL AND EXTERNAL CAROTID ARTERIES

31

The incision

An incision is made along the anterior border of the sternomastoid from just above the angle of the jaw, passing downwards for 7–9 cm. For simple ligation a shorter skin crease incision may be preferred.

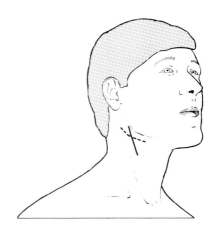

31

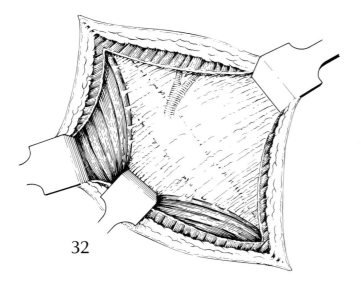

32

32

Dissection

The platysma is divided and the anterior border of the sternomastoid defined to allow retraction of the muscle away from the underlying vessels. The common facial vein is divided at the upper end of the incision and the vascular sheath opened.

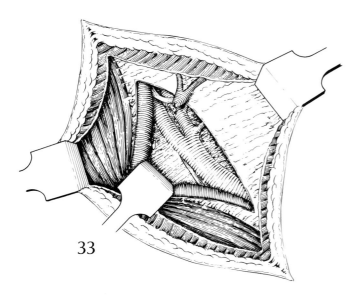

33

33

Exposure

The common carotid bifurcation usually lies much higher in the neck than is supposed. The two arteries lie close together beneath the angle of the jaw. Branches identify the external carotid, which is anterior and deeper. The hypoglossal nerve must be avoided as it crosses the vessels, and the vagus, superior laryngeal and sympathetic nerves which lie behind the bifurcation. The upper part of the internal carotid artery is difficult to expose; it runs deeply and is covered for the most part by the ascending ramus of the mandible. The sternomastoid can be detached from the mastoid process, which may itself be partly removed. The digastric muscle, the occipital artery and the styloid process are divided. This exposes the superficial aspect of the artery to some extent.

EXPOSURE OF THE AORTA ABOVE THE RENAL VESSELS

34

The incision

A thoracoabdominal incision is made along the line of the eighth rib and continued into the abdomen (*see Illustrations 8* and *9*), with the patient inclined backwards from the right lateral position. If only temporary control of the upper abdominal aorta is required during an operation on the distal vessel, a very long paramedian incision will suffice.

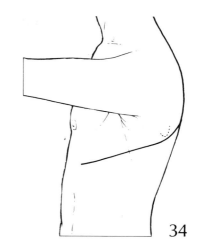

34

35

Deep dissection

The latissimus dorsi is divided. The chest is opened along the upper border of the eighth rib and the costal cartilage divided. The diaphragm is divided peripherally until the incision sweeps up to the aorta. The stomach, spleen and pancreas are swept forwards from the posterior abdominal wall to expose the aorta, the left kidney and the suprarenal gland. The visceral branches can be identified and controlled. Care must be taken in dividing intercostal vessels from which the spinal cord derives its blood supply. Temporary occlusion and hypothermia minimize the risk.

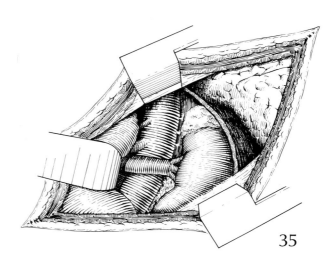

35

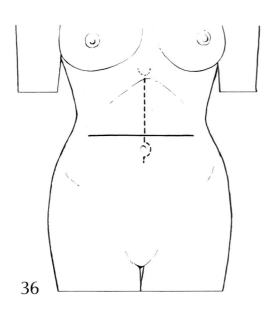

36

EXPOSURE OF RENAL ARTERIES

36

The incision

Either a midline upper abdominal[5] or a transverse incision above the umbilicus[6] gives adequate exposure.

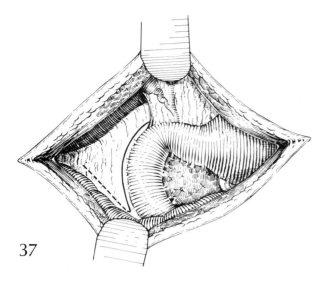

37

37–40

Deep dissection

On the right side, the peritoneum around the hepatic flexure of the colon is incised and the colon displaced downwards. The peritoneum on the right side of the duodenum is incised up to the free border of the lesser omentum. The duodenum can be displaced forwards and to the left, exposing the renal vessels, the vena cava and the aorta.

The left renal vessels are exposed by dividing the peritoneum lateral to the splenic flexure, continuing upwards behind the spleen. The spleen and colon can be displaced forwards and to the right to expose the left kidney and its vessels. The arteries lie behind the larger, more superficial renal veins.

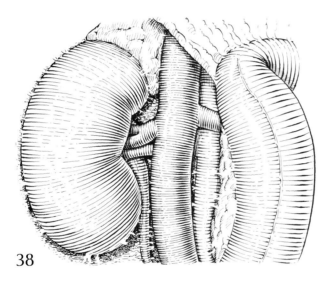

38

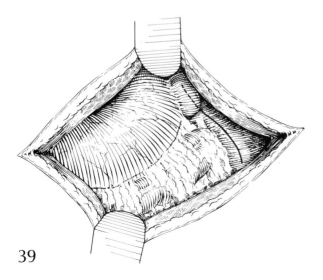

39

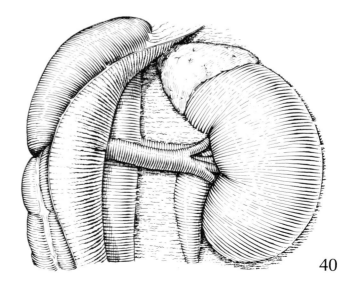

40

EXPOSURE OF SUPERIOR MESENTERIC ARTERY

41

The incision

A midline or high left paramedian incision is made and the peritoneal cavity opened.

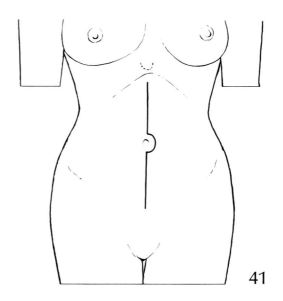

41

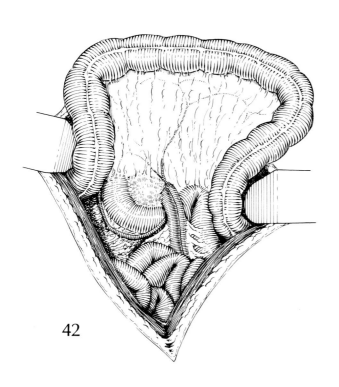

42

42

Deep dissection

The omentum and transverse colon are elevated and the posterior peritoneum incised. The superior mesenteric artery is seen where it emerges below the pancreas. The superior mesenteric vein lies on its right side. The origin of the vessel is exposed by upward dissection and retraction of the pancreas.

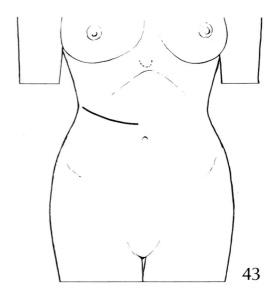

EXPOSURE OF INFRARENAL INFERIOR VENA CAVA

43

The incision

A transverse incision is made in the upper part of the right lumbar region.

43

44

Deep dissection

The oblique abdominal muscles and transversus are divided in line with the skin incision. The extraperitoneal space is entered and the peritoneum pushed to the left to expose the inferior vena cava. An alternative approach is to enter the peritoneal cavity, perform a Kocher man-oeuvre and retract the duodenum medially.

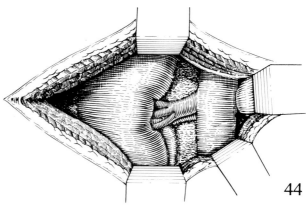

44

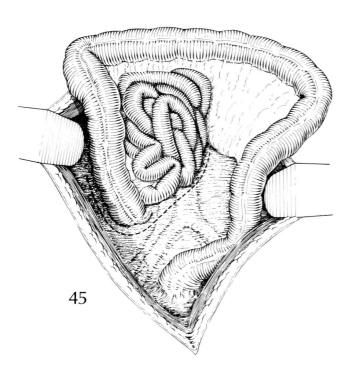

45

EXPOSURE OF ABDOMINAL AORTA BELOW RENAL VESSELS (TRANSPERITONEAL)

45

Incision and dissection

The incision is similar to that used to approach the superior mesenteric artery. Often it is sufficient to turn the small bowel across to the right side of the abdomen and to hold it there under a large abdominal pack with deep retraction. In very obese subjects, or where the aortic lesion is juxtarenal, it is better to mobilize the whole midgut loop by dividing the peritoneal reflection lateral to the right colon, continuing to the left to free the terminal ileum and small bowel mesentery. The intestines are then drawn up out of the abdomen and a plastic bag is placed over them.

EXPOSURE OF ABDOMINAL AORTA BELOW RENAL VESSELS (EXTRAPERITONEAL)

46

The incision

A long J-shaped incision runs along the left linea semilunaris and lateral to its upper half[7]. The patient's left side is lifted up on a sandbag. Alternatively, a transverse or more oblique incision as recommended by Rob[8] may be preferred, running from the tip of the left 12th rib downwards and across the lower abdomen.

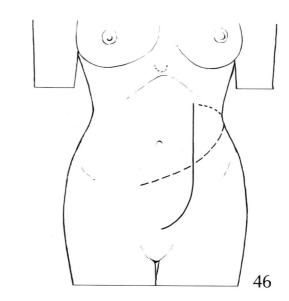

46

47

Dissection

The oblique and transversus muscles are divided in the same line over most of the central part of the incision. They are kept intact with their nerve supply at either end of the incision. The peritoneal sac is then wiped off the muscles. The aortic bifurcation and iliac arteries are exposed. Difficulty is most likely with the lower right iliac and the upper aorta. The inferior mesenteric artery is retracted with the peritoneum across the aorta to the right.

The ureter lies on the left of the aorta and inferior mesenteric artery and must be carefully avoided when extensive pathology is present.

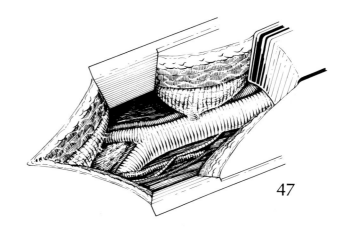

47

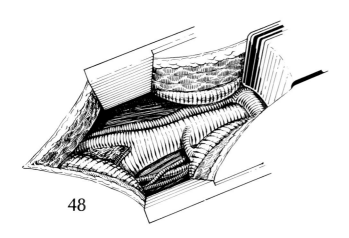

48

48

EXPOSURE OF ABDOMINAL AORTA BELOW RENAL VESSELS (BOTH ROUTES)

Whichever approach has been used the deep dissection is similar. The intestines are displaced to the right with mobilization of the terminal ileum, caecum and ascending colon as required. The aorta can be exposed as high as the left renal vein and the inferior mesenteric vessels displaced to the left. In an extraperitoneal approach these vessels are lifted forwards away from the aorta.

A large self-retaining retractor with deep blades is necessary for adequate exposure.

EXPOSURE OF THE COMMON ILIAC ARTERY (EXTRAPERITONEAL)

49

The incision

An oblique incision crosses the spinoumbilical line in its upper third.

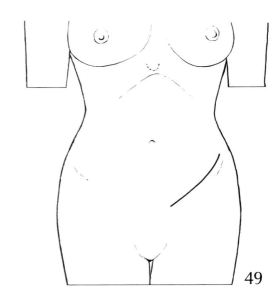

49

50

Dissection

The oblique and transversus muscles are divided in the same line. The peritoneum is carefully separated from beneath the transversus aponeurosis and the plane developed so as to displace the peritoneal sac medially.

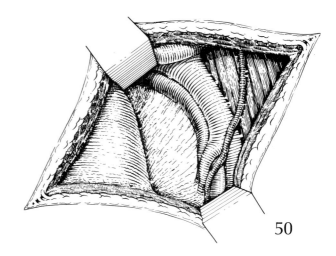

50

EXTRAPERITONEAL EXPOSURE OF EXTERNAL ILIAC ARTERY

51

The incision

An oblique incision is made in the iliac fossa extending from the midline to the anterior superior iliac spine.

51

52

Deep dissection

The posterior parietal peritoneum is pushed up under the medial edge of the incision. The external iliac vessels are found lying on the pelvic brim on the medial side of the psoas muscle. The obturator nerve lies under the vein in its upper part and the genitofemoral nerve on the muscle lateral to the artery. The ureter is seen crossing its origin.

This incision is suitable for renal transplantation, but is also of great value for controlling arterial inflow to the leg.

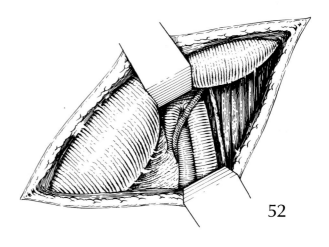

52

EXPOSURE OF COMMON FEMORAL ARTERY

53

The incision

A longitudinal incision allows adequate exposure of the common femoral artery, particularly of its deep branch, and can be extended if necessary. An extension laterally superior to the inguinal ligament allows elevation of the ligament to expose the distal external iliac artery.

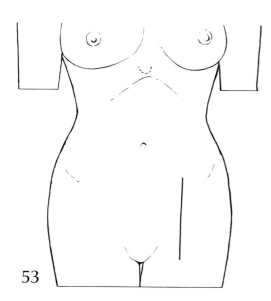

53

54

Superficial dissection

The termination of the long saphenous vein is exposed and retracted medially, dividing tributaries as required. The main vein should be preserved for grafting purposes. The superficial external pudendal artery is ligated as it passes between the saphenous and femoral veins.

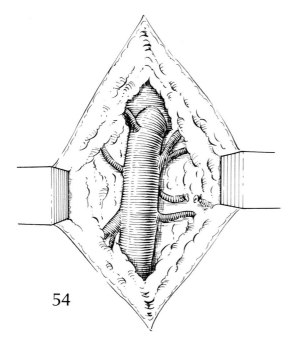

54

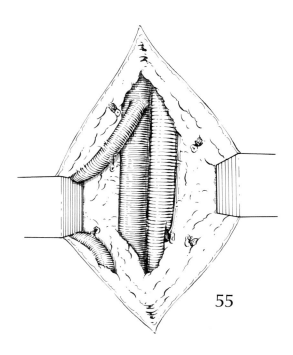

55

Deep dissection

The femoral sheath is opened to expose the common femoral vessels. The femoral nerve lies on the lateral side. The profunda femoris artery must be located with care. It arises from the posterior and lateral aspect of the common femoral artery. Its origin is closely related to the termination of the profunda femoris vein. A multiple origin or early branching of the vessel may cause difficulty.

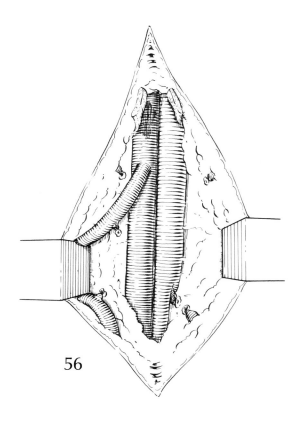

56

Iliofemoral junction

This can be exposed by an upward extension of the above dissection, by elevating or dividing the inguinal ligament. The deep epigastric vessels are preserved.

EXPOSURE OF SUPERFICIAL FEMORAL ARTERY IN HUNTER'S CANAL

57

The incision

This is made along the line of the anterior border of the sartorius muscle. The limb is slightly flexed and abducted, with a sandbag placed beneath the knee.

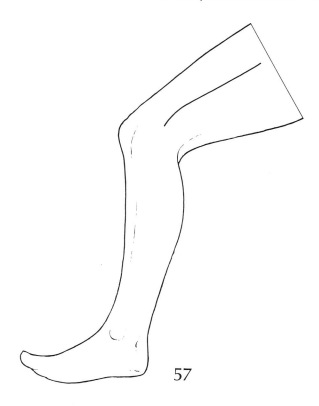

58

Superficial dissection

The saphenous vein is carefully preserved in the posterior flap. The fascia over the sartorius muscle is incised.

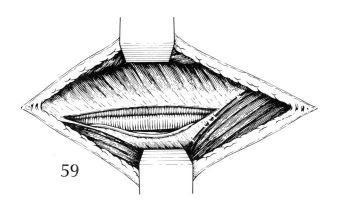

59

Deep dissection

The sartorius muscle is retracted backwards. The fascial roof of Hunter's canal is exposed and incised. The saphenous nerve is separated from the artery, which is then dissected from the underlying vein. Care is taken to preserve as many collateral vessels as possible.

EXPOSURE OF POPLITEAL ARTERY

The medial approach is used for most bypass operations, but the posterior approach is better for direct procedures such as the repair of arterial cysts or entrapment.

Medial approach (upper)

60

The incision

The patient is placed supine with the knee flexed over a sandbag. The line of the incision should run from four fingerbreadths above the adductor, opening downwards and backwards to a little behind the medial femoral condyle and avoiding the long saphenous vein.

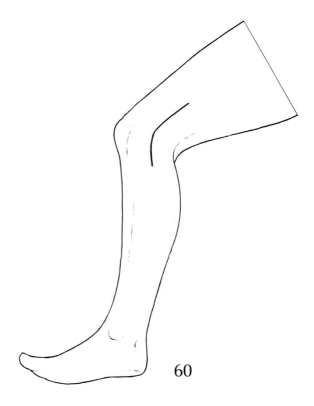

60

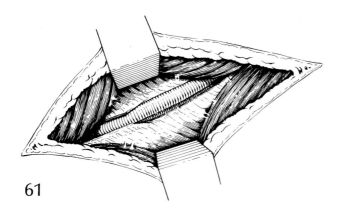

61

61

Dissection

The deep fascia is incised and the anterior border of the sartorius is defined. The muscle is displaced backwards to reveal the thicker aponeurosis of the adductor canal, running into the tendon of the adductor opening. The saphenous nerve leads the dissection to the artery. The fascia is incised to free it and the artery, which can then be followed downwards into the popliteal fat.

Medial approach (lower)

62

The incision

This is made along the posterior tibial border from the lower aspect of the medial condyle, avoiding the long saphenous vein[9].

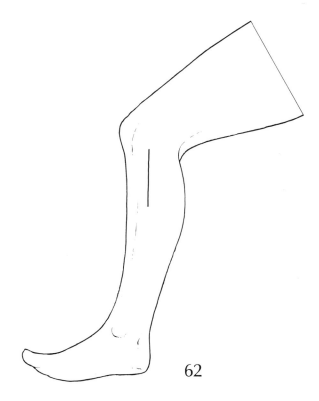

62

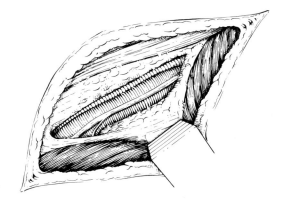

63

63

Dissection

The deep fascia, here very thick, is incised and the medial head of the gastrocnemius is displaced backwards. The loose popliteal fat is stroked free from the vascular bundle to reveal the vein, with the artery beneath it. Care should be taken not to damage the medial popliteal nerve. The bifurcation is obscured by the soleus arch and muscular veins, but by division of these the posterior tibial artery can be exposed.

Posterior approach

64

The incision

Recurrent ulceration and contraction often complicate the vertical incision which crosses the flexure at right angles. An S-shaped incision, with its upper limit medial, avoids this. The middle portion should run in the skin crease. A vertical incision is satisfactory, however, for exposing the lower portion of the popliteal vessels. Placed between the two heads of the gastrocnemius, it is commenced below the flexure and can be extended downwards to expose as much of the upper course of the posterior tibial vessels as may be necessary.

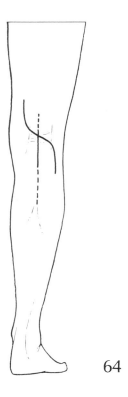

64

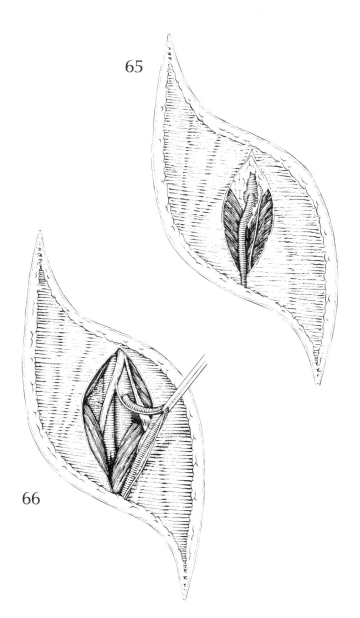

65

Superficial dissection

The short saphenous vein is followed through the popliteal fascia and the posterior cutaneous nerve is dissected aside. The fascia, the fibres of which run transversely, is split longitudinally to reveal the popliteal fat.

66

Deep dissection

The fat is cleared from the two popliteal nerves. Next the popliteal vein is found, usually via one of its deep tributaries, or perhaps by the short saphenous vein. The artery lies deeper still. It is crossed by a very constant leash of vessels, mainly some large veins from the medial head of the gastrocnemius; these must be divided. The short saphenous vein is preserved if possible.

EXTENSION OF EXPOSURE

Upwards

To reach the femoral vessels, the semimembranosus belly and tendon of semitendinosus are retracted or divided along the line of the artery. The tight hiatus in the adductor magnus is also cut through.

Downwards

The posterior tibial artery is readily exposed by splitting the gastrocnemius and soleus fibres in its line, and also the fascia which covers the vessels as they lie on the long deep flexors. A longitudinal incision through the interosseous membrane in line with the lateral border of the tibia will reveal an anterior tibial artery and its associated structures. These extensions of the posterior approach are limited and can be difficult. If long exposure is required the medial approach should be chosen.

Medial approach

The incision is centred at the site to be exposed, along a line similar to that used for a Scribner shunt. Separation and retraction of the calf muscles will expose the posterior tibial artery which is deep near the knee, becoming more superficial at the ankle[10]. The artery lies on the interosseus membrane near its origin. The anterior tibial artery can be approached through this membrane or from the front of the leg.

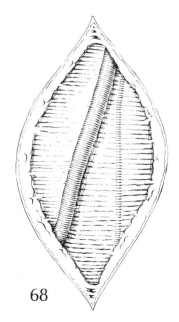

THE ARTERIOVENOUS SHUNT

67

The incision

To construct a shunt for access in haemodialysis the incision is centred 4–6 cm above the medial malleolus, 0.5 cm behind the posterior border of the tibia.

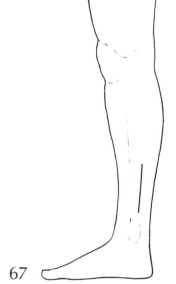

68

Dissection

The origin of the long saphenous vein lies in the superficial tissue in the anterior flap and the posterior tibial artery beneath the deep fascia directly under the incision. Limited mobilization of the vessels permits insertion of the Silastic cannula.

Postoperative care

Postoperative care depends upon the regular, detailed and careful observation of local and general signs. There must be continuity of responsibility to ensure accurate interpretation of the local and general circulation.

In the surgery of atherosclerosis it must be remembered that the disease is generalized. Hypovolaemia and hypotension must be stringently avoided. In all cases of major arterial surgery, postoperative monitoring of central venous pressure and a continuous electrocardiogram are recommended, in addition to the usual observations on pulse, blood pressure and respirations. Oxygen should be administered by mask or catheter to maintain maximal saturation. The urine output is best collected by catheter drainage over the first 24–28 hours.

Posture

The cerebral and coronary circulations take precedence over the peripheral circulation. If postoperative shock is present or the patient has not regained consciousness, head-down tilt is required. When the central circulation is adequate, dependency of an operated extremity promotes the local circulation.

Local signs

Immediately after operation, the state of the distal circulation must be established. In the extremities, the colour of the limb, the skin temperature, filling of the superficial veins and the pulses are all guides to adequate circulation.

Pulses

The distal pulses may not be felt immediately after an operation during which a limb artery has been clamped. They return following improvement in the general circulation and progressive local vasodilation. The latter can be encouraged before the closure of the arteriotomy by the injection of a vasodilator. Intravenous infusion of low molecular weight dextran is favoured by some surgeons to promote capillary circulation in the operated limb.

Skin temperature

After clamping the arterial supply, the distal part of the limb becomes pale and cold. The peripheral veins are collapsed. As recovery progresses the level of transition from warm to cold skin becomes more distal, with improvement in the colour and filling of the peripheral veins.

Sensory impairment

Numbness of the skin is a serious sign, though some skin sensation will often persist in parts of a limb which are on the same level as patches of established necrosis.

Complications
Haemorrhage

The use of heparin during operation and the presence of arterial suture lines require close observation of the operative site. The use of a vacuum drainage system gives an early indication of undue blood loss. The effect of heparin can be reversed at the end of the operation if necessary by the injection of protamine sulphate (protamine 2 mg neutralizes heparin 1 mg). If excessive haemorrhage occurs, re-exploration of the operative site is required.

Ischaemic muscle necrosis

The musculature of a limb is more sensitive to ischaemia than most other tissues. Prolonged ischaemia of the leg may cause necrosis of muscle, particularly in the anterior tibial compartment where the muscles are firmly enclosed by osseous and fascial boundaries. The presence of tenderness over this area and loss of dorsiflexion of the ankle demand early decompression. Delay in diagnosis or deferring active treatment will jeopardize recovery and lead to gangrene, ischaemic muscle contracture and an equinovarus deformity.

Swelling of the leg

Mild oedema of the foot and leg frequently follows operations on the femoral and popliteal vessels even in the presence of normal deep veins[11]. This disappears with increasing activity, and early mobilization should be practised whenever possible.

References

1. Henry, A. K. Extensile exposure applied to limb surgery. Edinburgh: Livingstone, 1945

2. Elkin, D. C. Exposure of blood vessels. Journal of the American Medical Association 1946; 132: 421–424

3. Elkin, D. C., DeBakey, M. E. eds. Vascular surgery in World War II. Washington: Office of the Surgeon General, 1955

4. Mustard, W. T., Bull, C. A reliable method for relief of traumatic vascular spasm. Annals of Surgery 1962; 155: 339–334

5. Morris, G. C., DeBakey, M. F., Cooley, D. A., Crawford, E. S. Autogenous saphenous vein bypass graft in femoropopliteal obliterative arterial disease. Surgery 1962; 51: 62–73

6. Owen, K. The surgery of renal artery stenosis. British Journal of Urology 1964; 36: 7–13

7. Helsby, R., Moossa, A. R., Aorto-iliac reconstruction with special reference to the extraperitoneal approach. British Journal of Surgery 1975; 62: 596–600

8. Rob, C. Extraperitoneal approach to the abdominal aorta. Surgery 1963; 53: 87–89

9. Jarrett, F., Berkoff, H. A., Crummy, A. B., Belzer, F. O. Femorotibial bypass grafts with sequential technique, clinical results. Archives of Surgery 1981; 116: 709–714

10. Hirsch, S. A., Jarret, F. S. Technique of femoropopliteal and femorotibial grafts using umbilical vein. Surgery, Gynecology and Obstetrics 1982; 155 (2): 247–249

11. Husni, E. A. The edema of arterial reconstruction. Circulation 1967; 35 (Suppl. 1): I-169–I-173

Illustrations by Kevin Marks

Arterial suture and anastomoses

H. H. G. Eastcott MS, FRCS
Honorary Consultant Surgeon, St Mary's Hospital, London, UK

A. E. Thompson MS, FRCS
Consultant Surgeon, St Thomas's Hospital, London, UK

Preoperative

Indications

Repair of a divided or injured major artery is usually preferable to tying its ends. This applies particularly in the lower limb. Trauma, surgical accident and the radical surgery of cancer, as well as the elective treatment of arterial lesions, require the surgeon to be familiar with methods of arterial suture. The methods illustrated will meet the requirements of the arterial operations shown in other sections.

Contraindications

Arteries are best not sutured in the presence of infection. Severe compound or crushing injury with loss of the main artery are indications for amputation, not arterial repair. Simpler procedures are similarly necessary in treating battle casualties when tactical considerations demand early evacuation. Some viscera almost always survive arterial ligation (for example, the left colon). Arterial reconstruction in such circumstances is superfluous.

Suture materials

Fine sutures on atraumatic needles are best for arterial anastomoses. Silk was used for many years but has now been replaced by manmade fibres, which are less traumatic to the vessel walls. Both braided and monofilament sutures are available in varying sizes (2/0 to 10/0). These sutures have the advantage that the anastomosis can be tightened easily by longitudinal tension. Care must be taken to avoid crushing the suture by careless use of instruments. It is necessary to use several throws in each knot to ensure that the knot is secure.

The operations

LATERAL SUTURE

1

This is a simple method of closing a longitudinal incision in the artery wall, such as exists after embolectomy or thromboendarterectomy. A simple continuous stitch is used, taking care that the needle passes through the full thickness of the arterial wall on each side of the anastomosis. Some narrowing of the vessel is always produced and the blood pressure tends to open the repair instead of tightening it, unlike the circumferential suture of an anastomosis.

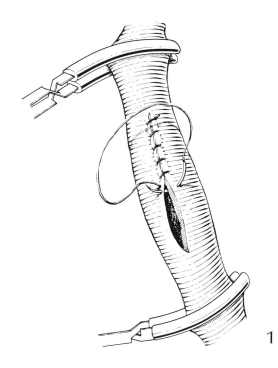

1

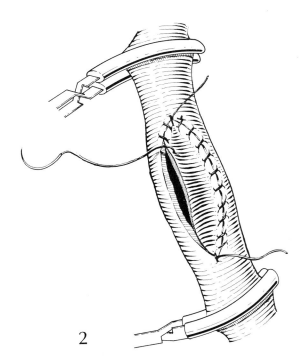

2

2

Where there is loss of substance of the arterial wall, and linear closure may narrow the vessel too greatly, resection and anastomosis or grafting are preferable. A vein patch graft is shown. An ovoid or rectangular patch should be used rather than a sharp-pointed elliptical patch which will narrow the vessel. Four stay sutures are placed and a continuous stitch used between the stays.

END-TO-END ANASTOMOSIS BY MODIFIED CARREL METHOD

3

Stay sutures

The ends of the vessels to be anastomosed are carefully cleared of excess adventitia. Inclusion of adventitia or other extraneous tissue in the suture line may promote thrombus formation. Everting horizontal mattress sutures are used as stay sutures to define the anterior and posterior aspects of the anastomosis.

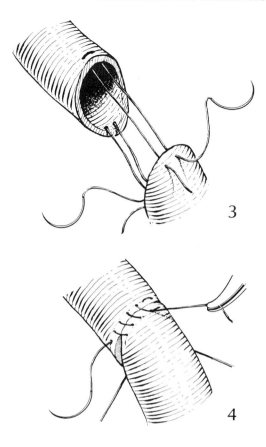

3

4

Continuous suture of anterior aspect

A simple continuous suture is placed along the anterior aspect at intervals of 1–2 mm, according to the size of the artery, and a similar distance from the edges which, if the wall is normal, will have already been everted by the stay sutures. These are held apart with sufficient tension to equalize the diameter of the ends of the vessels.

4

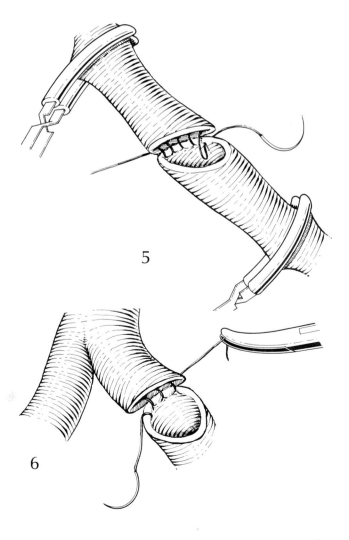

5

6

5

Rotation of anastomosis

The clamps and stay sutures are then used to rotate the anastomosis so that the posterior half can be seen and sutured in the same way. It is often possible to place the clamps in such a position that the anastomosis can be rotated without releasing them.

6

Single stitch method

If difficulty is anticipated in rotating the ends of the artery – near a large bifurcation, for example – a single continuous stitch is used. One supporting suture is placed nearest the operator and this is continued forwards from within the lumen, then back along the front of the anastomosis until the starting point is reached in an accessible position.

This method is particularly useful in diseased arteries which will not allow the smooth pull-up of the Blalock suture.

EVERTING MATTRESS SUTURE

This method still has some place in arterial surgery. It does evert the edges of the vessel and may therefore be chosen in circumstances where a second continuous suture is intended for haemostasis – for example in a healthy aorta. It is also useful in large arteries for ensuring haemostasis and a firm repair when suturing normal to diseased arteries.

Two everting mattress sutures are placed with the loop on the adventitia as shown in *Illustration 3*. Traction is exerted on them to equalize the diameter of the two ends.

7

A continuous everting suture is then placed, first anteriorly, then posteriorly by rotating the anastomosis. One stay suture is passed behind the anastomosis and the ends pulled in opposite directions.

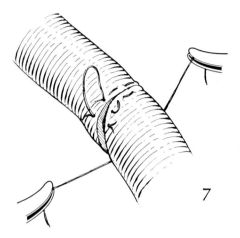

7

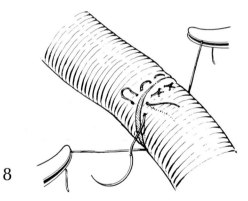

8

8

Use of interrupted sutures

Where growth of the anastomosis must be allowed for, as in coarctation of the aorta in children, interrupted everting mattress sutures may be used.

BLALOCK SUTURE

This is a valuable method of anastomosing normal or thin-walled arteries or veins when access to the posterior aspect of the anastomosis cannot be obtained by rotation. It is used in coarctation, Blalock's and Pott's operations, portacaval anastomoses and in the bypass type of arterial graft.

9

A continuous everting suture of polypropylene fibre is placed in the posterior half of the anastomosis with the loops on the adventitia. The ends are not tied.

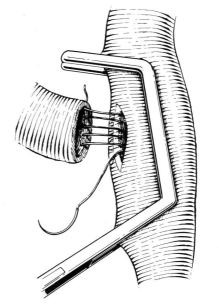

9

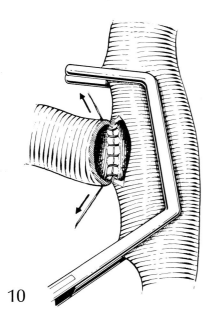

10

10

When this suture line is complete the ends are drawn together with steady traction and the edges are everted. It is then completed as a normal continuous everting stitch, maintaining the tension in the stitch throughout. The suture is finally tied to the free end.

SUTURING THE DISEASED ARTERY

Stronger material (2/0) may be used for suturing densely sclerotic or calcified vessels. Care must be taken so that the suture is not cut by a sharp plaque. A second, finer suture is recommended to ensure haemostasis.

11a & b

Fixation of plaque

If possible the lower limit of an arteriotomy or endarterectomy should be firmly sutured by several mattress sutures through the vessel wall, with the ties on the outer aspect. Unsecured plaques are liable to be dissected free by the subsequent bloodflow and to cause thrombosis.

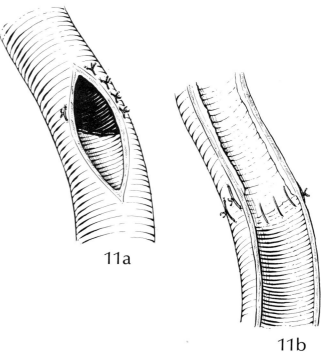

11a

11b

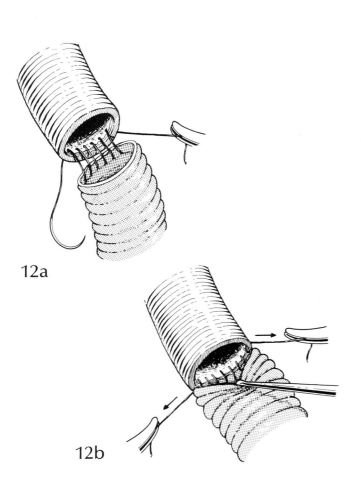

12a

12b

12a & b

Including plaques in end-to-end suture

The anastomosis can sometimes be made to include these plaques in the suture line. The needle should be passed through the plaque from within outwards to avoid loosening the plaques.

13

Including plaques in lateral suture

Often it is necessary to suture a synthetic graft to the side of a diseased artery, e.g. the femoral. It is particularly important to secure the plaques at its distal end where it may easily become loose. Interrupted sutures hold it well.

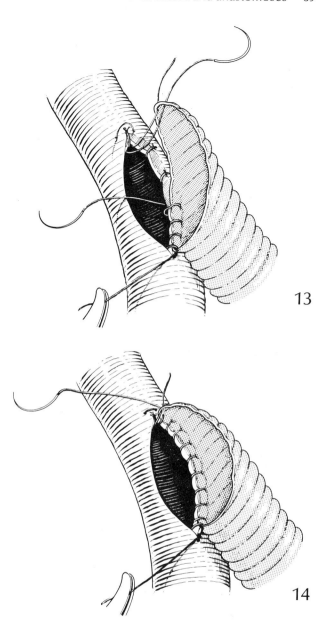

13

14

Completing lateral anastomosis to include plaques

Beginning at the proximal corner of the anastomosis a continuous suture of polypropylene is inserted from within the lumen. This effectively completes the approximation of the plaque to the arterial wall and the graft.

14

INVAGINATION OF GRAFT

A cloth graft or vein graft also may be sutured within the lumen of a diseased vessel using a continuous everting mattress suture. The bloodflow then tends to dilate the diseased vessel, reducing the tendency to strip plaques by longitudinal pressure.

RELEASE OF CLAMPS

While the artery is clamped the peripheral vessels are constricted. Early recovery of the circulation can be promoted by instillations of a vasodilator into the distal vessel before completing the anastomosis. The lower clamp is released first. This allows the air in the vessel to be expelled and the suture to take up the slack gently. It is customary to have some initial bleeding from the suture lines and the needle holes. This stops after applying steady pressure for 5–6 min over absorbent gauze. An inclination to add supplementary sutures should be resisted until an adequate period of pressure has been tried, as further stitch holes often increase rather than decrease the haemorrhage.

If haemorrhage is persistent, the possibility of the persistence of circulating heparin must be considered. One common practice is to reverse half the dose of heparin originally used with the appropriate amount of protamine sulphate (protamine sulphate 2 mg neutralizes heparin 1 mg). Rarely, a second continuous suture of reinforcement of a suture line with fascia, muscle or a cloth graft may be necessary.

Illustrations by Anita Matthews

Operative angiography

John J. Ricotta MD
Assistant Professor of Surgery, University of Rochester
School of Medicine and Dentistry, Rochester, New York, USA

Introduction

As vascular reconstruction has extended below the popliteal artery, operative angiography has become a necessity. Angiograms may be done either before reconstruction to define distal arterial anatomy more accurately, or after reconstruction to look for technical problems which might lead to early graft thrombosis. We have found intraoperative angiography to be a safe, relatively simple technique which adds little to operative time but often gives invaluable information.

Prereconstruction angiography

Accurate definition of the distal tibial vessels and the pedal arch is of great importance in distal popliteal and tibial reconstruction. Several authors have clearly shown that both early and late patency rates of tibial grafts are correlated with the anatomy of the pedal arch[1,2]. The arterial anatomy of the foot and calf can often be visualized preoperatively, especially when hyperaemia is induced[3], but this is not always possible. In some cases intraoperative angiography is required prior to revascularization to determine the optimal site of distal anastomosis[4].

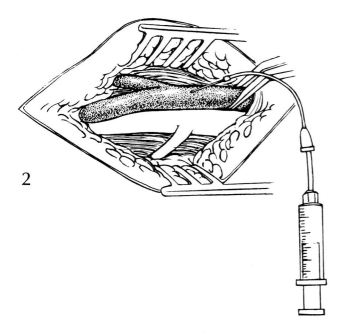

1

1

The common femoral artery is exposed in the standard fashion for femoral distal reconstruction. A 19 gauge needle is placed in the common femoral artery and the X-ray film is positioned under the calf to include the foot and ankle. This permits visualization of the popliteal trifurcation as well as the pedal arch. Papaverine hydrochloride 30 mg is injected into the common femoral artery to induce vasodilation and maximize distal visualization.

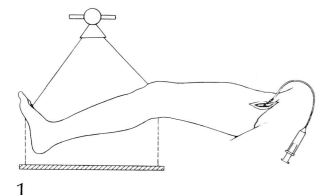

2

2

Following this, the common femoral artery is clamped proximally and 30 ml of full-strength diatrizoate sodium (Renografin 60) is injected into the distal common femoral artery. The arterial clamp is released and the radiograph taken immediately. The needle is left in the common femoral artery until the film is seen and judged to be adequate.

Postreconstruction completion angiography

Routine completion angiography has shown technical defects in 5–9 per cent of peripheral vascular reconstructions[5]. As the final arterial anastomosis is being completed, preparations are made for angiography. The X-ray film is placed in a sterile cover and then positioned directly under the leg at the area of interest, if a cassette table is not available.

3

A 21 gauge butterfly needle is placed in the proximal graft. Once again, papaverine hydrochloride 30 mg may be injected. Following this, the graft is clamped proximal to the needle puncture and 20 ml of dye is injected. The proximal clamp is released as the film is taken. A smaller needle and smaller dye dose are used here since injection is made directly into the graft itself with attention only to the area of distal anastomosis. After a satisfactory film is obtained, the needle is removed from the graft.

Occasionally a suture may be necessary at the puncture site, but this is rare when a 21 gauge needle is used. We prefer injecting the graft directly, since it allows better visualization of the distal anastomosis and avoids repetitive clamping of the common femoral artery.

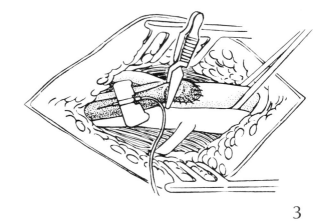

3

References

1. Dardik, H., Ibrahim, I. M., Sussman, B, *et al*. Morphologic structure of the pedal arch and its relationship to patency of crural vascular reconstruction. Surgery, Gynecology and Obstetrics 1981; 152: 645–648

2. O'Mara, C. S., Flinn, W. R., Neiman, H. L., Bergan, J. J., Yao, J. S. T. Correlation of foot arterial anatomy with early tibial bypass patency. Surgery 1981; 89: 743–752

3. Feins, R., Roedersheimer, R., Baumstark, A., Green, R. M. Predicted hyperemic angiography: a technique of distal arteriography in the severely ischemic leg. Surgery 1981; 89: 202–205

4. Scarpato, R., Gembarowicz, R., Farber, S. *et al*. Intraoperative prereconstruction arteriography. Archives of Surgery 1981; 116: 1053–1055

5. Liebman, P. R., Menzoian, J. O., Mannick, J. A., Lowney, B. W., LoGerfo, F. W. Intraoperative arteriography in femoropopliteal and femorotibial bypass grafts. Archives of Surgery 1981; 116: 1019–1021

Illustrations by Anita Matthews

Carotid endarterectomy

James A. DeWeese MD, FACS
Professor and Chairman, Division of Cardiothoracic Surgery,
University of Rochester Medical Center, Rochester, New York, USA

Preoperative

Symptoms

Arteriosclerotic disease of the carotid artery bifurcation is a recognized frequent cause of strokes. The classic symptoms associated with bifurcation disease are contralateral monoparesis or hemiparesis, dysphasia or amaurosis fugax. Symptoms such as dizziness, diplopia or drop attacks which are more frequently associated with vertebrobasilar disease may also occur. Partial or total occlusion of the vessel and reduced bloodflow may be responsible for some symptoms. The usual reason for the neurological deficits, however, is the embolization of portions of the atherosclerotic plaque or associated thrombus to the eye or brain. The symptoms may come and go within a few moments as a transient ischaemic attack (TIA) or transient blindness, described as amaurosis fugax. Complete recovery may occur within a few days and the episode is considered as a reversible ischaemic neurological deficit (RIND). Some patients show improvement but never fully recover (completed stroke). On the other hand, there may be continual worsening of symptoms (progressive stroke) with resultant severe permanent neurological deficits or death. There is a small group of patients who demonstrate significant fluctuation or 'waxing and waning' of their deficits within the first few days after onset (unstable stroke).

Evaluation

The presence of a bruit over the carotid bifurcation, particularly if it is localized or has a higher pitch or volume than other cervical bruits, suggests the presence of carotid stenosis. Unfortunately bruits are recognized in only 80 per cent of patients with significant disease. Other non-invasive diagnostic techniques are available and are of one of two types. There are those which are based on measuring haemodynamic changes which occur with a significant stenosis (50–60 per cent diameter narrowing) of the internal carotid artery. These methods include the determination of a decreased pressure in the ophthalmic artery (OPG-Gee), a delay in arterial pressure wave reaching the ophthalmic artery (OPG-Kirchner), or a reversal in bloodflow in an ophthalmic artery as demonstrated by a supraorbital doppler study. The second group of non-invasive techniques use continuous wave and pulsed doppler techniques or ultrasound B-mode scanning techniques to provide actual images of the vessels and their lesions.

Arteriography is the most definitive study for the determination of the extent and severity of the carotid artery lesion, as well as for identification of atherosclerotic involvement of other extracranial or intracranial vessels. Digital subtraction angiography which is rapidly improving will undoubtedly replace present angiographic techniques.

Indications

Carotid endarterectomy should be considered for individuals without medical contraindications and carotid stenosis who present with: amaurosis fugax; TIAs; RINDs; unstable strokes without significant neurological deficits; completed strokes (4 weeks after onset); or asymptomatic significant lesions in patients who have had contralateral carotid endarterectomies or who require other major operative procedures. Carotid endarterectomy should not be performed on patients with progressive strokes or recent completed strokes.

The operation

Cerebral protection

There are some patients who will suffer transient or permanent ischaemic brain damage from occlusion of one carotid artery. General anaesthetics decrease cerebral metabolic demands and are therefore preferred to regional anaesthetics. Indwelling shunts can be used to ensure bloodflow during carotid occlusion. Shunts may interfere with the performance of the endarterectomy and embolization of plaque or air may occur. Selective shunting is therefore preferred by the author. The need for a shunt can be determined by continuous monitoring of the patient's EEG. If this modality is not available, the back pressure in the occluded carotid artery can be measured: when it is greater than 30 mmHg, collateral circulation is able to protect the brain in almost all patients.

1

The incision

Following induction of anaesthesia, the head is hyperextended and tilted away from the operative side. The neck is prepared with antiseptic solution and an adhesive plastic drape used. The skin incision begins one fingerbreadth below the angle of the mandible anterior to the ear lobe and is carried along the anterior border of the sternocleidomastoid muscle and then along a skin crease, ending at the lower level of the thyroid cartilage in the midline.

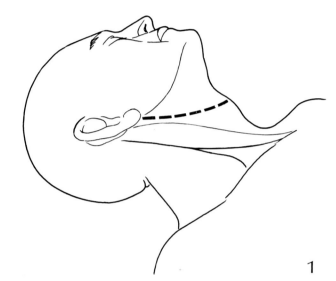

1

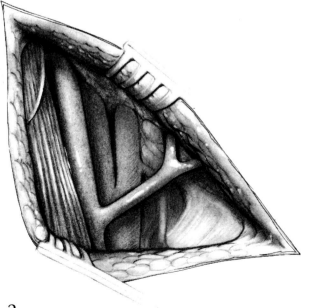

2

2

Exposure of carotid bifurcation

The platysma muscle is divided. The greater auricular nerve is identified in the posterior part of the incision and preserved. The dissection is then continued longitudinally over the palpable carotid artery. The common facial vein is identified as it crosses the carotid arteries to join the internal jugular vein.

3

Mobilization of carotid arteries

The carotid sheath is now opened and the common, internal and external carotid arteries identified and mobilized throughout the operative field. It is important to identify and preserve the hypoglossal nerve as it crosses the carotid vessels. The carotid sinus nerve is injected with a local anaesthetic or it may be divided if necessary. This prevents or corrects the bradycardia and hypotension which may follow stimulation of the nerve. The ansa hypoglossi branch of the hypoglossal nerve is identified and may be divided if necessary for complete mobilization of the carotid vessels. The superior thyroid artery is controlled with a double throw of a silk suture.

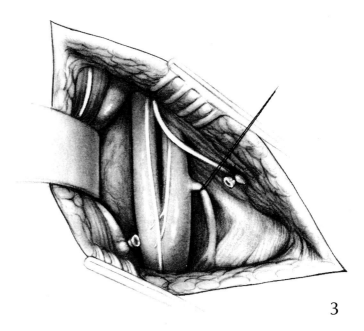

3

4

Trial occlusion of carotid arteries

The patient is given 5000 u of heparin intravenously. The common carotid, external carotid and superior thyroid arteries are occluded.

The arteries remain occluded for a period of 1 min, during which time particularly close attention is given to the monitoring of the patient's electroencephalogram. If any ischaemic changes are noted, the clamps are released and preparations made for the use of an indwelling shunt.

If EEG monitoring is not being used, the back pressure is measured. A 21 gauge needle is inserted into the internal carotid artery and the pressure recorded on a manometer or with a strain gauge connected to a recorder. If the recorded pressure is less than 30 mmHg, preparations are made for insertion of an indwelling shunt.

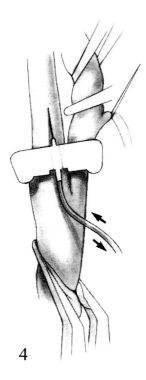

4

5

Arterial incision

A longitudinal incision is now made through the adventitia. The incision is made over the hardest portion of the palpable atherosclerotic plaque, but along the outer side of the carotid artery to avoid the loose adventitia in the region of the carotid body. The incision is not carried into the plaque but a plane of dissection established about the plaque. The incision is then carried down over the common carotid artery and up the internal carotid artery until the more normal bluish coloured media is identified. Stay sutures are placed in the edge of the arteriotomy and at the proximal end of the incision.

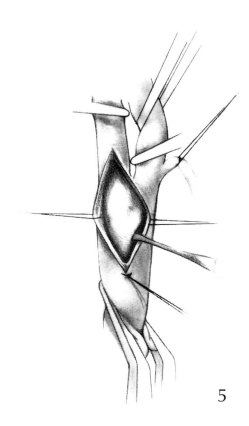

5

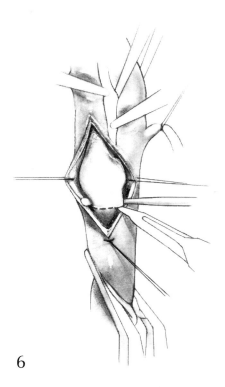

6

6

Mobilization of the plaque

A small blunt dissector is then used to mobilize the plaque more completely, beginning in the common carotid artery. A blunt dissector is carefully passed around the posterior border of the plaque which is elevated and then sharply cut. The dissector should be blunt and care taken not to pierce the thin adventitial wall during the mobilization of the plaque.

7

Endarterectomy of external carotid artery

The plaque is grasped firmly and the adventitial wall pushed away from it as the dissection continues into the external carotid artery. Resistance is met at the level of the superior thyroid artery, but gentle traction on the plaque and pushing of the dissection up to the external carotid artery finally results in a clean breaking away of the plaque from the outer wall of the artery.

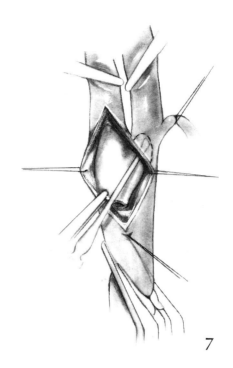

7

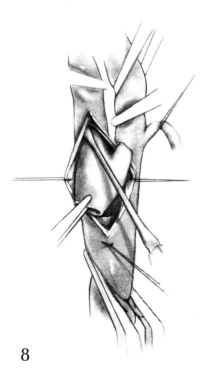

8

8

Completion of endarterectomy

There is continued firm traction of the plaque as the endarterectomy continues up the internal carotid artery. The artery is inverted as the wall is pushed away from the plaque with the dissector. The plaque finally becomes quite thin as it melts into the normal intima and usually separates cleanly from it. There is usually a normal seeming rim of intima and media adherent to the adventitia at the distal end of the endarterectomy.

9

Insertion of shunt

We prefer to complete the endarterectomy prior to insertion of the shunt. This rarely requires longer than 1 min. This is possible if the common carotid and internal carotid arteries are not occluded until after the arteriotomy is made through the adventitia. A plane of dissection is established, and stay sutures are placed in the proximal and distal ends of the arteriotomy.

A Silastic tube just smaller than lumen of the internal carotid artery is threaded up this vessel for about 4 cm and down the common carotid artery for a similar distance. Tapes or special clamps are then placed around the artery proximally and distally and these are closed tightly around the vessel. A suture is tied in the middle of the Silastic tube to expedite its removal and to prevent its embolization. The following steps of the endarterectomy are then completed, sometimes with difficulty because of the presence of the shunt.

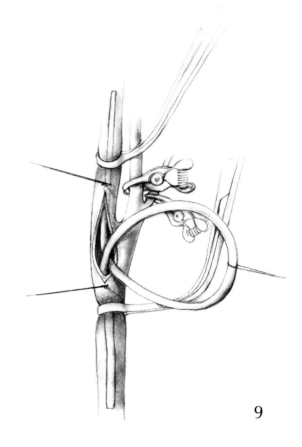

9

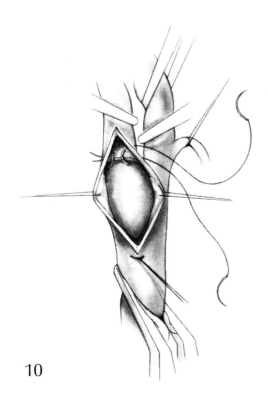

10

10

Distal tacking

It is important that the distal end of the endarterectomy be visualized. If necessary, the arteriotomy is extended. If there is any question about the adherence, tacking sutures are used to secure the layers and prevent continued dissection and development of flaps which could invert and occlude the vessel. Double-ended monofilament sutures are passed from within the vessel, with one suture passed through the full thickness of the remaining wall and the other through the adventitia. The stitch is tied on the outside of the artery.

11

Removal of all debris

After completion of the thromboendarterectomy it is important to remove all debris and loose tags from the lumen of the vessel. This is achieved by washing thoroughly with saline solution from a syringe and picking out any remaining loose fragments. The distal clamp is then briefly removed to flush out the occluded internal carotid artery. The clamp is reapplied. The clamp on the common carotid artery is also briefly removed in a similar fashion, then reoccluded and the vessel irrigated with saline.

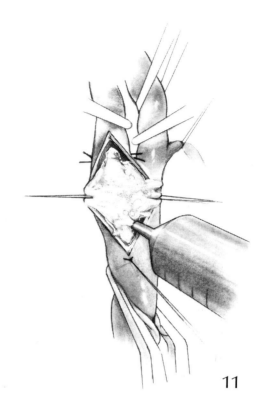

11

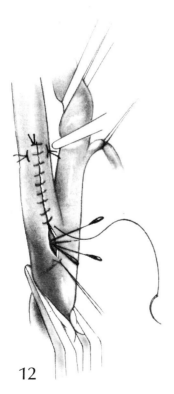

12

12

Closure of arteriotomy

Stay sutures have been placed in the proximal and distal end of the arteriotomy using fine monofilament sutures. Care is taken with the stay suture to anchor the intima to the arterial wall. The distal suture is then very carefully carried proximally, taking care to take fine bites and not to narrow the vessel. The over-and-over suture is then carried to the proximal arteriotomy.

13

Patch graft

In many patients a satisfactory closure can be achieved by simple arterial suture, but if it appears that such a closure will constrict the lumen of an artery or an incorrect plane of dissection was established, then a patch graft should be inserted. A short length of vein obtained from the arm or leg or a small oblong piece of prosthetic material is used. Stay sutures are placed in all four corners of the patch and an over-and-over stitch used to complete the suturing between the stays.

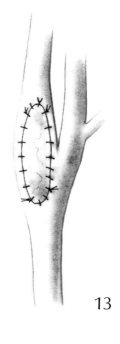

13

14

Removal of arterial shunt

Just before completion of the arterial closure or application of the patch, the shunt is removed. The distal end of the shunt is removed and the internal carotid artery occluded. The shunt is clamped and the proximal tape or clamp is then loosened, the shunt removed and the proximal artery clamped. The arterial closure is completed and all clamps are removed. The patient is then given protamine to neutralize the heparin.

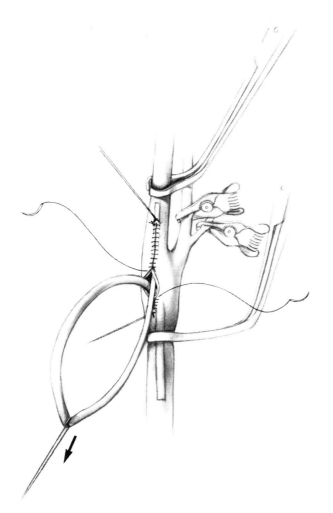

14

Postoperative care

The patient should be carefully observed for any neurological changes in the postoperative period, particularly in the first 12 hours. Should neurological changes occur, one of the tests which measures significant haemodynamic changes, such as the OPG-GEE test, should be performed. If there is evidence of occlusion of the vessel, the patient should be returned to the operating theatre for removal of the thrombus and correction of any technical faults. The most frequent findings are a distal intimal flap. This can be corrected either by extending the endarterectomy a short distance and placing tacking sutures if necessary, or by applying a patch graft for arteriotomy closure.

Recovery is usually rapid and most patients can be discharged from the hospital 4–5 days following the operation.

Complications

Postoperative hypertension

Hypertension frequently occurs in the early postoperative period and should be aggressively controlled with intravenous antihypertensive drugs. The hypertension may occur whether or not the carotid sinus nerves are bilaterally divided.

Peripheral nerve deficits

Traction on the hypoglossal nerve may result in deviation of the tongue to the side of the operation and function usually returns within a few weeks. Vocal cord paralysis secondary to trauma to the vagus nerve may occur and is also usually temporary. Compression of the submental branch of the facial nerve against the mandible produced by a retractor may result in weakness of the lower lip on the side of the lesion and is also usually temporary; patients almost always recover.

Late complications

False aneurysms may occur and are most frequently seen in patients with patch grafts or in those who have developed an infection. Late neurological complications are related to recurrence of disease at the site of the previous endarterectomy (which probably occurs in about 10 per cent of patients over a 5–10 year period). Patients may also experience progression of lesions in their contralateral carotid artery. Patients should be followed carefully at 6–12 month intervals and some type of noninvasive evaluation at that time would be helpful. There is some evidence that aspirin 325 mg daily and dipyridamole (Persantin) 75 mg three times daily might decrease both the occurrence of and the progression of atherosclerotic lesions.

Further reading

DeWeese, J. A., Rob, C. G., Satran, R. et al. Results of carotid endarterectomies for transient ischemic attacks five years later. Annals of Surgery 1973; 178: 258–264

DeWeese, J. A. Management of acute strokes. Surgical Clinics of North America 1982; 62: 467–472

DeWeese, J. A. In: Bergan, J. J., Yao, J. S. T. eds. Cerebrovascular insufficiency. New York, Grune & Stratton, 1983

Rob, C. G. The surgical treatment of stenosis and thrombosis of internal carotid, vertebral and common carotid arteries. Proceedings of the Royal Society of Medicine 1959; 52: 549–552

Rob, C. G. In: Beebe, H. G., ed. Complications in vascular surgery. Philadelphia: Lippincott, 1973

Rob, C. Occlusive disease of the extracranial cerebral arteries: a review of the past 25 years. Journal of Cardiovascular Surgery 1978; 19: 487–498

Thompson, J. E., Austin, D. J., Patman, R. D. Carotid endarterectomy for cerebrovascular insufficiency: long-term results in 592 patients followed up to thirteen years. Annals of Surgery 1970; 172: 663–679

Illustrations by Gillian Lee

Operations for occlusive disease of the vertebral artery

Anthony M. Imparato MD
Professor of Surgery and Director, Division of Vascular Surgery,
New York University Medical Center, New York, USA

Introduction

The realization that cerebral ischaemia results primarily from extracranial rather than intracranial arterial occlusive and stenotic lesions has been one of the major advances in surgery[1]. The lesions are surgically accessible, usually in the neck. The anatomical arrangement of the vertebral arteries, in which two vessels join to form a common basilar which then gives branches to the brainstem and the occipital lobes, together with the anatomical arrangement of the Circle of Willis, which permits interchange of blood between anterior and posterior circulations in 50–70 per cent of patients[2], renders operation upon the vertebral arteries much less common than upon the carotid bifurcations. In our series of 1600 operations, 5 per cent of patients have required operations upon the vertebral arteries.

The indications are precise and are clinical and radiographic. Clinical symptoms of brainstem ischaemia include ataxia, syncope, drop attacks without syncope, transient symptoms of paralysis or sensory disorders of a symmetrical nature and certain specific visual disorders. They appear to be due to interference with flow rather than due to embolization[3].

Unlike the frequently benign course of microembolization to the cerebral hemispheres from carotid plaques, those who embolize to the small brainstem arteries suffer such severe life-threatening disorders that they rarely appear for vascular reconstructive procedures. The question of whether brainstem ischaemia results in sudden death erroneously diagnosed as being due to coronary artery disease and myocardial ischaemia has been raised but has not been settled[4]. Only one vertebral of bilaterally involved vessels has had to be operated upon to relieve ischaemia, and then only after haemodynamically significant carotid lesions have been corrected without relief of brainstem symptoms[5,6,7].

Preoperative

Preoperative evaluation

Patients to be subjected to operation require cerebral angiographic studies to visualize the aortic arch, the origins of the four major extracranial vessels and the intracranial circulation as well. These studies can be performed by right brachial, left carotid and left brachial injection. More recently catheters have been passed to the aortic arch via the common femoral arteries, permitting selective opacification of arch branches. The recently introduced digital intravenous technique (DIVA) has been useful for screening the origins of the vertebral arteries but does not have sufficient resolution to allow definitive evaluations regarding operations. If the DIVA indicates the presence of vertebral ostial arterial lesions then retrograde catheter studies have been done to evaluate both vertebrals and to ascertain whether they join a patent basilar artery.

Indications

1

Vertebral stenosis

Vertebral stenoses of sufficient magnitude to interfere with brainstem circulation have usually been due to atherosclerosis of the subclavian artery. This rarely extends beyond the proximal 1–2 cm of the origin of the vertebral, distal to which the artery is smooth and thin walled.

2

Associated carotid stenosis

If haemodynamically significant carotid lesions (either greater than 50 per cent stenosis or associated with positive non-invasive haemodynamic studies such as the OPG-Gee) have been repaired, and symptoms persist, then in the presence of bilateral vertebral arterial stenoses the more stenotic of the two arteries has been treated surgically.

3

Carotid occlusion

On the other hand, occlusion of the carotid arteries and vertebral stenosis makes it necessary to proceed directly to an operation on the vertebral. Occasionally unilateral stenosis and contralateral atresia of the vertebral artery have necessitated operation.

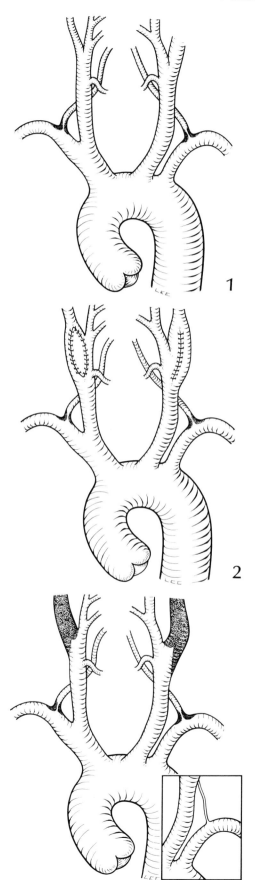

4

Vertebral occlusion

Bilateral occlusion at the origins of the vertebrals, extending to the intraosseous portions within the foramina transversaria, occurs infrequently but may require surgical intervention.

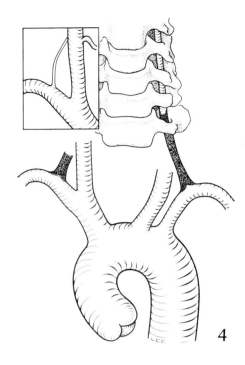

4

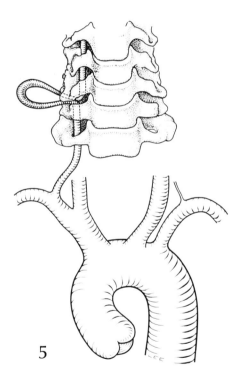

5

5

Vertebral herniation

Rarely, herniation of the artery between segments of the foramina transversaria have resulted in drop attacks on head turning, and this has required surgical relief. Very frequently marked tortuosity and kinking of the vertebral artery is associated with vertebral lesions and results in total occlusion of the kinked vertebral on head turning. The rarest lesion of all is bilateral occlusion of the vertebral arteries from the origins to the level of the second cervical vertebra, a lesion which can be approached surgically.

Preoperative preparation

Preoperative preparation is as for any other major operative procedure. The patient is informed of the possibility of a Horner's syndrome occurring postoperatively because of the proximity of the cervical sympathetic chain to the operative field. Paralysis of the ipsilateral hemidiaphragm may occur because of the need to retract the phrenic nerve. Continuous direct arterial monitoring and continuous electrocardiographic monitoring are performed. The spectre of stroke is ever present in any operative procedure upon the cerebral vessels but in a series of 90 operations upon the vertebral arteries there has been only one brain episode produced as a result of the operative procedure. Cervical block or general inhalation anaesthesia with endotracheal intubation can be employed.

The operations

6

The incision

The incision is started a third of the way between the manubrium sterni and the mastoid process at the anterior border of the sternocleidomastoid muscle, continued inferiorly and posteriorly parallel to the clavicle.

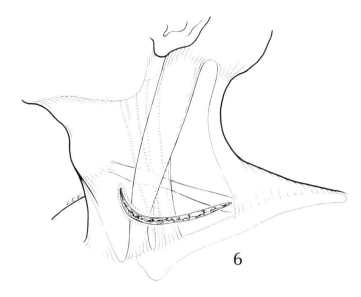

6

7

Division of muscles

The platysma muscle is divided, exposing the sterno-cleidomastoid muscle. The clavicular head of that muscle is divided.

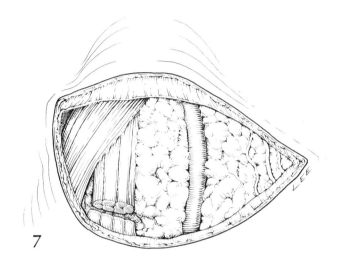

7

8

Mobilizing fat pad

The scalene fat pad overlying the major structures of interest is then dissected free, preserving its lateral portion. This permits it to be elevated off the deeper structures and used as a retractor of the phrenic nerve.

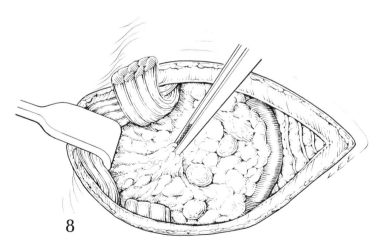

8

9

Exposure of arteries

The branches of the thyrocervical trunk then come into view, including the transverse cervical and the suprascapular arteries and veins. These are divided close to the thyrocervical trunk. The fascia over the phrenic nerve is incised. This nerve is dissected free and the scalene fat pad passed posteriorly, anteriorly and laterally around it, so that it is held out of the way by the fat pad.

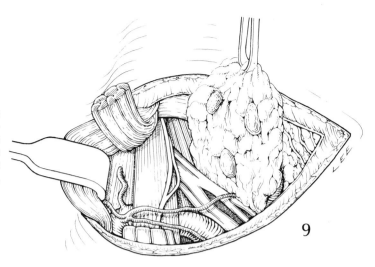

10

Exposure of vertebral artery

The anterior scalene muscle is divided close to the level of the clavicle and permitted to retract, exposing the subclavian artery which is dissected free to expose the internal mammary artery, the origin of the thyrocervical trunk, and the proximal portion of the vertebral artery which is cleared to its entrance into the foramina transversaria, dividing any overlying veins. The costocervical trunk on the posterior portion of the second part of the subclavian artery needs to be controlled to permit opening the subclavian artery without troublesome bleeding. Heparin (3000 u) is administered intravenously. The branch arteries are controlled with tapes and a soft non-crushing clamp is used to occlude the vertebral artery close to its entrance into the foramina transversaria. The subclavian artery is clamped proximally and distally with vascular clamps.

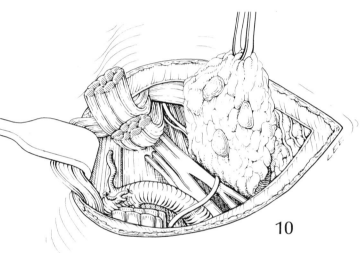

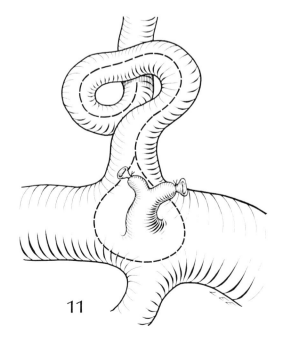

11

Arterial incision

The anterior wall of the subclavian artery, including the origin of the thyrocervical trunk, is outlined for excision and the incision is carried along the course of the vertebral artery to the last accentuated curve.

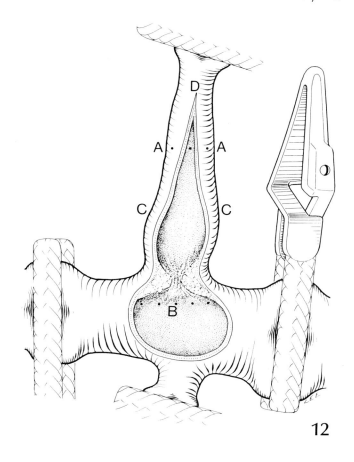

12

12

Unroofing plaque

Upon resection of the anterior wall of the subclavian artery and opening the anterior wall of the vertebral, the stenosing plaque is demonstrated at the origin of the vertebral.

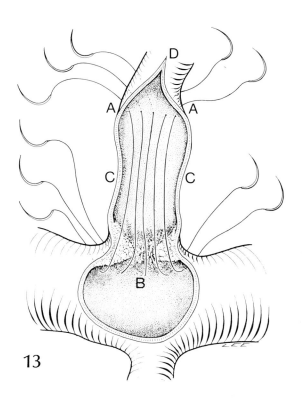

13

13

Plication

In order to get rid of the kink and to eliminate the subclavian plaque from the vertebral circulation, a plication procedure is performed.

14

Oversewing

Upon completion of the plication, the redundant portions of the plicated vertebral are oversewn.

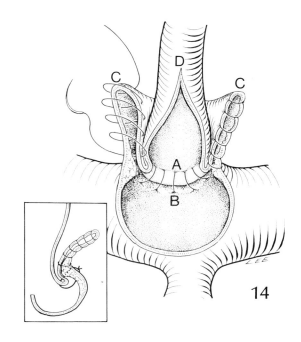

14

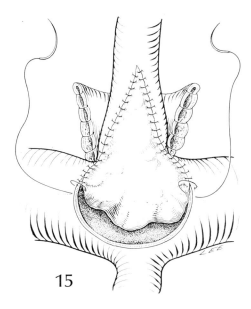

15

15

Vein patch

Closure is performed by employing a piece of autologous saphenous vein to close the vertebral arteriotomy and the opening in the subclavian artery. Flow is restored by flushing the system prior to complete closure and restoring flow first to the internal mammary and costo-cervical trunks, then to the upper extremity and lastly to the vertebral artery.

The wounds are usually closed with the elimination of all dead space, replacing the phrenic nerve without restoration of the anterior scalene muscle, re-uniting the cut ends of the clavicular head of the sternocleidomastoid muscle, and closing the remainder of the wound in layers without drainage.

ALTERNATIVE METHOD FOR CORRECTING REDUNDANCY

16

Arteriotomy

An arteriotomy is made of the vertebral artery and subclavian arteries.

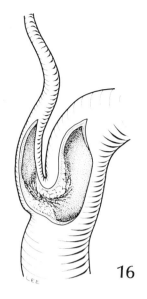

16

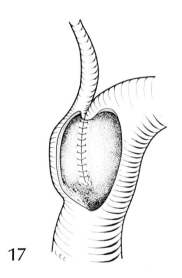

17

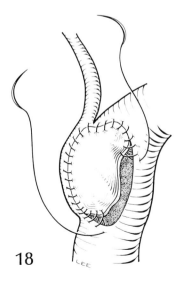

18

17

Anastomosis

A side-to-side anastomosis is performed between those two vessels.

18

Vein patch

Closure is accomplished with a vein patch.

VERTEBRAL TRANSPOSITION

19

A third method of correcting vertebral arterial stenosis[8–10] is shown, in which the vertebral artery is exposed in the groove medial to the anterior scalene muscle, dissected free from its origin to its entrance into the foramina transversaria, divided at its origin and then closed at the subclavian end. An incision is made into the common carotid artery. The vertebral artery is divided longitudinally to permit a spatula-like configuration to occur.

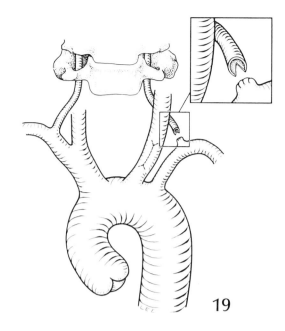

19

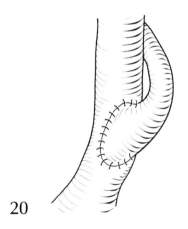

20

20

Anastomosis

An end-to-side anastomosis is performed to the carotid artery.

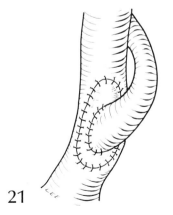

21

21

Alternative anastomosis

On occasions when the carotid artery is thick walled, a vein roof patch of autologous saphenous vein has been placed on the common carotid. The vein patch is used as the take-off for the vertebral artery.

22

CORRECTION OF HERNIATION

Surgery is possible for the unusual herniation of the vertebral artery between segments of the foramina transversaria. The vessel is exposed at the appropriate level. The foramina transversaria is unroofed, usually at two levels, correcting the acute kink in the vertebral artery to a gentle curve. This obviates the need for resection and reanastomosis of the vessel or replacement with an autologous vein graft. This procedure has been effective in relieving drop attacks with head turning.

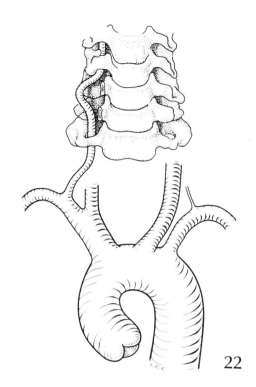

22

Postoperative care

Postoperative care is the same as for any patient undergoing major surgery. The antibiotics given prior to the creation of the neck incision are continued intravenously for a period of 48 hours. Heparinization is discontinued. Careful monitoring of the blood pressure is performed and any fall below an acceptable level of 100 mmHg is corrected with vasopressors.

As with all patients who have had cerebrovascular surgery, antiplatelet drugs are continued during the postoperative period in doses of aspirin 325 mg daily and dipyridamole 25 mg four times a day to obviate junctional anastomotic intimal hyperplasia which appears to result from the accumulation of thrombus at suture lines.

Patients are followed closely at yearly intervals. On occasion the patients who have suffered syncopal episodes have returned after several years with cardiac conduction difficulties requiring cardiac pacemaker implantation.

The follow-up of patients with vertebral arterial reconstructions has been excellent, with a stroke rate to the 14th year of 1 per cent per patient year of follow-up. Syncopal episodes, drop attacks and ataxia have been eliminated. Sometimes mild dizziness has persisted.

References

1. Hass, W. K., Fields, W. S., North, R. R., Kricheff, I. I., Chase, N. E., Bauer, R. B. Joint study of extracranial arterial occlusion II. Arteriography, techniques, sites and complications. Journal of the American Medical Association 1968; 203: 961–968

2. Alpers, B. J., Berry, R. G., Paddison, R. M. Anatomical studies of the circle of Willis in normal brain. Archives of Neurology and Psychiatry 1959; 81: 409–418

3. Hutchinson, E. C., Yates, P. O. Carotid-vertebral stenosis. Lancet 1957; 1: 2–8

4. Imparato, A. M., Riles, T. S., Kim, G. E. Cervical vertebral angioplasty for brain stem ischemia. Surgery 1981; 90: 842–852

5. Humphries, A. W., Young, J. R., Bevan, E. G., Lefevre, F. A., de Wolfe, V. G. Relief of vertebrobasilar symptoms by carotid endarterectomy. Surgery 1965; 57: 48–52

6. Blaisdell, W. F., Clauss, R. D., Galbraith, J. G., Imparato, A. M., Wylie, E. J. Joint study of extracranial arterial occlusion as a cause of stroke IV. A Review of surgical considerations. Journal of the American Medical Association 1969; 209: 1889–1895

7. Imparato, A. M., Lin, J. P. T. Vertebral arterial reconstruction: internal plication and vein patch angioplasty. Annals of Surgery 1967; 166: 213–221

8. Berguer, R., Andaya, L. V., Bauer, R. B. Vertebral artery by-pass. Archives of Surgery 1967; 111: 976–979

9. Edwards, W. H., Mulherin, J. L. The surgical approach to significant stenosis of vertebral and subclavian arteries. Surgery 1980; 87: 20–28

10. Powers, S. R., Drislane, T. M., Iandoli, E. W. The surgical treatment of vertebral artery insufficiency. Archives of Surgery 1963; 86: 60–64

Treatment of occlusion of branches of the aortic arch and subclavian arteries

James A. DeWeese MD, FACS
Professor and Chairman, Division of Cardiothoracic Surgery,
University of Rochester Medical Center, Rochester, New York, USA

Introduction

Atherosclerotic lesions of the extracranial cerebral vessels, as in many major arteries, occur at the site of bifurcations. Lesions of the innominate, left common carotid or left subclavian arteries occur at the origin of these vessels from the arch of the aorta. The lesions actually begin within the aorta as plaques which encircle the origins of the vessels and then extend for short distances along their walls. Lesions of the right subclavian and right common carotid artery begin at their bifurcating origin from the innominate artery and both vessels may be involved. Diaphragm-like lesions are occasionally found in the mid-portions of either subclavian artery. All of the lesions are quite localized unless thrombosis occurs, in which case the occlusions extend to the first distal major branch. Occlusions of the subclavian arteries proximal to the origin of the vertebral artery may result in retrograde flow down the vertebral artery to supply the subclavian arteries, a 'subclavian steal'. Arm motion may accentuate the flow. A significant occlusion of the innominate artery may result in a similar retrograde flow in the right common carotid and vertebral arteries. The plaques may also become ulcerated and may become the source for emboli.

Preoperative

Indications[1]

There is extensive collateral supply to the brain and arm and multiple stenotic or even occlusive lesions may be present without symptoms. Operations are indicated for significant symptoms of upper extremity arterial insufficiency or for cerebral ischaemia. Significant signs and symptoms of upper extremity arterial insufficiency include claudication interfering with work or other activities or ischaemic lesions involving the fingers or hand. Cerebral symptoms may also be secondary to diminished flow or embolization. Symptoms related to exercise usually occur in the presence of multiple lesions with decreased perfusion. The target area may be the carotid distribution and consist of unilateral visual loss, dysphasia or hemiparesis. Bilateral visual disturbances, drop attacks or ataxia indicate decreased perfusion of the vertebrobasilar system.

Embolization from ulcerating lesions of the innominate or common carotid arteries may produce classic transient ischaemic attacks of ipsilateral amaurosis fugax, dysphasia or contralateral hemiparesis. Vertebrobasilar symptoms may occur secondary to embolization from ulcerations of the subclavian or vertebral arteries. It should be appreciated that, with occlusion of the right subclavian artery, retrograde thrombosis may result in the presence of potential emboli in the origin of the right carotid artery.

Diagnosis

Bruits, differential arm pressures and noninvasive studies of the cerebral circulation may provide some information regarding the lesions responsible for symptoms. Carefully performed selective angiograms are necessary, however, for the accurate demonstration of the site and extent of the lesion and the planning of the appropriate arterial reconstruction.

The operations

There are various methods available for the management of these lesions. Endarectomy is the most direct approach and may be used to manage most lesions which can be approached through the neck. Grafts which bypass lesions in line with normal flow are preferred for the treatment of lesions of the proximal innominate and common carotid arteries in good-risk patients. Extrathoracic remote bypass procedures are reserved for poor-risk patients and for cases where a direct approach would be difficult technically because of previous direct arterial reconstructions. The transposition of arteries to normal adjacent arteries is occasionally possible. If the indication for the operation is embolization, and bypass procedures are used, it is important that the proximal diseased artery is sacrificed.

Operations for lesions of the innominate artery

1a, b & c

Operations for the treatment of lesions of the innominate artery are endarterectomy (*a*), aortoinnominate bypass (*b*) and axilloaxillary bypass (*c*). Endarterectomy of the proximal innominate artery, using the same principles as described later in operations for left subclavian lesions, may be performed through a median sternotomy. The extension of the lesion along the wall of the aorta, however, may complicate the application of a side clamp which provides access to the entire lesion. Therefore, the aortoinnominate bypass is preferred for most patients. Axilloaxillary bypasses are reserved for poor-risk patients or special situations.

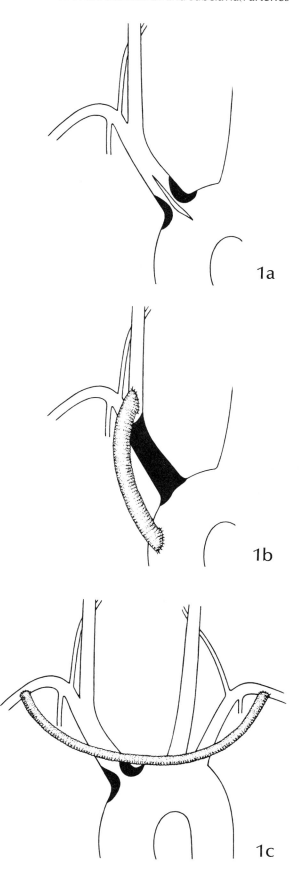

AORTOINNOMINATE BYPASS

2

The incision

The incision passes down the anterior border of the right sternocleidomastoid muscle to the suprahyoid notch and is carried down the middle of the sternum.

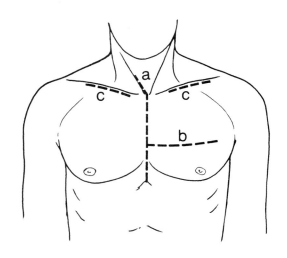

2

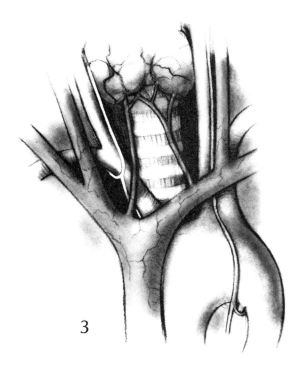

3

3

The sternum is divided in the midline. The lobes of the thymus are separated. The pericardium is opened longitudinally. The innominate artery is identified superior to the innominate vein and the inferior and middle thyroid branches of the right innominate vein are divided. The carotid and subclavian arteries are mobilized, taking care to identify the vagus nerve as it descends along the carotid artery. The recurrent laryngeal branch of the nerve must be carefully preserved as it passes around the subclavian artery.

4

Occlusion of aorta

Aqueous heparin in doses of 5000–7500 u is administered intravenously. The ascending aorta is partially occluded with a side-clamp. Before incision it is important to determine that the side-clamp is actually occluding the sometimes thickened and calcific ascending aorta. This can be accomplished by pressing out the blood through the occluding blades of the clamp and observing whether blood returns through the blades. Inserting an 18 gauge needle into the occluded portion of the aorta will also identify an incomplete occlusion.

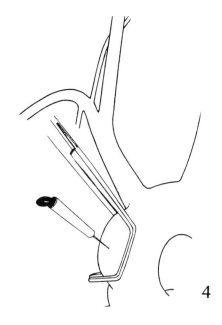

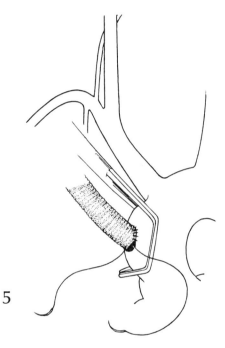

5

Proximal anastomosis

A small button of aorta is excised. An 8–10 mm plastic graft is then cut obliquely and sutured end-to-side to the aorta, using a 4/0 monofilament suture and a continuous everting running stitch.

6

Distal anastomosis

The innominate, carotid and subclavian arteries are then occluded and the distal anastomosis is performed. Usually the anastomosis is made to the distal innominate and proximal carotid artery. Before completion of the distal anastomosis, great care is taken to evacuate all air from the graft. The head of the operating room table is lowered and the carotid clamp is released, filling the graft and allowing the air to escape through the untied suture line. The carotid is again occluded and the suture tied. The subclavian clamp and aortic clamps are then released before finally re-releasing the carotid clamp.

After bleeding is controlled, protamine sulphate is administered intravenously. Two plastic chest catheters are left beneath the sternum and brought out through stab wounds, attached to suction, and the wounds closed. Prophylactic antibiotics are administered preoperatively and for 5 days postoperatively.

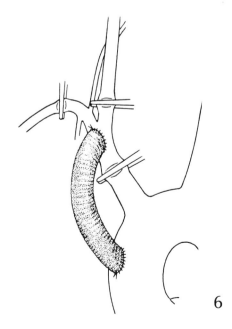

Operations for lesions of the subclavian artery[3]

7a–e

Operations for treatment of most lesions of the subclavian artery can be performed through extrathoracic incisions. They include right subclavian endarterectomy (a), repositioning of the subclavian artery (b), carotid to subclavian artery bypass (c) and axilloaxillary bypass (d). An endarterectomy of the left subclavian artery requires a thoracic approach (e). Repositioning of the subclavian artery presents some problems in exposure and tailoring of the cut end of the subclavian artery to reach the carotid artery. Endarterectomy may be difficult if the lesion extends distally. Axilloaxillary bypass requires two incisions and violates the arterial supply of the opposite limb. We therefore prefer a carotid to subclavian artery bypass for the management of most of these lesions.

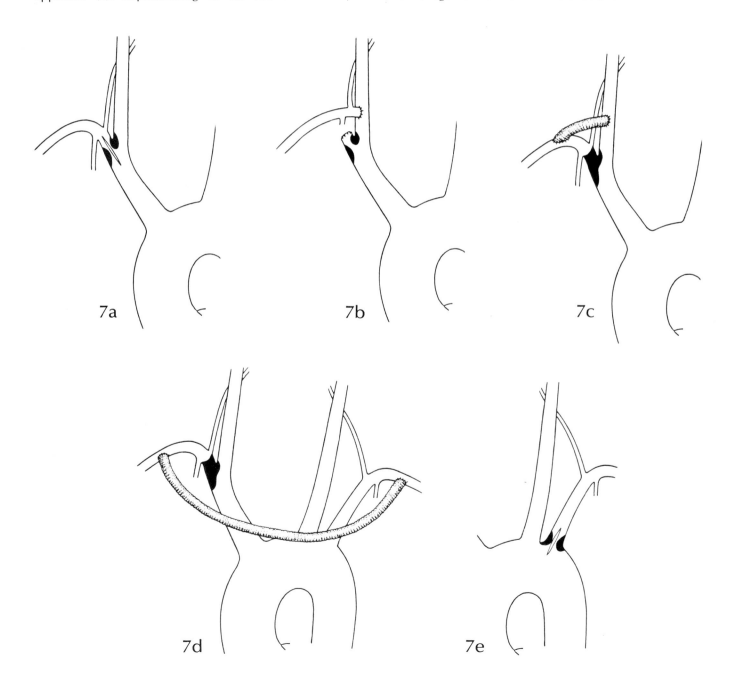

7a

7b

7c

7d

7e

CAROTID TO SUBCLAVIAN BYPASS[4, 5, 6]

8

The incision

The incision is made 1 cm above and parallel to the clavicle, beginning at its midpoint and extending medially to the suprasternal notch. Extension down and through the sternum to the level of the 4th interspace may be necessary. The incision is carried through the sterno-cleidomastoid muscle and both sternohyoid and sterno-thyroid muscles are also divided.

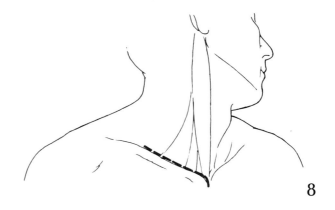

8

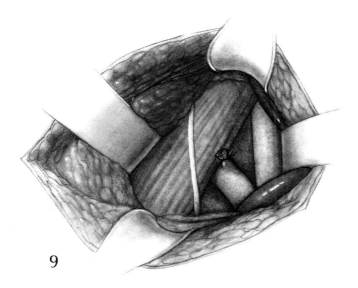

9

9

Mobilizing fat pad

The prescalene fascia is incised and the fat pad swept upwards and laterally to expose the scalenus anticus muscle and phrenic nerves. The subclavian vein is mobilized and retracted medially to expose the common carotid artery, taking care to preserve the vagus nerve.

10

Exposure of arteries

The phrenic nerve is identified and preserved. The scalenus anticus muscle is divided. The subclavian artery is mobilized medially. The thyrocervical trunk is taped or ligated. Heparin is administered.

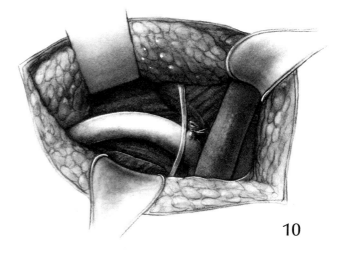

10

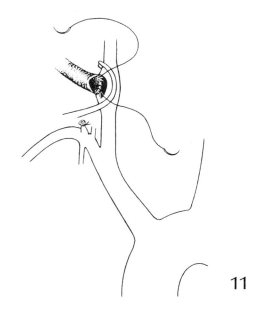

11

Proximal anastomosis

The common carotid artery is partially occluded and an arteriotomy made. A 6–8 mm Dacron graft is preclotted and the posterior half of an end-to-side anastomosis performed. If the carotid artery is large, a partial occlusion clamp does not complicate the performance of the anterior half of the anastomosis. If the artery is small, however, the carotid is totally occluded for the short time required to complete the anastomosis.

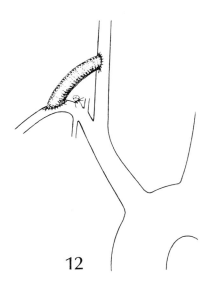

12

Distal anastomosis

The distal anastomosis is performed to the subclavian artery beyond the divided thyrocervical trunk. We have preferred knitted Dacron grafts for these short bypasses. In our hands the long-term patency of the Dacron grafts has surpassed that of autogenous vein, possibly because of the contained space in which they lie[5,6]. Endarterectomy is best performed through a thoracotomy and is reserved for young, good-risk patients with stenotic lesions.

LEFT SUBCLAVIAN ENDARTERECTOMY

13

The incision

The long-term results of endarterectomy of the subclavian artery have been excellent and should be considered in young, good-risk patients[5,6]. The incision begins at the suprasternal notch, extends down the middle of the sternum and then laterally through the left 3rd interspace (*see Illustration 2, incision b*). The lung is retracted downwards and the mediastinal pleura incised over the proximal left subclavian and carotid arteries and the adjacent aorta. A 3–4 cm length of phrenic and vagus nerves is mobilized so they can be retracted easily.

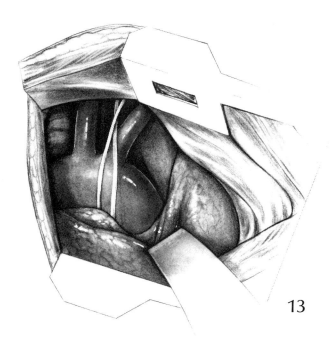

13

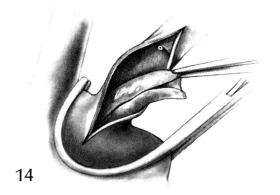

14

14

Endarterectomy

Heparin is administered intravenously. An angulated side-clamp is applied which partially occludes the aorta at least 1 cm away from the origin of the subclavian. The subclavian artery is occluded at least 2 cm distal to the palpable plaque and extended into the aorta and also 1 cm beyond any visible plaque in the subclavian artery. A longitudinal incision is made over the plaque. A plane of dissection is established and an endarterectomy performed.

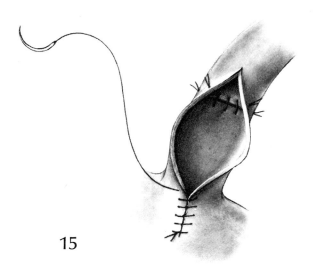

15

15

Tacking and closure

Care is taken to cut the proximal and distal ends of the plaque flush with the level where the intima becomes tightly adherent to the media. Mattress tacking sutures are placed distally through any intimal flaps and tied outside the artery. The arteriotomy is carefully closed with a fine suture as a continuous stitch. Care is taken to evacuate any air before completing the closure. Protamine is given and the wounds closed. A chest catheter is inserted and placed on continuous suction for 18 hours.

AXILLOAXILLARY BYPASS

16

The incision

Axilloaxillary bypass may become the preferred operation in patients with previous cervical incisions or following failure of other reconstructions. An incision is made 1 cm inferior to and parallel to the clavicle from its midportion to the palpable head (*see Illustration 2, incision c*). The pectoralis major muscle is divided in the direction of the fibres. The clavipectoral fascia is divided to expose the pectoralis minor muscle which is retracted laterally. The axillary artery is identified superior to the axillary vein. The first part of the axillary artery extends from the clavicle to the medial border of the pectoralis minor muscle. It has one branch, the supreme thoracic, which may either be controlled or ligated. The thoraco-acromial and lateral thoracic arteries arise from the second part of the axillary artery, which lies behind the pectoralis minor muscle. These branches are also controlled or ligated. The anterior thoracic nerve, 1–2 mm in diameter, crosses the second part of the axillary artery and can be retracted laterally.

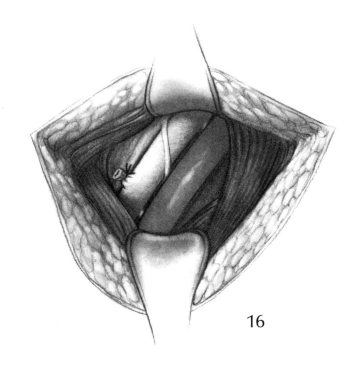

16

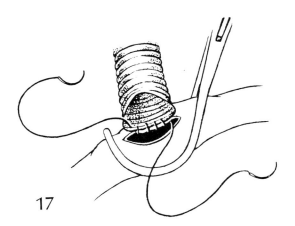

17

17

Anastomosis

Heparin is administered. The artery is occluded with a single clamp, which elevates the artery out of the wound. An 8 mm preclotted knitted Dacron graft is anastomosed end-to-side to the inferior edge of the artery, using a fine suture and a continuous stitch beginning posteriorly and tied anteriorly. The clamp is intermittently released until there is no further oozing of blood through the graft wall. Any clot is removed. A similar incision is made over the opposite axillary artery, the graft tunnelled between the two incisions with a long clamp taking care that no twist occurs. A similar anastomosis is then performed. Care is taken to evacuate air before tying the suture. Protamine is administered and the wound closed.

Operations for lesions of the common carotid artery

18a, b & c

Operations for lesions of the common carotid arteries include endarterectomy (a), aortocarotid bypass (b) or subclavian to carotid bypass (c). The operation for a left carotid endarterectomy is essentially the same as that for the left subclavian artery and is performed through a modified trapdoor incision. The aortocarotid artery bypass would be performed through the same type of incision and adhere to the same technique as described for an aortoinnominate bypass. The subclavian to distal common carotid artery bypass is preferred for occluded carotid arteries.

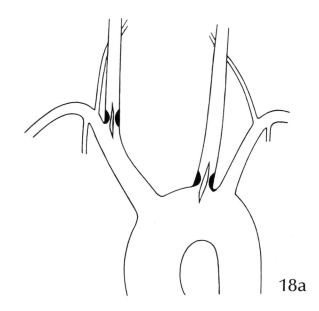

18a

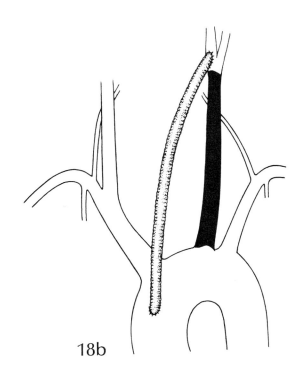

18b

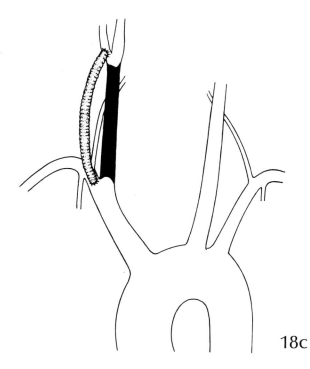

18c

SUBCLAVIAN TO DISTAL CAROTID ARTERY BYPASS[8]

19

The incision

The patient is supine with the head hyperextended but not turned. An incision is made along the anterior border of the sternocleidomastoid muscle from the angle of the jaw to the suprasternal notch.

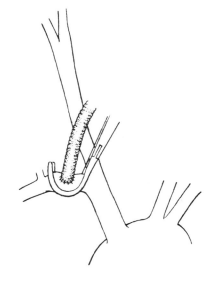

19

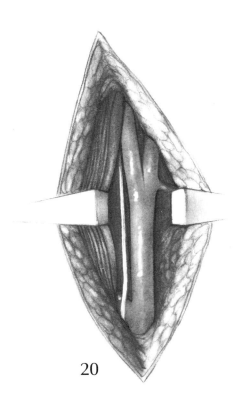

20

20

Exposure of arteries

The carotid artery is exposed near the lower part of the incision and the dissection is carried down the lateral border of the carotid artery until the innominate artery on the right side and the aorta on the left side can be identified. The origins of the subclavian arteries are then exposed, taking care to preserve the vagus nerve.

21

Proximal anastomosis

Heparin is given. The artery is occluded with a single clamp and an 8 mm preclotted knitted Dacron graft anastomosed to the superior edge of the vessel.

21

22

Distal anastomosis

The distal end of the graft is anastomosed to the proximal internal carotid artery bulb. Air is carefully evacuated before completing the anastomosis. Protamine is administered. The wound is closed.

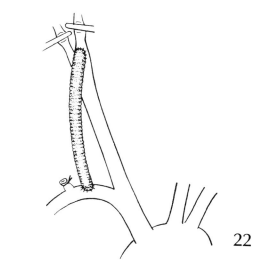

22

23

Operation for multiple occlusive lesions of the aortic arch[2]

Patients with multiple lesions may be treated in many ways. Some of the lesions can be treated through the same incisions, such as combined lesions of either the right or left carotid and subclavian arteries or of the subclavian and vertebral arteries. For lesions of the proximal innominate and left carotid and/or subclavian arteries, aortoinnominate bypasses with side-arms to the other vessels in either right or left neck can be performed. Ingenious and complicated extrathoracic bypasses have also been performed. Bypasses from the femoral artery to axillary arteries have been described for bypass of innominate or subclavian lesions.

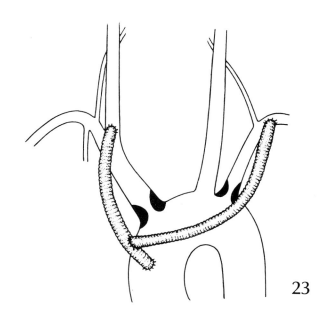

23

References

1. Wylie, E. J., Effeney, D. J. Surgery of the aortic arch branches and vertebral arteries. Surgical Clinics of North America 1979; 59: 669–680

2. Crawford, E. S., DeBakey, M. E., Morris, G. C., Jr, Howell, J. F. Surgical treatment of occlusion of the innominate, common carotid, and subclavian arteries: a 10-year experience. Surgery 1969; 65: 17–31

3. Ehrenfeld, W. K., Chapman, R. D., Wylie, E. J. Management of occlusive lesions of the branches of the aortic arch. American Journal of Surgery 1969; 118: 236–243

4. Diethrich, E. B., Garrett, H. E., Ameriso, J., Crawford, E. S., El-Bayar, H., DeBakey, M. E. Occlusive disease of the common carotid and subclavian arteries treated by carotid-subclavian bypass. Analysis of 125 cases. American Journal of Surgery 1967; 114: 800–808

5. Resnicoff, S. A., DeWeese, J. A., Rob, C. G. Surgical treatment of the subclavian steal syndrome. Circulation 1970; 41–42 Suppl: II147–II151

6. Gerety, R. L., Andrus, C. H., May, A. G., Rob, C. G., Green, R., DeWeese, J. A. Surgical treatment of occlusive subclavian artery disease. Circulation 1981; 64 Suppl.: II228–II230

7. Myers, W. O., Lawton, B. R., Ray, J. F. III., Kuehner, M. E., Saulter, R. D. Axillo-axillary bypass for subclavian steal syndrome. Archives of Surgery 1979; 114: 394–402

8. Podore, P. C., Rob, C. G., DeWeese, J. A., Green, R. M. Chronic common carotid occlusion. Stroke 1981; 12: 98–100

Illustrations by Anita Matthews and Robert Wabnitz

Treatment of dissecting thoracic aortic aneurysms

James A. DeWeese MD, FACS
Professor and Chairman, Division of Cardiothoracic Surgery,
University of Rochester Medical Center, Rochester, New York, USA

Introduction

The pathological process is best described as a dissecting haematoma within the media of the aorta rather than an aneurysm. It is only when the haematoma communicates with the aortic lumen and blood flows through this second channel that aneurysmal dilatation develops. This second channel also distorts the intima, causing compression of the lumen, and can occlude branches of the aorta. Smaller branches may be sheared off by the dissection.

Classically the patients present with severe chest and back pain. They may have central neurological deficits secondary to occlusion of extracranial vessels or be paraplegic from involvement of the anterior spinal arteries. They may be oliguric or anuric from renal artery occlusion. Ischaemia of an extremity secondary to peripheral arterial compression is commonly seen. The dissection may loosen the support of the cusps of the aortic valve, allowing prolapse and aortic insufficiency. Rupture through the thin adventitia may occur into the pericardial, pleural or abdominal cavities. The mortality rate in untreated patients is 50 per cent within 48 hours, 70 per cent within 1 week and 90 per cent at 3 months.

Preoperative

Initial treatment

Almost 90 per cent of patients with dissecting haematomas are hypertensive. Except for patients who have suffered rupture, the initial therapy should be aggressive drug control of the hypertension with the intravenous administration of trimethaphan or nitroprusside and propanolol. The parenteral administration of reserpine or methyldopa (Aldomet) should begin at the same time. Guanethidine and oral preparations of propranolol, reserpine and Aldomet may be useful later. The systolic blood pressure must be significantly lowered, preferably below 120 mmHg. Close monitoring of the arterial pressure requires an intra-arterial line. Indwelling nasogastric tubes and urinary catheters are usually necessary. Endotracheal tubes or tracheostomies and assisted ventilation may be required for the control of tracheobronchial secretions in heavily sedated patients[1].

1

Diagnostic procedures

The diagnosis of dissection may be suspected or demonstrated with echocardiography or computerized axial tomography scans, but angiography is usually required to prove the diagnosis. Only angiography can demonstrate a patent second channel and establish the sites of communication of the aortic lumen with this second channel. The extent of the dissection can also be demonstrated. It is of practical importance to know if it includes both ascending and descending aorta (Type I), ascending aorta only (Type II) or descending aorta only (Type III)[2].

Indications

Patients with Type I, II, and III dissections require immediate operations if rupture has occurred. Significant aortic insufficiency, cardiac tamponade, or the occlusion of major arteries is an indication for operations on Type I and II dissections. The operation is preferably delayed until the hypertension is under control and for at least 2 weeks, if possible. The operative mortality for patients operated on within 2 weeks of onset is twice that for later operations[1]. Patients with Type III dissections require operation if major vessels are occluded and also if a patent second channel results in progressive aneurysmal dilatation. The entire extent of the disease can rarely be resected. The operation is designed to obliterate the intimal tear which allows communication between the aortic lumen and second channel. At the same time, the second channel is circumferentially obliterated, preventing progression of the dissection.

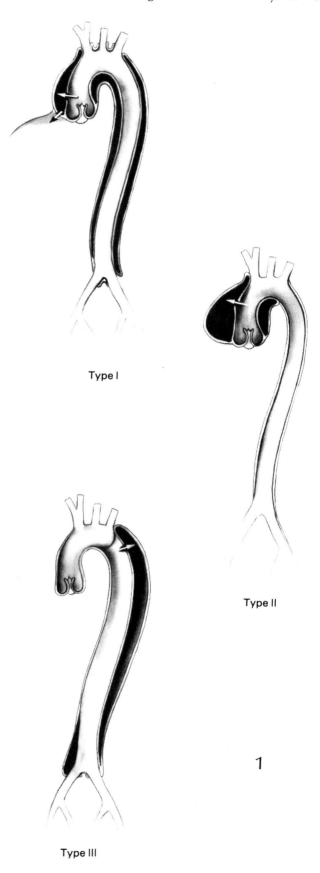

Type I

Type II

Type III

1

Operation for Types I and II

2

Division of aorta

Operations on Type I and II dissections require total cardiopulmonary bypass (*see* chapter on 'Treatment of intrathoracic aneurysms and thoracoabdominal aneurysms', pp. 111–122). Hypothermia and cardioplegia are used. The aorta is partially divided about 2.5 cm (1 inch) distal to the coronary arteries. The intimal tear is usually found at this level and the aortotomy is completed through the tear if possible. Catheters are then inserted into one or both coronary artery orifices for instillation of cardioplegic solution.

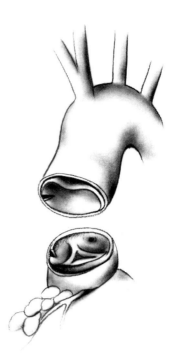

2

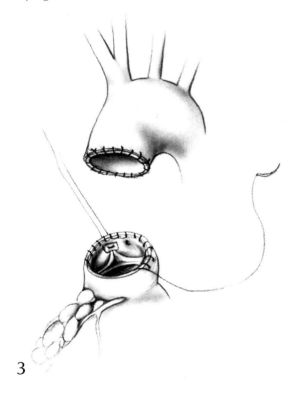

3

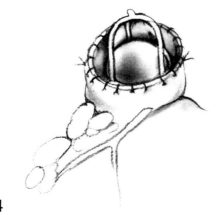

4

3

Obliteration of second channel and suspension of valve

The dissection usually involves only a portion of the circumference of the vessel. The separated intima and adventitia are reapproximated and the remaining circumference of the vessel strengthened by a continuous over-and-over stitch of a fine 4/0 or 5/0 monofilament suture on a fine needle.

The aortic valve leaflets usually appear normal, but the intima and attached commissure and cusp are unsupported. The commissure is resuspended by placing a mattress stitch through a pledget, through the aortic wall and then through a second pledget over which it is tied.

4

Aortic valve replacement

The aortic valve may be deformed as a result of coexisting disease or in the presence of a chronic dissection. The valve may then be excised and replaced with an artificial valve. Mattress sutures over pledgets are used to secure the valve in a subcoronary position.

In the presence of a chronic dissection and an aneurysmal aorta, the valve and an attached graft may be inserted within the aorta as described in the chapter on 'Treatment of intrathoracic aneurysms and thoracoabdominal aneurysms', pp. 111–122.

5

Reapproximation of aorta

If the aorta has an acceptably thick adventitia and is mobile so that the ends can be brought together without tension, it may be merely reapproximated. A 1–3 cm cuff of a synthetic plastic graft is placed around the ends of the aorta. A continuous mattress stitch of 3/0 or 4/0 monofilament plastic suture is placed through all layers to evert the edges. Great care must be taken in placing these stitches to avoid leaving suture holes or needle tears in the thin intima. A second layer of fine sutures is placed using an over-and-over continuous stitch.

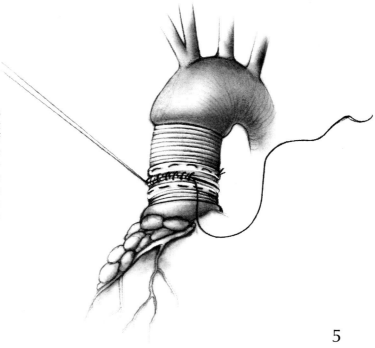

5

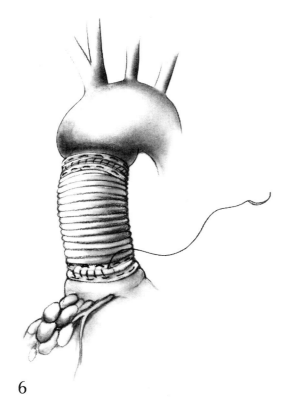

6

6

Insertion of graft

A graft is inserted if the dissection is sharply localized proximal to the innominate artery so that it can be totally excised, or if the edges of the divided aorta cannot be reapproximated without tension. A woven plastic tube graft is anastomosed end-to-end to the ends of the excised or divided aorta. An everting mattress stitch of 3/0 suture through a plastic cuff with a second over-and-over continuous stitch of 4/0 suture is used at each end. Any anastomotic leaks or suture holes must be controlled before the patient is taken off cardiopulmonary bypass. These leaks cannot be controlled when the aorta is distended by normal arterial pressures.

7

Insertion of intraluminal sutureless prosthesis

An intraluminal sutureless prosthesis is now available and useful in certain situations. The prosthesis consists of a plastic graft into which rigid plastic or metal grooved rings are incorporated at each end. Tapes are passed around the aorta proximal to the innominate artery and distal to the coronary arteries. A longitudinal aortotomy is preferred. The cuffs of the graft are fixed in place with horizontal mattress sutures passed through the graft and all layers of the aortic wall. Two of the proximal sutures are positioned 2 cm distal to the coronary artery orifices to avoid coronary artery obstruction.

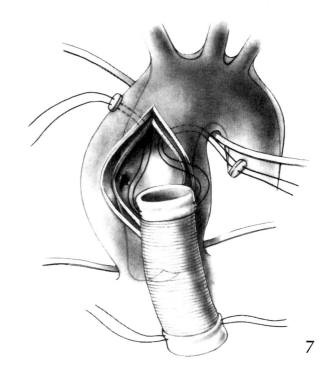

7

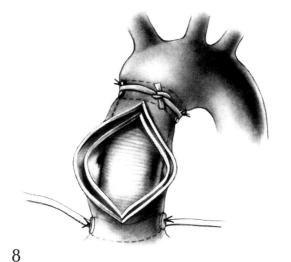

8

8

Fixation of prosthesis

The tapes which encircled the aorta are now tied over the ring. Additional sutures may be placed through the tape, aortic wall and the plastic covering the ring to prevent migration of the graft. The aortic clamps are removed and the aortotomy closed.

Operation for Type III

9

Exposure of descending aorta

Operations on Type III dissections require left heart bypass (*see* chapter on 'Treatment of intrathoracic aneurysms and thoracoabdominal aneurysms', pp. 111–122). A left thoracotomy is performed. The mediastinal pleura is incised to expose the transverse aortic arch, the subclavian artery and the descending thoracic aorta. The first two or three pairs of intercostal arteries are carefully mobilized and taped. After left heart bypass has been initiated, the aorta and subclavian artery are clamped.

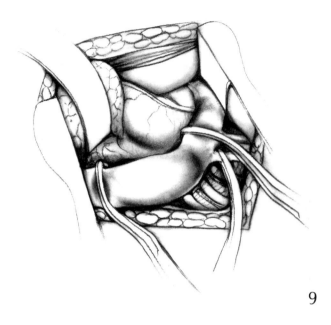

9

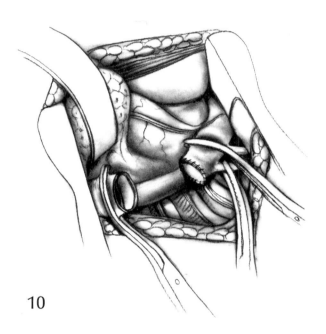

10

10

Division and oversewing of aorta

The aorta is divided at the level of the ligamentum arteriosum. The intimal tear allowing communication between the aortic lumen and second channel is usually found at this level. The ends of the aorta are then oversewn circumferentially to approximate the intima and media which obliterates the second channel.

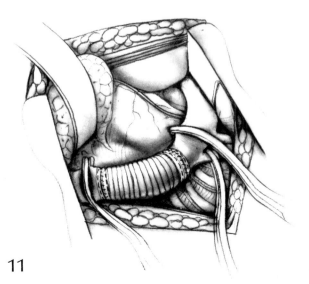

11

11

Insertion of grafts

Unless the aorta is very mobile, a woven graft is interposed between the cut oversewn ends of the aorta. A 3 cm cuff of a woven Dacron graft is placed around both ends. A continuous mattress stitch using a 3/0 monofilament suture with a fine needle is used to approximate the graft and aorta. The suture is passed through graft, aorta and the short cuff of graft. An over-and-over continuous stitch of fine suture is then run as a second layer. When this first anastomosis is completed the clamp is removed, allowing the graft to fill. The anastomosis, particularly its posterior half, is carefully inspected for leaks. The second anastomosis is completed and the graft and aorta carefully covered with pleura.

12

Insertion of intraluminal prosthesis

A sutureless intraluminal prosthesis can be used if the intimal tear is at least 2 cm distal to the left subclavian artery. The ringed graft is fixed in place with horizontal mattress sutures which pass through the prosthesis and all layers of the aortic wall. The externally placed tapes are then tied over the grooved rings and the aortotomy is closed.

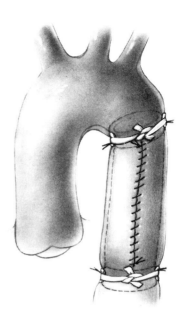

12

Postoperative care

It is just as important to maintain the systemic arterial pressure in the normotensive range following operation as it was prior to operation to protect suture lines and to prevent progression of the dissection.

Endotracheal intubation with assisted ventilation is required for at least 18 hours following operation to allow for improvement in mechanics of respiration and gaseous diffusion.

The status of oxygenation, blood volume and ventricular function is followed closely and controlled with appropriate medications and fluids by the monitoring of blood gases, atrial pressures, systemic arterial pressure and cardiac output.

Prophylactic antibiotics are indicated.

References

1. Wheat, M. W. Treatment of dissecting aneurysms of the aorta: current status. Progress in Cardiovascular Disease 1973; 16: 87–101

2. DeBakey, M. E., McCollum, C. H., Crawford, E. S., et al. Dissection and dissecting aneurysms of the aorta: twenty-year follow-up of five hundred twenty-seven patients treated surgically. Surgery 1982; 92: 1118–1134

Further reading

Ablaza, S. G. G., Ghosh, S. C., Grana, V. P. Use of a ringed intraluminal graft in the surgical treatment of dissecting aneurysms of the thoracic aorta. Journal of Thoracic and Cardiovascular Surgery 1978; 76: 390–396

Dureau, G., Villard, J., George, M., Deliry, P., Froment, J. C., Clermont, A. New surgical technique for the operative management of acute dissections of the ascending aorta. Journal of Thoracic and Cardiovascular Surgery 1978; 76: 385–389

Lemole, G. M., Strong, M. D., Spagna, P. M., Karmilowicz, N. P. Improved results for dissecting aneurysms intraluminal sutureless prosthesis. Journal of Thoracic and Cardiovascular Surgery 1982; 83: 249–255

Illustrations by Diane Elliott, Anita Matthews and Robert Wabnitz

Treatment of intrathoracic aneurysms and thoracoabdominal aneurysms

James A. DeWeese MD, FACS
Professor and Chairman, Division of Cardiothoracic Surgery,
University of Rochester Medical Center; Rochester, New York, USA

Preoperative

Indications

Fusiform or saccular aneurysms may occur in the ascending aorta, arch aorta and descending thoracic aorta, as well as its major branches. The usual causes are arteriosclerosis, lues and trauma. Dissecting aneurysms occurring in the presence of cystic medial necrosis present unusual problems in diagnosis and treatment and will be discussed elsewhere.

Surgical treatment should be considered whenever the diagnosis is made, since in general the lesions are progressive to rupture and death. Surgical treatment becomes imperative in the presence of pain secondary to erosion of the spine or compression of nerves. Other indications include: phrenic nerve or recurrent laryngeal nerve involvement; compression or erosion of the trachea or oesophagus; and rupture[1,2].

Contraindications

Age alone is not a contraindication to surgery. In fact, the lesions are most commonly found in patients over 60 years of age. Arteriosclerotic heart disease, chronic lung disease or other significant medical illnesses may contraindicate surgery in the asymptomatic patient.

Special preparations

For elective operations patients are admitted to hospital 2–7 days prior to surgery for a final medical evaluation. Attention should be directed towards improvements of the respiratory tract, particularly in those with chronic lung diseases. Smoking should be discontinued. Hyperventilation exercises should be prescribed. Bronchodilators, secretagogues, detergents, positive pressure breathing and even prophylactic antibiotics may be indicated.

Special techniques

When the thoracic aorta is clamped, special equipment is needed to prevent left ventricular failure and to ensure adequate circulation to the heart, brain, kidneys and viscera. The bypass procedures vary according to the site of clamping and will be discussed separately.

Special techniques for suturing the thoracic aorta are also necessary. The diseased thoracic aorta is more friable than the abdominal aorta or peripheral arteries. The simpler techniques of anastomosis used for the abdominal aorta, therefore, may be unsatisfactory in the thoracic aorta. Bleeding from suture lines or through needle holes is further accentuated by the fact that the patient is best heparinized for the bypass procedures and until the catheters used for the bypass procedures are removed. For these same reasons woven, not knitted grafts are preferred.

The operation

ANEURYSMS OF ASCENDING THORACIC AORTA[3, 4]

1

Total cardiopulmonary bypass with coronary perfusion

Resection of an aneurysm of the ascending thoracic aorta requires clamping of the aorta proximal to the innominate artery. Total cardiopulmonary bypass is necessary. The vena cavae are cannulated through the right atrium with a single or double catheter. Venous blood is thereby returned to a pump oxygenator and heat exchanger. The left ventricle is vented with a catheter. Arterialized and cooled blood is then returned to the femoral artery for retrograde perfusion of the visceral, renal and cranial arteries. A separate line from the pump oxygenator leads to the coronary arteries which are cannulated through a longitudinal incision in the base of the aorta. Alternatively a cold cardioplegic solution with or without blood is perfused into the right and/or the left coronary artery.

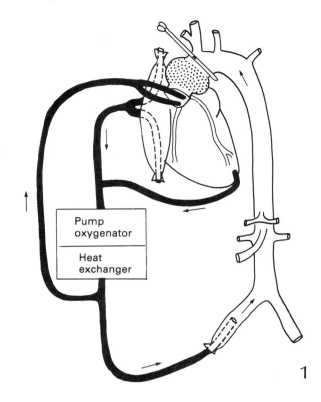

1

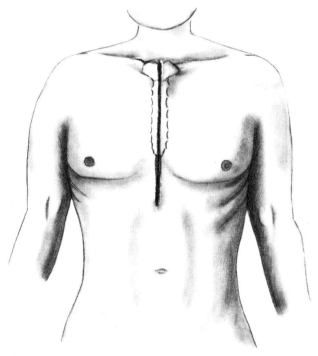

2

Median sternotomy incision

Beginning just below the supraclavicular notch a longitudinal incision is made along the entire length of the sternum beyond the xiphoid process. The sternum is then split longitudinally with an oscillating saw. To establish haemostasis, it is advisable to use cautery for cutting the periosteum and bone wax to control marrow bleeding.

2

3

Exposure of aorta and heart

The pericardium is incised longitudinally after dividing the thymus. It is advisable to avoid entering either pleural space. The innominate vein is carefully retracted superiorly. The aorta is mobilized under direct vision to avoid injuring the pulmonary artery. Catheters are inserted into the vena cava through the right atrium for the return of venous blood to the pump oxygenator. A catheter has been placed in the femoral artery through an incision in the groin for the return of arterialized blood from the pump oxygenator.

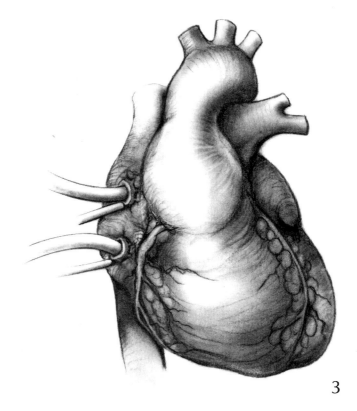

3

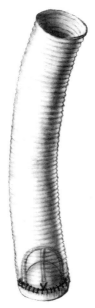

4

4

Preparation of artificial valve and graft

Aneurysms of the ascending aorta are usually associated with aortic valvular insufficiency. An artificial valve replacement as well as the insertion of a woven Dacron graft is therefore usually required. An appropriate-sized valve is sutured to the end of the Dacron tube using a continuous suture.

5

Cardiopulmonary bypass and excision of aortic valve

The patient is placed on cardiopulmonary bypass and the body temperature lowered. A left ventricular sump is inserted. A longitudinal incision is made in the aneurysm without excision of any of the aortic wall. The aortic valve leaflets are excised at least 3 mm from the annulus. Small catheters are inserted into the orifices of the right and left coronary arteries for perfusion of whole blood with or without a cold cardioplegic solution.

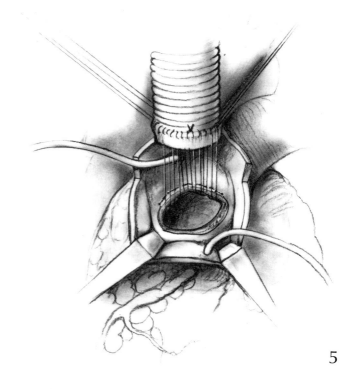

5

6

Seating of artificial valve

Mattress stitches of a 1/0 braided plastic suture are placed through the annulus of the aorta and the base of the artificial valve which has been sutured to the graft. When all the sutures have been placed, the valve is glided down the sutures and seated in the aortic annulus.

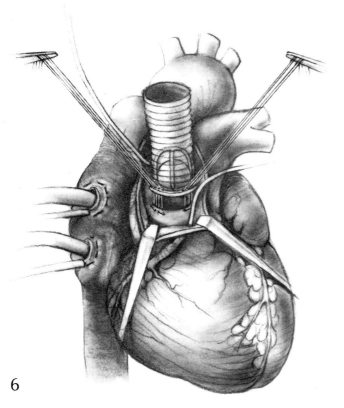

6

7

Distal anastomosis

Holes, 1 cm in diameter, are cut out of the Dacron tube at the estimated level of the coronary orifices. The coronary perfusion catheters are repositioned to pass through these holes and the distal end of the graft is then sutured to the posterior wall of the aorta from within. A mattress stitch is placed directly posteriorly, taking generous bites of the aortic wall.

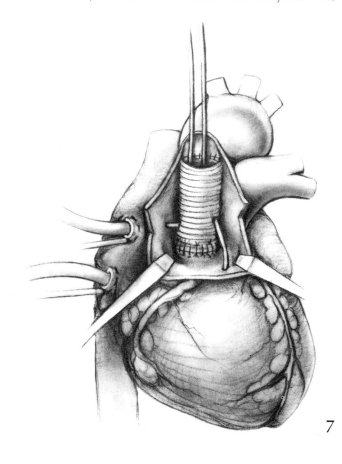

7

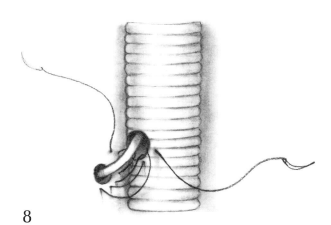

8

8

Suturing of new coronary orifices

The edges of the holes in the graft are now approximated to the aortic wall 2–3 mm from the coronary orifices. This is all accomplished from within the aorta using a continuous stitch and taking generous bites of the aortic wall.

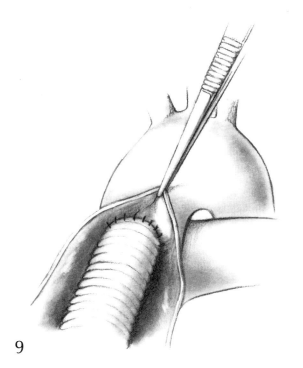

9

Completion of distal anastomosis

An over-and-over continuous stitch is then brought around both sides of the graft and the sutures are tied anteriorly. Both the proximal and distal anastomoses have been made from within the aorta.

9

10

Closure of aorta

Strips of Teflon felt 1.5 cm are placed along the edges of the aortotomy. A horizontal mattress stitch of 0/0 silk suture is placed through the felt pad about 2 cm from the edge of the aortotomy. A second layer is made, using a continuous stitch, about 1 cm from the edge of the aortotomy. The patient is then slowly taken off cardiopulmonary bypass, taking care to evacuate air from the aorta and heart before the heart contracts forcefully.

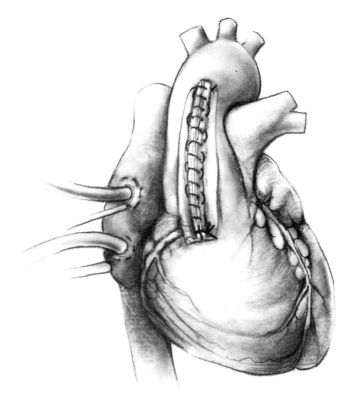

10

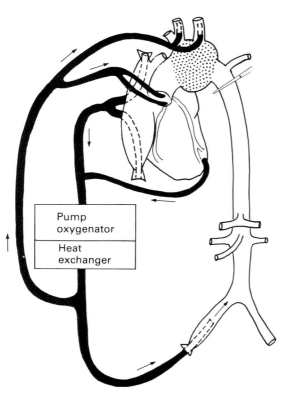

11

ANEURYSMS OF THE AORTIC ARCH[5]

11

Cardiopulmonary bypass, coronary perfusion and cerebral perfusion

The resection of aneurysms of the aortic arch involving the origins of the innominate and left carotid artery require occlusion of the thoracic aorta distal to these important cerebral vessels. In addition to perfusion of the coronary arteries, it is advisable to perfuse the cerebral vessels. This perfusion is accomplished by the insertion of catheters from the oxygenator into the appropriate vessels[5].

12

Exposure and preparations for excision

The initial steps are the same as those used for treatment of aneurysms of the ascending aorta. A median sternotomy incision is made and cardiopulmonary bypass with hypothermia is instituted. The thoracic aorta is occluded distal to the aneurysm. The innominate, left carotid and left subclavian arteries are also occluded. The innominate and left carotid artery can be cannulated with catheters from the pump oxygenator and cerebral perfusion can be started.

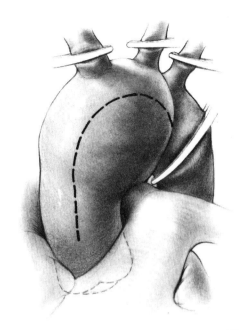

12

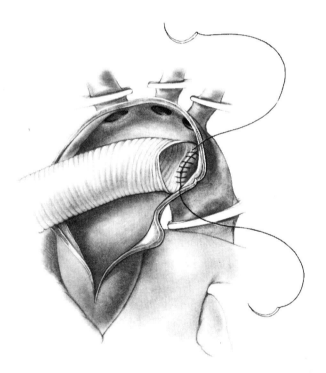

13

Aortotomy and distal anastomosis

A longitudinal aortotomy is made through the aneurysm, extending to within 2 cm of normal aorta proximally and distally. It is advisable to instill cold whole blood and/or cardioplegic solution into the right and/or left coronary artery. A woven Dacron graft the size of the normal aorta is selected. The distal anastomosis is performed with a continuous stitch using monofilament suture which is passed deeply through the cuff usually found at the junction of the aneurysm and normal aorta.

13

14

Anastomosis to arch vessels

Blood flow is re-established to the branches of the aortic arch from within the aneurysm sac. A hole is made in the graft which will encircle the orifices of all three of the branches. The edges of the incised graft are now approximated to the aortic wall around the three orifices using a continuous stitch, taking deep bites with a monofilament suture.

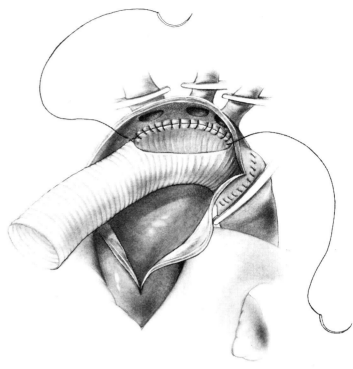

14

15

Proximal anastomosis

Air is evacuated from the arch vessels and graft by the sequential release of the clamps on the left carotid, innominate, left subclavian and distal aortic vessels. The graft is then clamped proximal to the innominate artery. The proximal anastomosis is then performed to the cuff of normal proximal aorta within the aneurysm sac. After release of the clamp and evacuation of air from the graft the aneurysm sac is closed over the graft with a continuous mattress stitch using monofilament suture over plastic felt followed by a continuous stitch using similar suture material.

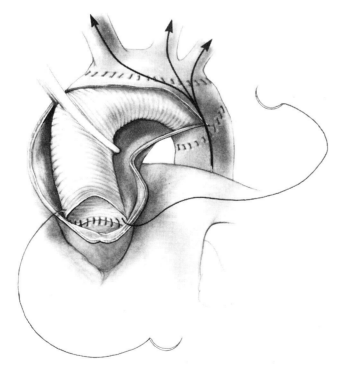

15

ANEURYSMS OF THE DESCENDING THORACIC AORTA

Occlusion of the descending thoracic aorta may result in a proximal hypertension with left ventricular failure and possible cerebral haemorrhage and a distal hypotension with possible renal and hepatic failure.

16

Left heart bypass provides a means for the controlled equalization of proximal and distal pressures. Inclusion of a heat exchanger in the circuit allows cooling of the body for further protection of the kidneys and spinal cord. The rate of flow required to equalize the pressures is usually between 1500 and 2000 ml/min but accurate monitoring of both the proximal and distal pressures is necessary to guarantee adequate distal perfusion. The proximal catheter can be inserted into the left subclavian artery, transverse aortic arch or apex of the left ventricle, but the left atrium is the most satisfactory site. The distal catheter is inserted retrogradely into the femoral artery or descending aorta[2]. In some instances it is possible to use a heparinized plastic tube for bypass[6].

For shorter periods of aortic occlusion it may be possible to control proximal hypertension and improve distal perfusion pharmacologically[7].

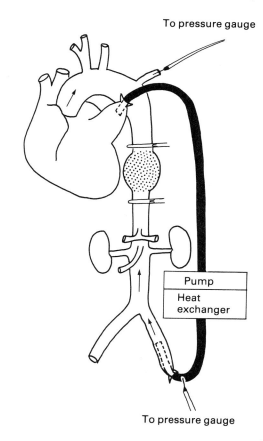

To pressure gauge

Pump

Heat exchanger

To pressure gauge

16

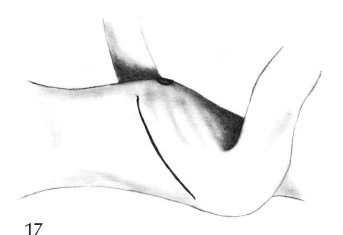

17

17

The incision

With the patient in a lateral position with the left side up, an incision is made along the course of the 5th rib beneath the nipple and tip of the scapula. The latissimus dorsi muscle and the posterior portion of the serratus anterior muscle are divided. The serratus anterior and pectoral muscles are then divided anteriorly to the nipple line. The chest is entered through the 4th or 5th intercostal space. Additional exposure can be obtained by division of the necks of the adjacent ribs posteriorly or by removal of the rib.

18

Exposure and preparation for left heart bypass

The lung is retracted anteriorly and downwards. The phrenic nerve, vagus nerve, subclavian artery and thoracic aorta are visualized. The pericardium is incised longitudinally just anterior to the phrenic nerve to expose the left atrial appendage. A purse-string suture of heavy silk is placed around the appendage and the tip excised. A catheter is inserted through the appendage and connected by plastic tubing to the pump and heat exchanger which, in turn, is connected to a catheter inserted into the femoral artery through a groin incision.

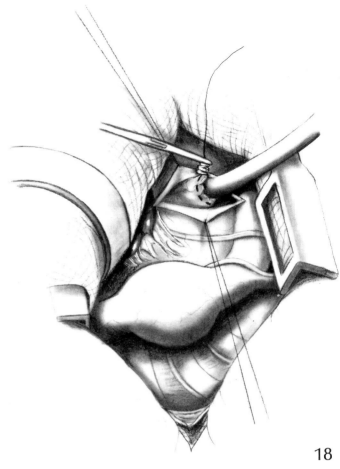

18

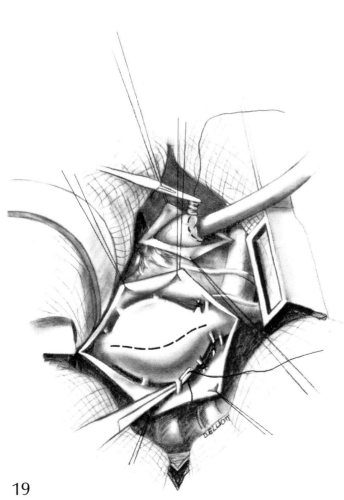

19

19

Dissection of aorta

The mediastinal pleura is incised over the aneurysm and to normal aorta proximally and distally. Under careful direct vision the proximal and distal aorta is mobilized. Intercostal arteries just proximal and distal to the aneurysm are carefully dissected free, ligated in continuity and divided. It is important to sacrifice only those intercostal arteries which must be divided since the important spinal arteries may arise from the intercostals.

20

Management of aneurysm

After the patient is heparinized, the aorta is occluded proximally and distally at the same time that left heart bypass is begun. Acute traumatic aneurysms are opened transversely. In some instances end-to-end anastomosis can be performed. In others short grafts are inserted. Chronic aneurysms do not need to be removed. Longitudinal aortotomy is made and a graft inserted within the aneurysm sac.

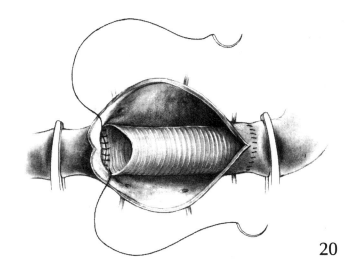

20

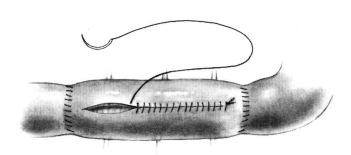

21

21

Closure of aneurysm sac

The aneurysm sac is then closed over the graft using a continuous stitch with a 2/0 suture. The patient is given protamine to counteract the heparin after bypass is discontinued and the catheters in the atrium and femoral artery are removed. If possible the pleura is approximated over the graft. The wound is closed in layers after inserting a catheter through the 7th interspace for postoperative drainage of the pleural space.

THORACOABDOMINAL ANEURYSM[7]

22

Aneurysms involving the lower thoracic aorta and the suprarenal abdominal aorta require thoracic incisions, through the 5th to 8th interspace, which extend into the abdominal cavity. The aorta is occluded and the aneurysm sac opened longitudinally. Vigorous back-bleeding from visceral or renal arteries can be controlled with balloon catheters. The proximal and distal and branch arterial anastomoses are made within the aneurysm sac as described in this chapter (*see also* chapter on 'Treatment of abdominal aortic aneurysms', pp. 123–135).

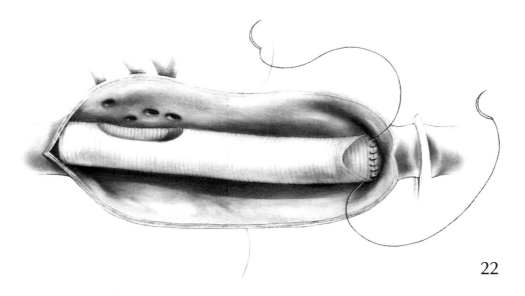

22

Postoperative care

These patients all require careful post-thoracotomy management. Catheters are inserted into the thoracic cavity and mediastinum, brought through stab wounds and connected to negative pressures of 10–20 cmH$_2$O to ensure drainage of blood and expansion of lungs during the first 2–3 postoperative days. Oxygen by mask is recommended during the first 1–2 days. Atelectasis is prevented by hyperventilation and vigorous physiotherapy. The use of prophylactic antibiotics is recommended.

No anticoagulants are administered postoperatively. The patient receives heparin during the operation, when on bypass or when major vessels are clamped, but protamine is administered to reverse this effect before the wound is closed.

References

1. Joyce, J. W., Fairbairn, J. F., Kincaid, O. W., Juergens, J. L. Aneurysms of the thoracic aorta: a clinical study with special reference to prognosis. Circulation 1964; 29: 176–181

2. Plume, S., DeWeese, J. A. Traumatic rupture of the thoracic aorta. Archives of Surgery 1979; 114: 240–243

3. Houser, S., Mijangos, J., Sengupta, A., Zaroff, L., Weiner, R., DeWeese, J. A. Management of fusiform ascending aortic aneurysms. Annals of Thoracic Surgery 1980; 30: 70–75

4. Edward, W. S., Kerr, A. R. A safer technique for replacement of the entire ascending aorta and aortic valve. Journal of Thoracic and Cardiovascular Surgery 1970; 59: 837–839

5. Crawford, E. S., Snyder, D. M. Treatment of aneurysms of the aortic arch: a progress report. Journal of Thoracic and Cardiovascular Surgery 1983; 85: 237–246

6. Wolfe, W. G., Kleinman, L. H., Wechsler, A. S., Sabistoa, D. C. Heparin-coated shunts for lesions of the descending thoracic aorta: experimental and clinical observations. Archives of Surgery 1977; 112: 1481–1487

7. Crawford, E. S. Thoraco-abdominal and abdominal aortic aneurysms involving renal, superior mesenteric, and celiac arteries. Annals of surgery 1974; 179: 763–772

Treatment of abdominal aortic aneurysms

James A. DeWeese MD, FACS
Professor and Chairman, Division of Cardiothoracic Surgery,
University of Rochester Medical Center, Rochester, New York, USA

Introduction

Aneurysmal degeneration of major arteries has attracted the attention of physicians for many centuries. The enlargement of some aneurysms with erosion of the chest wall or fistulization into the oesophagus, intestine, or cava dramatizes the lethal nature of the problem. The most common location of aneurysm is in the abdominal aorta beginning below the renal arteries and ending above the bifurcation. The common iliac and internal iliac vessels may also be aneurysmal but the external iliac is usually spared. Aneurysms infrequently involve the proximal abdominal aorta, being even less common here than in the descending thoracic region. Some patients have polyaneurysmal disease with additional involvement of the common femoral and popliteal arteries.

Operative procedures

Dubost is credited with initiating the modern era of management of abdominal aortic aneurysms when in 1951 he resected an aneurysm and replaced it with a homograft[1]. Within a few years significant experiences with resections of aneurysms were reported[2,3,4]. A variety of materials were evaluated but Dacron remains the graft of choice. Alternative methods for the treatment of abdominal aortic aneurysms such as ligation, wrapping or wiring have been abandoned. For the patient with very serious medical problems, ligation of the iliac arteries, thrombosis of the aneurysm and performance of an axillobifemoral graft can be considered[5].

Symptoms

Patients may have aneurysms of considerable size without symptoms. Some patients feel the aneurysm and report that their heart has dropped into the stomach. Others note pulsation when leaning against a firm object, such as a desk top. Some complain of postprandial fullness. Many aneurysms are first discovered on a routine physical examination or at the time of radiological examination for an unrelated problem. Unfortunately the first symptoms may precede frank rupture very closely. These symptoms are usually a deep aching and then sharp abdominal pain frequently radiating to and settling in the flank or back. Depending on the site of the largest retroperitoneal haematoma, the initial diagnosis may be appendicitis, cholecystitis, perforated ulcer, diverticulitis or renal colic. The presence of postural hypotension or shock supports the diagnosis of rupture.

Preoperative

Indications for operations

Patients with painful symptoms require immediate operation. Asymptomatic patients with proven aneurysms should have an elective operation unless they have significant medical contraindications. There has been an attempt to relate size of aneurysm to risk of rupture. Unfortunately, even small aneurysms may rupture[6]. The mortality rate for patients with ruptured aneurysms who reach the operating room is still 50 per cent in most hospitals. The mortality rate for patients undergoing elective resection is approximately 5 per cent[7]. Therefore, even though an aneurysm is less than 6 cm in diameter, the patient should be evaluated for a possible elective operation. Patients with historical or ECG evidence of coronary artery disease require the most careful evaluation. The postoperative mortality rates as a result of myocardial infarction is significantly higher in patients with known coronary artery disease (2 per cent versus 9 per cent)[8].

Preoperative evaluation

Prior to an elective operation it is advisable to obtain an intravenous pyelogram. It can provide information regarding the relationship of the aneurysm to the renal arteries, reveal a horseshoe kidney and provide baseline evaluation of renal anatomy and function. Ultrasonography may be of help in diagnosing or following the size of an aneurysm but has not been routinely useful to us in evaluating the extent of the aneurysm. Computerized axial tomography may be useful in determining the extent of the aneurysm. CAT and aortography, however, are reserved for patients with associated arterial occlusive disease or suspected suprarenal involvement on the basis of the presence of a palpably high aneurysm or widened descending thoracic aorta on a radiograph of the chest.

Preoperative preparation

Patients undergoing elective operation are hydrated with 1500–2000 ml of a balanced electrolyte solution during the 12 hours prior to surgery. Broad spectrum antibiotics are administered intravenously preoperatively and during the first 4 postoperative days. At least 4 units of whole blood should be available. Patients with ruptured aneurysms are cautiously transfused preoperatively to avoid hypertension and increased bleeding. After the patient has been anaesthetized, a nasogastric tube is inserted and the patient is kept on gastric suction until the bowel regains normal activity, usually 3–5 days. A urinary catheter is inserted for constant monitoring of urine flow during the first 48 hours after operation. The radial artery is cannulated for continuous monitoring of blood pressure and intermittent monitoring of blood gases. A central venous pressure line is inserted for constant monitoring of pressures for routine operations. The use of flow-directed, balloon-tipped catheters which allow measurement of both right and left heart pressures and the cardiac output is useful for monitoring high risk patients. Patients with ruptured aneurysms should have preoperative, intraoperative or postoperative placement of these monitoring devices.

Anaesthesia

General anaesthesia with an endotracheal tube is required. It is advisable to prepare and drape patients with ruptured aneurysms prior to induction of anaesthesia. Optimal management of the patient during the operation is dependent on close cooperation between the surgeon and anaesthesiologist. Myocardial depression occurs during anaesthesia and is then aggravated by aortic clamping[9]. Continuous monitoring of systemic arterial pressure, intracardiac pressures and cardiac output permit maintenance of optimal cardiac performance, particularly during the critical periods of clamping, declamping and blood loss. Preload can be increased by infusion of appropriate non-colloidal or colloidal fluids or reduced by appropriate diuretic or drug. Inotropic drugs may be used intelligently, particularly in combination with drugs which decrease after load. Clamping and declamping should be done slowly to allow appropriate pharmacological manipulations[10].

The operations

THE INFRARENAL ABDOMINAL AORTA

Except in the rarest of circumstances, the functional replacement of the abdominal aorta with a plastic graft is the operation of choice for treatment of an abdominal aortic aneurysm. It is not necessary to remove the aneurysm sac itself. Rather, the sac is opened longitudinally and the anastomoses performed from within by suturing the graft to the cuff found at the junction of the aneurysm and aorta. The aorta may or may not be partially or completely transected. This more simplified method of operative management has decreased dissection, blood loss and complications, and has been at least partially responsible for the decreased mortality rate for the operative management of abdominal aortic aneurysms. The operative mortality rates for elective operations now is approximately 5 per cent. On the other hand, mortality rates for patients urgently operated on for symptomatic but unruptured aneurysms is 12–20 per cent in most reported series[7,11].

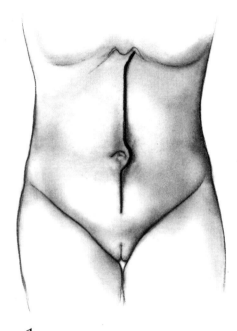

1

1

The incision (midline)

For most aneurysms a long midline incision is made. The supine patient is prepared and draped from the nipples to the midthigh. The incision begins at the base of and to the left of the xiphoid process. It is carried downward and around the umbilicus and ends at the symphysis pubis. Care is taken to make the incision exactly in the midline by following the decussations of the fibres of the rectus sheath.

An extraperitoneal approach should be considered in patients with a history of peritonitis or extensive intra-abdominal operations (see chapter on 'Aortoiliac reconstruction', pp. 136–151).

2

High proximal control of aorta

If the aneurysm extends to the renal arteries or if the aneurysm has ruptured, proximal control is best obtained above the level of the renal arteries. The transverse colon and stomach are retracted downward, the lesser omentum incised and the aorta exposed by bluntly separating the right and left crus of the diaphragm. A large vascular clamp is applied, taking care not to injure the coeliac artery. More immediate control can be obtained by compressing the aorta against the lumbar spine with a retractor. Alternatively a large balloon catheter can be introduced through an incision or tear in the aneurysm and positioned in the suprarenal aorta and distended.

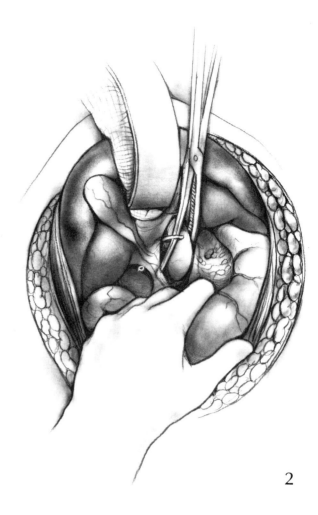

2

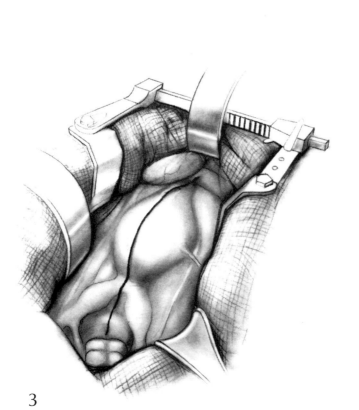

3

3

Exposure of aneurysm

The patient is hyperextended. The small intestine is mobilized superiorly and to the patient's right side and protected by moist pads or within a plastic bag. Moist pads and retractors are used to pack away the duodenum and large bowel. A self-retaining chest retractor with long blades is quite useful. The posterior peritoneum is incised beginning at the ligament of Treitz, carried distally to the right of the midline to avoid the mesenteric artery and vein, and over the sacral promontory in the midline.

4

Infrarenal control of aorta

The ligament of Treitz is incised superiorly to the pancreas, allowing separation of the duodenum from the mesenteric vein. The left renal vein is dissected away from the aorta and the left gonadal vein may be divided. A plane of dissection is established immediately adjacent to the adventitia of the aorta distal to the left renal artery. Using careful sharp and blunt dissection, the aorta is mobilized sufficiently to allow it to be lifted from the lumbar spine. Encircling it with a tape only increases the risk of bleeding from lumbar veins or arteries and is not necessary.

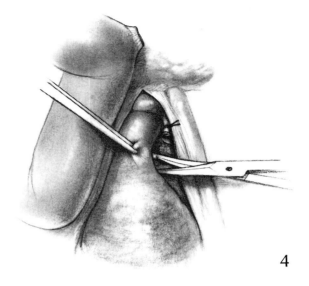

4

5

Ligation of inferior mesenteric artery

If the inferior mesenteric artery is immediately visible it is mobilized at its origin. A proximal and two distal ligatures are placed before dividing the artery. It is important that the ligatures do not occlude the first large left colic branch. If no pulsations can be felt in the sigmoid mesentery after ligation of the inferior mesenteric artery, if the vessel is unusually large or if the left colon appears ischaemic, the stump of the vessel should be carefully preserved and implanted into the side of the graft.

6

Clamping of aorta

The granular tissue over the iliac veins is incised and the ureter identified. Using sharp and blunt dissection, the artery and frequently adherent iliac veins are exposed but not separated.

Heparin sodium in 5000–7500 unit amounts is administered intravenously. After 1 minute the aorta and both iliac arteries are occluded with vascular clamps. It is not necessary to encircle the iliac arteries or aorta but it is important that the dissection be extensive enough to allow the vessels to be elevated and the posterior structures pinched by the approximated thumb and index finger.

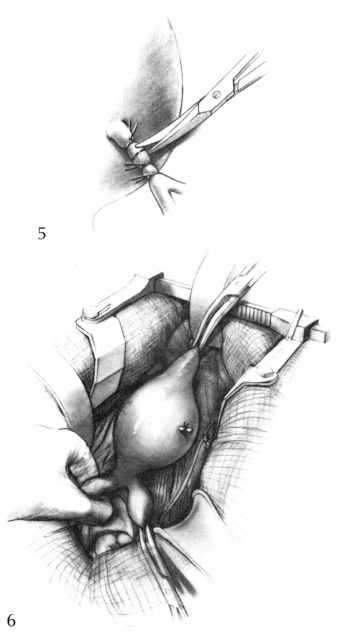

5

6

7

Aortotomy

It is helpful to establish the extent of the aortotomy by cauterizing the adventitia with a broad blade. The final incision will be midline and longitudinal over the bulk of the aneurysm. Superiorly, where the aorta becomes of more normal calibre, there will be a transverse 'T' extension of the incision to encompass 30–50 per cent of the circumference of the aorta. If the iliac arteries are aneurysmal or stenotic, the incision will extend longitudinally along the anterior surface. If the bifurcation of the aorta is relatively normal, a transverse 'T' extension is made at that level. A partial aortotomy is made and a plane of dissection is established either between media and intima or between the intima and old thrombus, which is almost always found within the aneurysm. When the lumen is entered, the remainder of the aortotomy is rapidly completed along the course of the cauterized aorta.

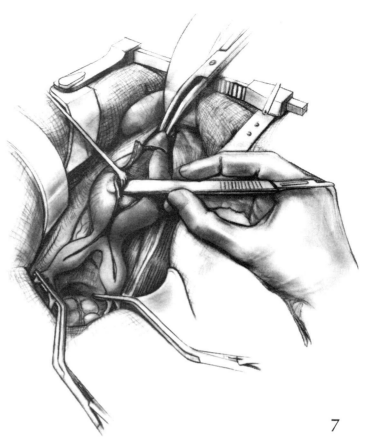

7

8

Removal of aneurysm contents and control of lumbar arteries

The thrombus and, if possible, the atherosclerotic intima are removed from within the aneurysm. Most of the lumbar arteries are usually thrombosed. Bleeding from the patent vessels is controlled with mattress or figure-of-eight stitches of 2/0 suture. Atherosclerotic plaques must be debrided away before attempting to suture these vessels. If the inferior mesenteric artery was not previously identified and is patent, it can also be controlled from within the aneurysm.

8

9

Proximal anastomosis – suturing posterior half

To avoid extensive mobilization of the aorta the posterior half of the proximal anastomosis can be performed from within the aneurysm. The body of the bifurcated woven graft is usually much longer than needed and must be cut before beginning the anastomosis. Usually a distinct ridge can be identified where the aorta becomes aneurysmal. A deep mattress stitch is placed through this ridge and carried through the midpoint of the posterior edge of the graft as an everting stitch, and the suture is tied. The posterior suture is then run around both sides of the graft as a continuous everting over-and-over stitch. It is important that each bite of the stitch be made through the entire thickness of the wall of the aorta.

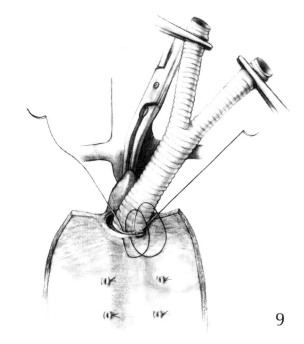

9

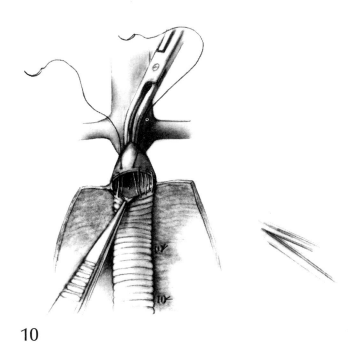

10

10

Proximal anastomosis – suturing anterior half

As the posterior stitch is carried anteriorly it is important to place the sutures under direct vision at the transition zone between the intact and incised aorta to avoid tearing the adventitia. In addition it is frequently necessary to remove calcified arteriosclerotic plaques in order to place stitches, which leaves a thin aortic wall for suturing. It then becomes very important to use smaller needles and stitches of equal depth in the aortic cuff to avoid tearing.

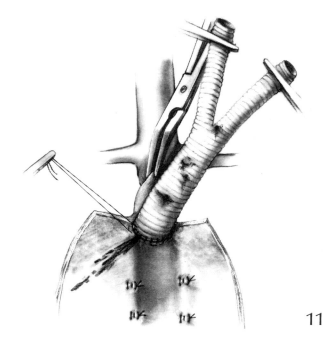

11

11

Testing the proximal anastomosis

Regardless of whether woven or preclotted knitted grafts are used, it is important to test the anastomosis and control bleeding through the graft interstices after completion of the proximal anastomosis. The limbs of the graft are occluded and the proximal clamps slowly released. Any significant bleeding between sutures is controlled with mattress stitches. The graft is then allowed to fill, the clamp occluded and the graft allowed to sit until there is no further bleeding through the interstices.

12

Distal aortic anastomosis

It is possible to use a tube graft and make the distal anastomosis just proximal to the bifurcation in about 66 per cent of the patients. The anterior wall of the aorta was divided with the original distal transverse 'T' incision. The posterior wall of the aorta is carefully inspected before cutting the bifurcated graft. Calcified arteriosclerotic plaques are debrided and a test stitch passed through the wall of the aorta to be sure that it will be possible to make an anastomosis at that level. The graft is then gently stretched and cut. It is important not to overstretch the graft, since it may be necessary later to elevate it if bleeding occurs from the posterior anastomotic suture line. The posterior part of the anastomosis is begun by placing a deep stitch through the ridge between normal and aneurysmal aorta. The suture is then passed from outside to the inside of the graft and continued as an over-and-over stitch around one-half the circumference of the graft. The original end of the suture is passed from inside to outside of the graft and continued as an over-and-over stitch to join the first suture, and the two ends are tied.

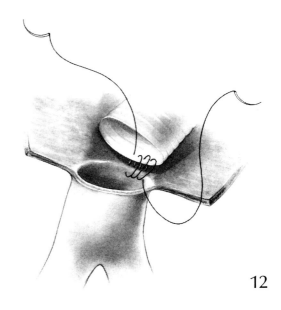

12

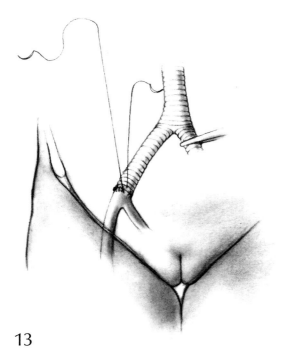

13

13

Anastomosis to the iliac artery

When the proximal iliac arteries are severely diseased, a bifurcation graft is used. One limb of the graft is occluded with a non-crushing vascular clamp. The opposite limb is then cut to the length necessary to reach the site of the distal anastomosis. A suction catheter is introduced into the limb and loose thrombi removed. It is preferable to make the anastomosis to the common iliac artery end-to-end if possible. If the common iliac is severely diseased and the external iliac artery soft-walled, the anastomosis should be made end-to-end to the external iliac artery. The internal iliac artery is divided and the distal end oversewn.

14

End-to-end anastomosis

With any end-to-end anastomosis it is advisable to pass the suture from inside to the outside of the diseased artery to tack loose intima. The suture is passed from outside the graft to inside of the graft at the end of the anastomosis opposite the surgeon. It is then run as an over-and-over stitch from inside the anastomosis. It is continued around the entire circumference of the artery and tied to the original suture. If there is a disparity in the size of the artery and graft it is helpful to place a stay suture through the midpoint of the circumference of both the artery and graft to assist in accurate approximation of the two ends.

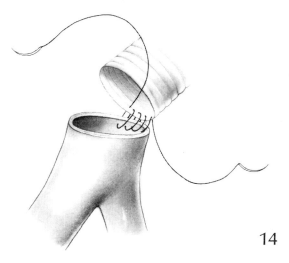

14

15

Preparation for distal anastomosis to common femoral artery

After completing the anastomosis of one limb of the graft, the distal clamp is removed, allowing retrograde filling of the graft. The clamp on the opposite limb is then removed and the limb with the completed anastomosis is occluded as the proximal clamp is removed to flush any debris from the graft. Flow is gradually restored to the leg with the completed anastomosis while carefully monitoring the blood pressure. Sudden drops in blood pressure can be expected unless the clamps are slowly and intermittently removed over a 5–10 minute period. If it is necessary to carry the craft to the groin, a clamp is passed from the groin incision over the femoral artery and retroperitoneally to the sacral promontory. The limb of the graft is carefully orientated and passed to the groin.

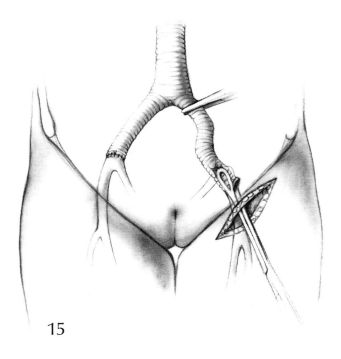

15

16

Oversewing common iliac artery

It is important carefully to oversew the common iliac artery since in the presence of a patent external iliac artery there will be abundant retrograde flow and systemic pressure in the stump of the divided common iliac artery. If there is calcified plaque in the common iliac artery a short endarterectomy is performed. Stay sutures are then placed in opposite sides of the artery about 1 cm from the cut end and tied. A continuous mattress stitch is made from the first stay suture to the other and the suture tied. One end of the tied suture is run as a continuous over-and-over stitch back to the first stay suture and tied.

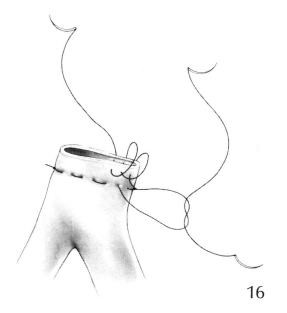

16

17

Distal anastomosis to common femoral artery

The common femoral artery is mobilized from the inguinal ligament to the profunda femoris artery. An end-to-side anastomosis is made to the occluded common femoral artery (*see* chapter on 'Aortoiliac reconstruction', pp.136–151). Backflow from the femoral artery is checked prior to completion of the anastomosis. If the backflow is unsatisfactory, a Fogarty thrombectomy catheter is passed distally and any thrombi removed (*see* chapter on 'Arterial embolectomy', pp. 201–206). Flow is also gradually re-established to this limb. Protamine sulphate is then administered intravenously in doses of 1 mg for each 100 units of heparin sodium given when the vessels were clamped.

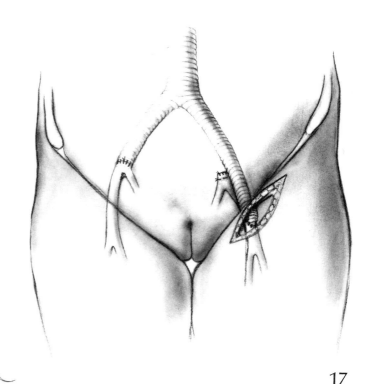

17

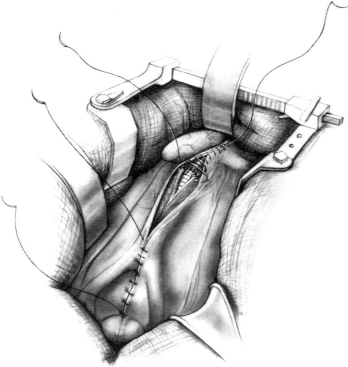

18

18

Closure of peritoneum and aortic wall

In order to avoid aortoenteric fistulae it is important to separate the graft and particularly the anastomoses from direct contact with the duodenum and jejunum. Bleeding from the cut edge of the aneurysm sac is first controlled with cautery and suture ligatures. A stay suture is placed at each end of the incision. The peritoneum and the edge of the aneurysm sac, where appropriate, are then approximated with a single-layer continuous stitch of 0 chromic catgut. As the superior peritoneal stitch reaches the level of the cut aneurysm sac, the tip of the edge of the sac is included in a stitch which is then passed through the adventitia of the aorta, the opposite tip of the edge of the sac and finally the peritoneum. The stitch is continued and tied to the inferior suture.

Suprarenal abdominal aortic aneurysms

Suprarenal aortic aneurysms usually involve the lower thoracic aorta as well but may be confined to the abdominal aorta. These dumb-bell shaped aneurysms may be suspected on the basis of a preoperative aortogram or CAT scan but on occasion are an unexpected finding at operation. If the infrarenal cuff of the aneurysm is narrow and the suprarenal component thick walled, it may be judicious to resect and replace only the infrarenal portion. The suprarenal aneurysm can then be carefully followed and resected through a thoracoabdominal approach if it becomes symptomatic.

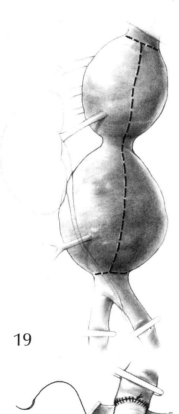

19

19

Exposure

The infradiaphragmatic suprarenal aneurysm may be resected through an extended abdominal incision. The left rectus muscle is divided in the epigastrium and the incision carried out through the 9th interspace. The left posterior gutter peritoneum is incised to enter the retroperitoneum. The spleen, stomach, pancreas, left colon and left kidney are retracted medially.

20

20

Insertion of graft

The aorta is clamped above and below the aneurysm. A longitudinal incision is made 3 cm posterior to the origin of the left renal artery. The clot is removed and any bleeding lumbar arteries are oversewn or included in the anastomosis of the aortic wall to the graft. The proximal aortic anastomosis is performed from the inside as previously described. The origins of two or more of the right renal, coeliac, superior mesenteric and left renal arteries may be close to one another in a relatively thick-walled portion of the aneurysm. The left renal artery is frequently 2–3 cm away. An elliptical button which is large enough to encircle adjacent origins of the arterial branches is cut out of the graft. Back bleeding from the branches may be controlled with balloon catheters if necessary.

21

Anastomosis of aortic wall to graft[12]

The posterior edge of the opening in the graft is sutured from inside the graft to the aorta posterior to the origins of the vessel. The continuous stitch is carried around the anterior edge of the graft opening anterior to the origins of the vessels. It is important to include all layers of the aortic wall in these sutures and to place the suture line close to the origin of the vessels without narrowing the orifices. In this way a minimal amount of the dilated weakened aorta is included in the anastomosis. When all of the anastomoses of the aortic wall to graft are completed the graft is flushed. The proximal aortic clamp is released and the graft clamped distal to the aortic wall anastomoses while the distal anastomosis to the infrarenal aorta is completed.

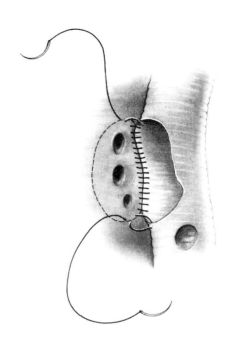

21

Special postoperative care

Monitoring

It is advisable to continue careful continuous monitoring of the patient for at least the first 24–48 hours postoperatively and longer if the patient is unstable. Intra-abdominal bleeding can be recognized by falling central venous, intracardiac or systemic arterial pressures, decreased urinary output and increased girth of the abdomen, which is recorded hourly with a tape measure. It is important to maintain systemic arterial pressures and central pressures within normal limits to prevent decreased cardiac output or left ventricular strain and thereby maintain myocardial oxygenation. In high risk patients endotracheal intubation and assisted respiration is continued for 18 hours to ensure adequate myocardial and cerebral oxygenation and prevent atelectasis. Urinary output is monitored carefully for the first 48 hours and assisted with diuretics or increased fluids as indicated from monitoring devices.

Pulmonary

Vigorous pulmonary therapy is instituted when the patient awakes from anaesthesia. Turning from side-to-side, 'cupping' the chest, deep breathing exercises and assisted coughing are all important. The incision is large and may be painful. Judicious use of narcotics and holding a firm object to the wound makes coughing easier. Early ambulation on the first or second postoperative day also assists the mechanics of respiration.

Paralytic Ileus

This follows nearly every abdominal aortic operation and should be treated by gastric aspiration with an indwelling tube until intestinal mobility has been re-established.

References

1. Dubost, C., Allary, M., Oeconomos, N. Resection of an aneurysm of the abdominal aorta. Archives of Surgery 1952; 64: 405–408

2. DeBakey, M. E., Crawford, E. S., Cooley, D. A., Morris, G. C., Jr, Royster, T. S., Abbott, W. P. Aneurysm of abdominal aorta. Analysis of results of graft replacement therapy one to eleven years after operation. Annals of Surgery 1964; 160: 622–639

3. Rob, C. G., Eastcott, H. H. G., Owen, K. The reconstruction of arteries. British Journal of Surgery 1956; 43: 449–466

4. Vasko, J. S., Spencer, F. C., Bahnson, H. T. Aneurysm of the aorta treated by excision. Review of 237 cases followed up to seven years. American Journal of Surgery 1963; 105: 793–801

5. Leather, R. P., Shah, D., Goldman, M., Rosenberg, M., Karmody, A. M. Nonresective treatment of abdominal aortic aneurysms: use of acute thrombosis and axillofemoral by-pass. Archives of Surgery 1979; 114: 1408–1409

6. Darling, R. C., Messina, C. R., Brewster, D. C., Ottinger, L. W. Autopsy study of unoperated abdominal aortic aneurysms. The case for early resection. Circulation 1977; 56 (Suppl. 2): II,–161–164

7. Hicks, G. L., Eastland, M. W., DeWeese, J. A., May, A. G., Rob, C. G. Survival improvement following aortic aneurysm resection. Annals of Surgery 1975; 181: 863–869

8. Hertzer, N. R. Fatal myocardial infarction following abdominal aortic aneurysm resection. Annals of Surgery 1980; 192: 667–673

9. Bush, H. L., LoGerfo, F. W., Weisel, R. D., Mannick, J. A., Hechtman, H. B. Assessment of myocardial performance and optimal volume loading during elective abdominal aortic aneurysm resection. Archives of Surgery 1977; 112: 1301–1306

10. Babu, S. C., Sharma, P. V. P., Raciti, A., et al. Monitor-guided responses. Operability with safety is increased in patients with peripheral vascular disease. Archives of Surgery 1980; 115: 1384–1386

11. McCabe, C. J., Coleman, W. S., Brewster, D. C. The advantage of early operation for abdominal aortic aneurysm. Archives of Surgery 1981; 116: 1025–1029

12. Crawford, E. S. Thoraco-abdominal and abdominal aortic aneurysms involving renal, superior mesenteric, and celiac arteries. Annals of Surgery 1974; 179: 763–772

Aortoiliac reconstruction: thromboendarterectomy, bypass graft

John J. Ricotta MD
Assistant Professor of Surgery, University of Rochester
School of Medicine and Dentistry, Rochester, New York, USA

James A. DeWeese MD, FACS
Professor and Chairman, Division of Cardiothoracic Surgery,
University of Rochester Medical Center, Rochester, New York, USA

Introduction

Occlusive disease of the aorta and iliac arteries is one of the most common problems encountered by the vascular surgeon. Patients may present with claudication involving the hips, thighs or calves. Occasionally patients will develop rest pain or frank tissue necrosis, most often when complete aortic occlusion has occurred. Operation is indicated to preserve ischaemic limbs, prevent tissue loss or improve symptoms of claudication. Mortality of aortoiliac reconstruction in good risk patients is less than 5 per cent, early relief of symptoms is found in 85–90 per cent of patients and good long-term (10 year) results are seen in 66–80 per cent of patients[1–7].

A variety of operative procedures has been developed to treat aortoiliac occlusions, including thromboendarterectomy, aortoiliac or aortofemoral bypass, and extra-anatomical bypass techniques. The first two procedures, thromboendarterectomy and aortic bypass grafts will be described in this chapter. Currently, bypass techniques are practised most frequently, endarterectomy usually being reserved for those patients with segmental lesions confined to the aorta and common iliac arteries. Direct comparisons of these two techniques is difficult since patient groups are usually not identical; however, reported results are good with both approaches. The results of several representative large series are presented in *Table 1*. The best results are achieved in those patients with claudication and a patent superficial femoral artery[6]. Late thromboses are often associated with progression of disease distal to the inguinal ligament.

Table 1 Results of aortoiliofemoral reconstructions

Authors	No. of patients			Early patency (%)		Late patency (5 Yr) (%)	
	Bypass	*Endarterectomy*	*Total*	*Bypass*	*Endarterectomy*	*Bypass*	*Endarterectomy*
Minken et al. (1965)[1]	119	92	211	80	91	87	83
Duncan, Linton and Darling (1971)[4]	102	240	342	91	93	~91	~87
Brewster and Darling (1978)[5]	341	241	582	98	98	90	87
Martinez, Hertzer and Bevan (1980)[7]	376	0	376	98	–	88	–
Crawford et al. (1981)[3]	not stated*	949	95	–	87	–	

*Vast majority of patients received bypass grafts

Thromboendarterectomy

Thromboendarterectomy was the earliest operation performed for treatment of aortoiliac occlusive disease. The technique of open endarterectomy was developed by Dos Santos[8] while the semiclosed procedure was refined by Cannon, Kawakami and Barker[9]. Although thromboendarterectomy has the advantage of avoiding prosthetic material the dissection is more time consuming than that required for bypass grafting and the more extensive dissection may be associated with increased blood loss. Disturbances in sexual function in males may attend dissection of the anatomical plexus at the aortic bifurcation[10]. Currently, thromboendarterectomy is reserved for those patients with localized occlusions of the aorta and common iliac arteries. If disease extends into the extenal iliac arteries, which is often the case, bypass grafting is preferred. In cases of aortic hypoplasia, bypass is preferred over endarterectomy. Endarterectomy may occasionally be used in re-establishing arterial continuity in a contaminated field or in the presence of an established graft infection[11]. The aorta and iliac vessels may be approached through a transabdominal or retroperitoneal approach. The retroperitoneal approach will be described here and has the advantage of lower morbidity and a shortened convalescence[12]. However, with the standard retroperitoneal approach, exposure of the aorta and iliac arteries is somewhat limited. This is satisfactory for thromboendarterectomy but more extensive exposure is usually needed for placement of a bypass graft. Aortofemoral bypasses are best performed through a transabdominal approach or an extended retroperitoneal exposure, both of which will be described later.

STANDARD RETROPERITONEAL APPROACH

Position of patient

The patient is positioned with the left side slightly elevated (30–45°). This is achieved by use of a rolled sheet or a sandbag placed under the left flank. Breaking the table in the 'jack-knife' position will give additional exposure.

1 & 2

The incision

The incision is begun 5–8 cm (2–3 inches) below the umbilicus at the midline and extends superiorly and laterally to the tip of the 12th rib. The anterior rectus sheath is incised and the rectus muscle is retracted medially or occasionally partially transected for additional exposure. The external oblique, internal oblique and transversus abdominus muscles are incised along the line of incision.

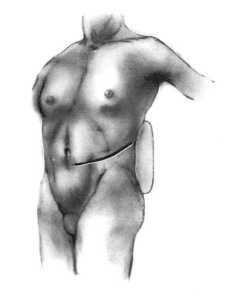

1

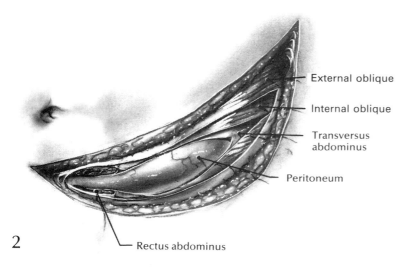

External oblique

Internal oblique

Transversus abdominus

Peritoneum

Rectus abdominus

2

3

Exposure of the aorta and iliac vessels

The retroperitoneal space is entered and the peritoneum and its contents are displaced medially using a gauze pack. As in lumbar sympathectomy, the retroperitoneal fat is left posteriorly and care is taken to keep the plane of dissection above the psoas major muscle. The ureter is displaced medially with the peritoneum. In this way, the aorta and iliac vessels are visualized. Additional exposure is gained by dividing the inferior mesenteric artery. From this point on, the procedure is identical to the transperitoneal approach.

At the conclusion of the operation, the muscle layers are individually reapproximated using running absorbable suture. The rectus sheath is closed with interrupted suture, and the skin is closed in the usual fashion.

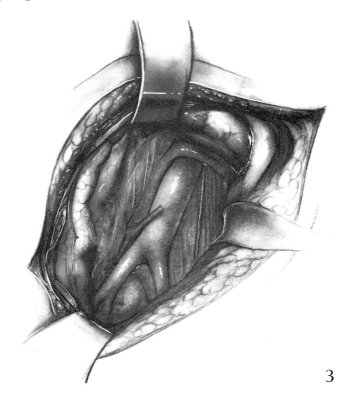

3

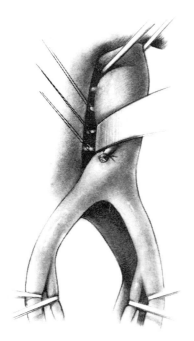

4

4

Mobilization of the aorta and iliac vessels

Completion of thromboendarterectomy requires extensive mobilization of the aorta and iliac arteries including their tributaries. Mobilization should extend 2–3 cm proximal and distal to the known area of disease and may include the distal abdominal aorta, common external and internal iliac arteries, middle sacral and lumbar arteries. The smaller arteries can be controlled by Pott's ties or small bulldog clamps.

5

Arterial incision

A longitudinal incision is made throughout the length of the proposed thromboendarterectomy. The incision is carried into the vessel lumen. For most endarterectomies two incisions are required as shown. The incision should be carried beyond the plaque to be removed so that the distal intima can be inspected. The preaortic autonomic plexus which lies on the left side of the aortic bifurcation is easily damaged at this point. Every effort should be made to spare as many of these nerve fibres as possible to preserve normal sexual function in the male.

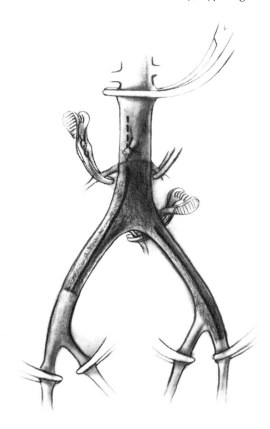

5

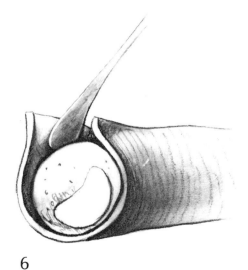

6

6

Thromboendarterectomy

The plane of cleavage is identified just deep to the intima. This plane is developed using a clamp or endarterectomy spatula. The dissection is carried circumferentially throughout the diseased segment. The inner core is divided proximally and distally with scissors and the plaque is removed. Endarterectomy may be facilitated by dividing the plaque proximally early in the procedure to aid in developing the cleavage plane.

7

Treatment of the distal intima

This is the critical step in the operative procedure. Endarterectomy should be ended distally where the plaque becomes attenuated. This is usually just distal to the aortic or common iliac bifurcation. The intima is usually most adherent at these levels. The intima should be cut flush so that no loose flaps remain.

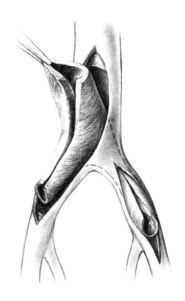

7

8

Securing the intima

Following transection of the intima, it is inspected closely and the area irrigated with heparinized saline solution. If the intima is loose at its distal cut margin, it should be anchored to the vessel with a series of interrupted mattress sutures tied outside the vessel. After inspecting the distal operative site, the entire endarterectomy is flushed with heparinized saline to remove any loose debris and thrombus.

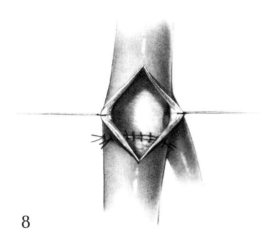

8

9

Closure of the arteriotomy

The arteriotomies are then closed with running 4/0 or 5/0 Prolene suture. Before tying down the suture line clamps are momentarily released proximally and then distally to flush out debris and thrombus. The suture line is then secured and the distal clamp is released to test the arterial closure for leakage. Any leakage points are repaired with interrupted 5/0 suture. If only slight bleeding occurs when the clamps are removed it can usually be controlled with a gauze pack and pressure. Use of liquid thrombin or microcrystalline collagen may also be helpful in these cases.

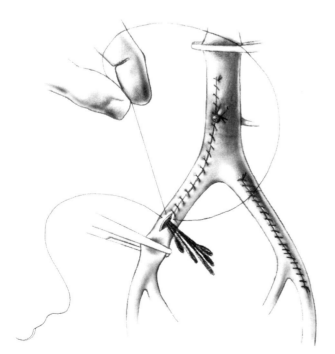

9

10

Patching the arteriotomy

If the endarterectomized artery is felt to be small, the lumen can be enlarged by closing the arteriotomy with a Dacron patch. A single elliptical patch is used for the aorta, or two separate patches may be required if it is desirable to extend into both iliacs. Woven Dacron is our preferred material although polytetrafluorethylene may also be used. The ends of the patch should be squared off so that the artery is noticeably widened after the patch is completed.

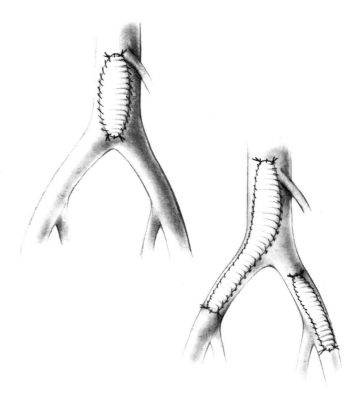

10

11

Eversion endarterectomy

The two common alternatives to open endarterectomy are eversion endarterectomy and the semiclosed endarterectomy using loop strippers. With eversion endarterectomy, the vessel is completely transected and rolled back on itself. Stay sutures are used on the vessel to facilitate traction. The inner core is then removed under direct vision. Following this the ends of the vessel are reanastomosed using continuous 5/0 Prolene suture. This technique is useful in the proximal internal iliac or superficial femoral arteries for relatively short occlusions. It has been combined with standard aortofemoral endarterectomy by Inahara to treat extensive aortoiliac disease[13].

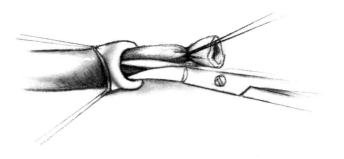

11

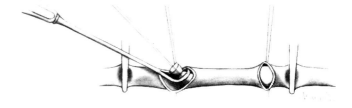

12

12–15

Semiclosed method of endarterectomy

The semiclosed method of endarterectomy involves use of a ring stripper under direct vision and passed blindly throughout the diseased segment[9]. The artery is exposed and mobilized proximal and distal to the diseased area. Transverse incisions extending two-thirds of the circumference of the vessel are made to allow introduction of the ring stripper under direct vision. The endarterectomy plane is established and the distal inner core is transected. This is transfixed with traction stitches which are then passed through the ring of the stripper. Traction is applied to the inner core and the stripper is advanced proximally. For long occlusions, multiple arteriotomies may be required. When the proximal limit of the endarterectomy is reached, the intima is again carefully divided so that a flap is avoided. The specimen is removed by traction through the distal incision. The endarterectomized segment is flushed with heparinized saline to remove loose fragments and the arteriotomies are closed using running 5/0 Prolene suture. This technique is particularly applicable in the external iliac and superficial femoral arteries. It may also be combined with proximal endarterectomy for extensive aortoiliac lesions.

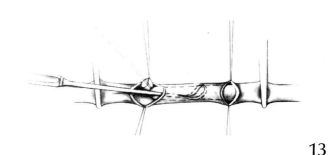

13

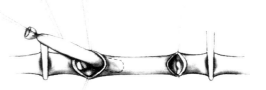

14

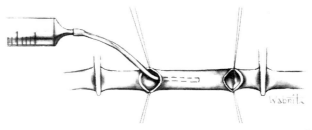

15

Aortoiliac and aortofemoral bypass graft

This is the most common type of reconstruction for aortoiliac occlusive disease. A wide variety of graft materials is used, but our preference is knitted or woven Dacron. The distal anastomosis may be carried to the common iliac, external iliac or femoral arteries. There is some evidence that in occlusive disease aortofemoral bypass is to be preferred over aortoiliac bypass as a more durable operation[14].

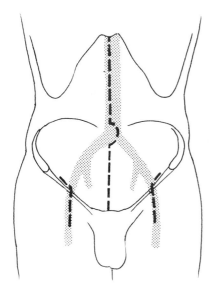

16

16

The incision

The transabdominal approach is most commonly used for bypass grafting. The incision we prefer is a long midline extending from xiphoid to pubis although a left paramedian and even a transverse incision are employed by some surgeons. When the graft is to be carried to the femoral arteries, these are exposed by a longitudinal incision beginning above the level of the inguinal ligament and extending down over the femoral artery low enough to expose the common femoral bifurcation. Additional proximal exposure of the distal external iliac artery can be gained by curving the incision laterally parallel to the inguinal ligament. The ligament can be retracted superiorly and the artery exposed, often without transecting the ligament.

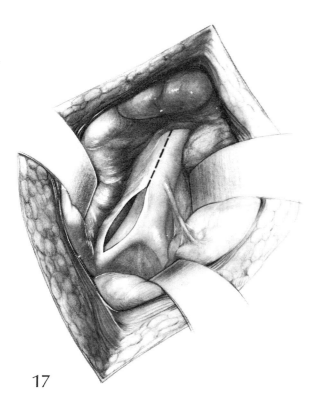

17

17

Exposure of the abdominal aorta

The retroperitoneum is entered by incising the retroperitoneal attachments of the duodenum and retracting this structure to the right of the midline. The lymphatics overlying the aorta are divided between ligatures or clips. The preaortic tissues are divided until the left renal vein is visualized. This usually marks the upper limits of the aortic dissection. During the proximal aortic dissection, care should be taken to identify the inferior mesenteric vein which is usually to the left of the midline. This is preserved and retracted laterally with the mesentery. The infrarenal aorta is dissected free from the vena cava and surrounding tissues and encircled with a tape. Usually 2–3 cm of aorta need to be dissected for the proximal anastamosis to be performed. One or more pairs of lumbar arteries may be sacrificed at this point. When obtaining proximal control of the aorta, care must be taken to avoid injury to the vena cava or lumbar veins.

18

Mobilization of the renal vein

In especially high lesions additional exposure can be gained by mobilizing the left renal vein and retracting it superiorly. Occasionally the vein may need to be divided, although this is unusual when operating for occlusive disease. If this is necessary, the left renal vein should be divided close to the vena cava and the cut end oversewn with running Prolene suture.

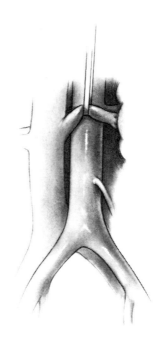

18

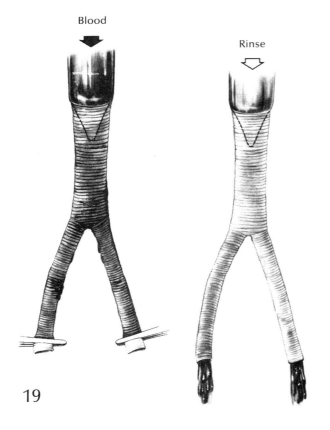

19

19

Clotting the graft

After control of the aorta is obtained, the prosthetic graft must be preclotted prior to implantation. This step is always necessary when a knitted Dacron graft is used, although it is not as important when the less porous woven grafts are employed. Preclotting serves two purposes: to seal the graft effectively against leakage and to provide a smooth fibrin lining at the blood-graft interface.

Prior to systemic heparinization 100 ml of fresh blood are withdrawn from the aorta or vena cava and placed in a basin. An appropriately sized graft is selected for use. The graft should be isodiametric or slightly smaller than the artery for aortic reconstruction. One end of the graft is clamped and fresh blood is forced through the graft using a catheter-tipped or bulb syringe. This procedure is continued until leakage through the prosthesis is minimal. The prosthesis is then flushed with heparinized saline to remove any loose debris.

20

Making the tunnel

Following removal of blood for clotting the retroperitoneal tunnel is made using blunt dissection. Tunnelling is accomplished using finger dissection from the abdominal and femoral incisions. The tunnel begins in the abdomen behind the ureter and directly over the iliac artery. In the groin, the plane is found immediately over the femoral artery. Tunnelling is completed bluntly and a long vascular clamp is guided through the tunnel from below upwards. A Dacron tape is left in the tunnel. The patient is then anticoagulated with intravenous heparin (100–150 u/kg). The arteries are clamped distally first to avoid embolization, and the prosthesis is inserted. At this point, the inside of the prosthesis is inspected and any loose fibrin or clot is removed using forceps or flushing techniques. After completion of the proximal anastomoses, the graft will be filled with blood to test for leakage and then flushed with blood to remove debris prior to performing the distal anastomosis.

Proximal anastomosis

The proximal anastomosis may be end-to-end or end-to-side. There is evidence to suggest that proximal end-to-end anastomosis gives a slightly better long-term patency and this is our preferred technique. When there is extensive aortic calcification, end-to-end anastomosis is preferred since this allows more accurate removal of any loose plaque that results from clamping.

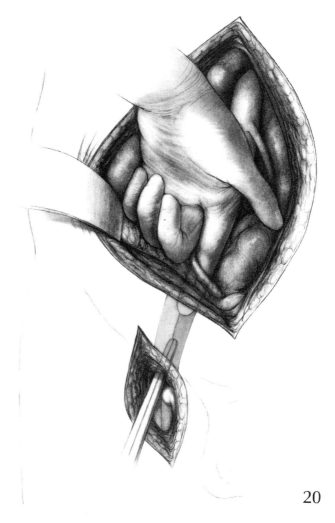

20

End-to-end technique

21a & b

The aorta is clamped proximal and distal to the area proposed for anastomosis and the aorta is transected. The distal end of the aorta is oversewn with a double layer of 3/0 or 4/0 Prolene. A preclotted graft of appropriate size is then anastomosed to the cut end of the aorta using a running 3/0 or 4/0 Prolene suture. The anastomosis is begun on the posterior wall of the aorta with a mattress suture which is tied. The two ends of the suture are then continued around posteriorly and anteriorly to complete the suture line.

Alternative techniques include placing two equidistant sutures to bisect the anastomosis or using interrupted mattress sutures for the posterior aortic wall or the entire circumference of the anastomosis. While these methods have their advocates, we have not found them particularly advantageous in the usual aortic reconstruction.

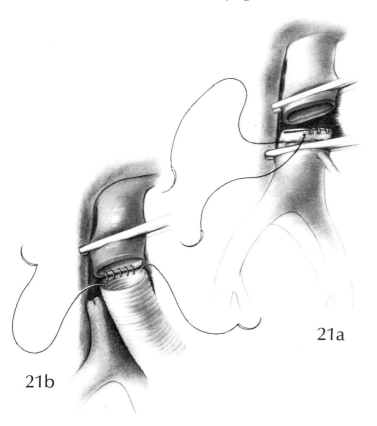

21a

21b

22

Testing the proximal suture line

At this point, the limbs of the aortic graft are clamped and the aortic clamp briefly removed to allow the graft to fill with blood. Following this, the graft is reclamped close to the suture line and the aortic clamp again released to test anastomotic integrity. Bleeding from needle holes is usually controlled with pressure. However, any large leaks are best repaired with interrupted sutures at this point. Once the suture line is secure, a cuff of graft may be placed over the limbs of the bifurcation graft and brought proximally to cover the anastomosis. This is particularly helpful when the aortic cuff is friable, and has been used routinely by some surgeons with the hope of decreasing aortoenteric fistulae.

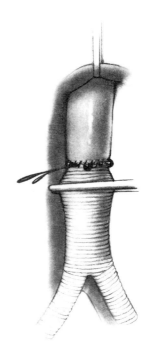

22

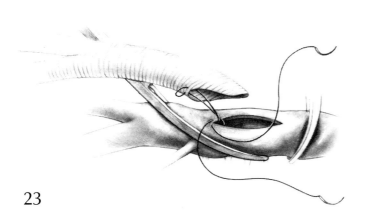

23

23

End-to-side technique

End-to-side anastomosis is preferred in patients with a small aorta. It may also be used in patients where the aortic segment to be used is soft and disease free. The exposure of the aorta is identical to that already described. A side-biting partial occlusion clamp may be used; however, two aortic occlusion clamps are preferred since this allows better exposure of the arteriotomy. The upper clamp is applied in the standard fashion above the level of anastomosis. The lower clamp is applied from below in the axis of the aorta to occlude the lumbar vessels as well as the distal aorta. End-to-side anastomosis does not require mobilization of the posterior aortic wall. An elliptical incision is cut in the graft and the suture is begun at the distal aorta and the 'heel' of the graft. This is begun as a mattress suture which is tied and then carried up each side. One suture is carried around the apex of the graft so that this critical area can be completed under direct vision. Suturing should always proceed from inside out on the artery to avoid raising a flap of intima. When the anastomosis is complete, it is tested as described for the end-to-end anastomosis.

Distal anastomosis

24

The distal anastomosis may be performed to the common iliac, external iliac or common femoral artery. While there are some advantages to avoiding an anastomosis in the groin (lower incidence of wound problems and avoiding an area of flexion), the long-term patency of aortofemoral grafts may be superior to that of aortoiliac grafts when performed for occlusive disease[14]. For this reason the distal anastomosis is usually carried to the common femoral artery. Since progressive disease is frequent in the superficial and common femoral arteries, we feel it is important to bring the femoral anastomosis low on the common femoral artery over the orifice of the profunda femoris. A long vascular clamp is pulled through the tunnel with the umbilical tape previously placed. Each limb of the graft is grasped and pulled down into the groin, care being taken not to twist it. The distal end of the graft is carefully bevelled for the distal anastomosis. The graft should be cut in an 'S' shape with heavy scissors. The distal end should be tailored to accommodate the distal arteriotomy. The distal anastomosis can then be performed.

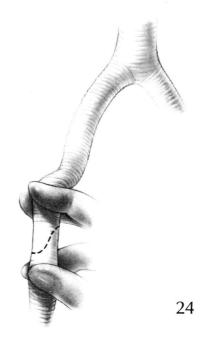

24

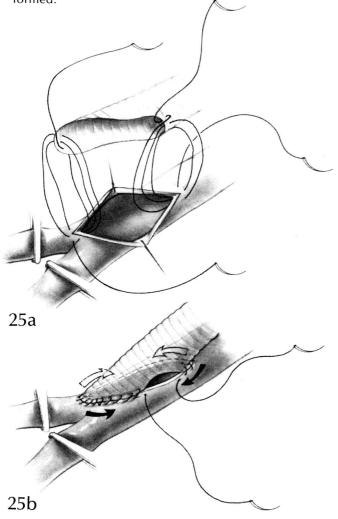

25a

25b

25a & b

Technique of distal anastomosis

The technique of distal anastomosis is the same in the iliac and femoral arteries. A segment of artery is isolated between clamps and a longitudinal arteriotomy made. In the femoral artery the origins of the superficial and deep femoral arteries are dissected free and these arteries are clamped. As stated above, the incision should extend down to the common femoral bifurcation so that the profunda orifice is visualized. If the superficial femoral artery is occluded or there is disease at the profunda orifice, the arteriotomy can be extended down the profunda femoris and the distal anastomosis can be extended as a tongue over the deep femoral artery, forming a profundoplasty. The anastomosis is begun by placing double-ended 5/0 or 6/0 Prolene sutures at each corner of the graft. These are carried from the inside to the outside of the artery. With the graft suspended, three or four sutures are placed at each corner under direct vision. The sutures are then drawn taught, the graft brought down to the artery, and the anastomosis completed by running sutures placed toward the middle of the suture line from each apex. This technique permits optimal visualization of the corner stitches which is important to avoid compromising both inflow and outflow. In an alternative technique, a mattress suture is placed at the heel of the graft and then run around the top of the graft under direct vision.

26

Flushing the graft

Flushing the graft is an important procedure prior to completion of the anastomosis. A routine technique for graft flushing includes: antegrade flushing down each limb of the graft prior to completion of each anastomosis and retrograde flushing of any clot or debris from the distal arterial tree combined with the use of the Fogarty embolectomy catheter, if necessary, to retrieve any distal thrombus. Upon completion of one anastomosis, the graft is flushed and an occluding clamp is placed on the free limb of the graft just distal to its bifurcation. Flow is restored gradually to the opposite limb. The patient should be closely monitored for drop in blood pressure during unclamping, and if this occurs, the limb should be reclamped. Under conditions of prolonged ischaemia, acidosis may develop in the legs and systemic acidosis may result with reperfusion. If this is anticipated, sodium bicarbonate should be administered prior to unclamping.

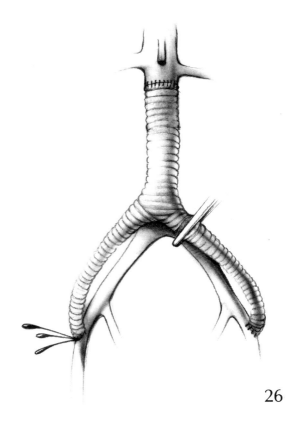

26

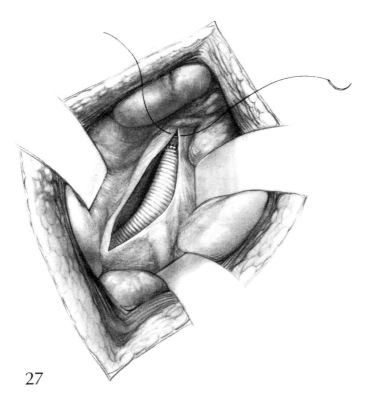

27

Closure

27

Following insertion of the graft, the retroperitoneum is closed. The purpose is to separate the intestine, especially the duodenum, from contact with the aortic prosthesis. The retroperitoneal incision is approximated with a running absorbable suture. A double-layer closure has been suggested to separate more effectively the aorta from the abdominal viscera[14]. Every attempt is made to leave the mobilized duodenum free rather than to reattach it to its retroperitoneal position. If necessary, an omental pedicle may be placed between the aorta and the bowel to provide further coverage.

The groin wounds are closed meticulously in layers. At least two subcutaneous layers are employed. Haemostasis and avoidance of lymphatic leaks are of utmost importance in prevention of wound complications. Subcuticular closure of the skin avoids transcutaneous sutures in the groin.

28

Reimplantation of the inferior mesenteric artery

In most patients, the inferior mesenteric artery can be sacrificed with impunity but in a small number collateral circulation is inadequate. A large 'meandering artery' seen on preoperative arteriography may help to identify these patients. Larger arteries ($\geq$ 5mm), especially those without backbleeding, are more likely to require reimplantation. If reimplantation is necessary, a button of aortic wall with the inferior mesenteric artery at its centre is excised and sewn onto the side of the graft. At operation, the inferior mesenteric artery may be tested by temporary occlusion. During this time, the colour of the intestine is observed and Doppler flow can be studied in the inferior mesenteric artery and along the antimesenteric border of the intestine[16].

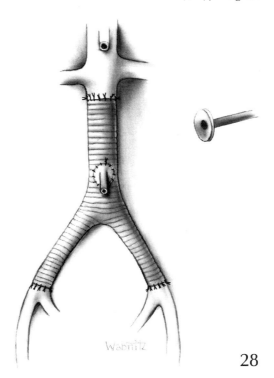

28

EXTENDED RETROPERITONEAL APPROACH TO THE AORTA

29

Occasionally atherosclerotic lesions may involve the aorta at or above the level of the renal arteries. In these instances, the suprarenal aorta must be controlled. This is possible using an extended extraperitoneal approach[17]. The patient is placed in the left lateral thoractomy position and his shoulders are secured with wide tape. The hips are left free and rotated as much as possible so that they are parallel with the operating table. The table is moved to a jack-knife position to extend the flank exposure. The surgeon stands at the patient's back and the table can be rotated toward or away from the operator to facilitate exposure. With the hips rotated and free, easy access to the groin is possible. Use of an orthopaedic 'bean bag' to stabilize the patient after positioning is quite helpful. The incision is made 2–3 cm below the umbilicus, beginning at the lateral border of the rectus abdominus and extending upward between the 11th and 12th ribs. In most cases, a rib need not be removed. Care must be taken to avoid entering the pleura at the superior portion of the incision. The oblique and transverse abdominal muscles are divided in line with the incision and the retroperitoneal space is entered. The peritoneum is bluntly dissected anteriorly as described earlier (see 'Thromboendarterectomy'), and the aorta is visualized. The plane of dissection is posterior to the left kidney.

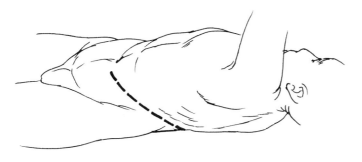

29

30

Dissection of the aorta

Dissection of the aorta begins along the vertebral column and continues posteriorly. The most important landmark is the left renal artery which should be identified early. The aortic dissection should proceed posterior to this vessel. Lymphatics and lumbar vessels are ligated in continuity as necessary with 3/0 silk ligatures. Dissection can be carried up to the diaphragm and if necessary to the lower thoracic aorta by dividing some of the diaphragmatic crus. This allows the aorta to be clamped in a disease-free area. No attempt should be made to dissect the aorta circumferentially from this approach since this could result in troublesome venous bleeding. The vessel is mobilized enough to allow placement of a larger vascular clamp above the level of disease and below the renal arteries.

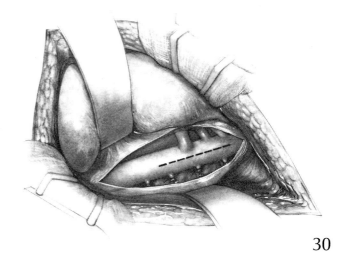

30

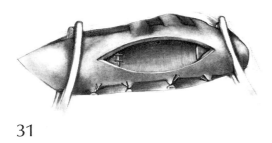

31

31

Endarterectomy of the suprarenal abdominal aorta

The aorta is incised posterior to the renal artery. An endarterectomy plane is established at this point. Backbleeding from the renal and superior mesenteric and iliac arteries is controlled with Fogarty balloon catheters. If necessary, endarterectomy of the renal and visceral arteries may be carried out at this point. After the aortic segment has been endarterectomized, the repair proceeds in one of two ways. If the distal aorta is normal, the arteriotomy may be closed with 5/0 Prolene after the distal intima has been secured to avoid dissection.

32

Endarterectomy with aortofemoral bypass

When there is extensive aortoiliac disease this procedure may be combined with standard aortofemoral bypass. The endarterectomy is extended into the proximal cuff of the infrarenal aorta (without extending the arteriotomy) which is then transected 2–3 cm below the renal arteries. The aortotomy is closed with a running 5/0 Prolene suture and the transected endarterectomized aorta is reclamped below the renal arteries. Following this, a standard end-to-end aortofemoral graft is placed. Once again, however, 4/0 or 5/0 Prolene on a fine needle is used for the proximal suture line. Fine sutures and use of felt pledgets to buttress the aortic closure diminish bleeding problems. The aorta is usually clamped above the renal arteries for no more than 30–45 minutes, and this is tolerated without ill effects in most patients. Following completion of the reconstruction, the wound is closed in layers. If the pleura has been entered, it is closed around a 20 Fr red rubber catheter which is then removed. The muscle layers are then closed individually using running No. 0 or No. 1 absorbable suture. Scarpa's fascia is closed with a 3/0 running suture and the skin is approximated in the usual fashion.

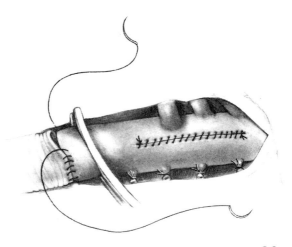

32

Complications

Vasculogenic impotence

Much attention has been directed recently to pelvic ischaemia as a contributing factor to impotence[18]. This has re-emphasized the importance of good blood supply to the hypogastric arteries. If there is history of difficulty with attaining or maintaining an erection coupled with evidence of occlusive disease of the common or internal iliac arteries, the diagnosis of vasculogenic impotence should be entertained. While impotence by itself is a controversial indication for arterial reconstruction, when this condition exists in a patient undergoing aortoiliac reconstruction for other reasons, attention should be given to improving hypogastric blood supply. This can be achieved by endarterectomy of the common or internal iliac arteries using techniques previously described or by adding a side-to-side anastomisis at the level of the common iliac bifurcation when performing an aortofemoral bypass. As mentioned previously, attention to the preaortic anatomical plexus will help prevent retrograde ejaculation.

Postoperative care

Most patients undergoing aortic surgery are monitored in the intensive care unit during the early postoperative period. Attention should be directed toward supporting intravascular volume, diagnosis of bleeding and maintenance of optimal cardiac function. Use of intra-arterial lines, measurements of central venous and pulmonary wedge pressure as well as cardiac output have greatly facilitated this. These measures combined with use of vasoactive drugs, including afterload reduction, have significantly decreased operative mortality and allow us safely to extend indications for surgery in these patients.

References

1. Minken, S. L., DeWeese, J. A., Southgate, W. A., Mahoney, E. B., Rob, C. G. Aortoiliac reconstruction for atherosclerotic occlusive disease. Surgery, Gynecology and Obstetrics 1968; 126: 1056–1060

2. Malone, J. M., Moore, W. S., Goldstone, J. The natural history of bilateral aortofemoral bypass grafts for ischemia of the lower extremities. Archives of Surgery 1975; 110: 1300–1306

3. Crawford, E. S., Bomberger, R. A., Glaeser, D. H., Saleh, S. A., Russell, W. L. Aortoiliac occlusive disease: Factors influencing survival and function following reconstruction operation over a 25-year period. Surgery 1981; 90: 1055–1067

4. Duncan, W. C., Linton, R. R., Darling, R. C. Aortoiliofemoral atherosclerotic occlusive disease: Comparative results of endarterectomy and Dacron bypass grafts. Surgery 1971; 70: 974–984

5. Brewster, D. C., Darling, R. C. Optimal methods of aortoiliac reconstruction. Surgery 1978; 84: 739–748

6. Sumner, D. S., Strandness, D. E. Aortoiliac reconstruction in patients with combined iliac and superficial femoral arterial occlusion. Surgery 1978; 84: 348–355

7. Martinez, B. D., Hertzer, N. R., Bevan, E. G. Influence of distal arterial occlusive disease on prognosis following aorto-bifemoral bypass. Surgery 1980; 88: 795–805

8. dos Santos, J. C. Sur la désobstruction des thromboses arterielles anciennes. Mémoires de l'Académie de chirugie 1947; 73: 409–411

9. Cannon, J. A., Kawakami, I. G., Barker, W. F. The present status of aortoiliac endarterectomy for obliterative atherosclerosis. Archives of Surgery 1961; 82: 813–825

10. May, A. G., DeWeese, J. A., Rob, C. G. Changes in sexual function following operation on the abdominal aorta. Surgery 1969; 65: 41–47

11. Ehrenfeld, W. K., Wilbur, B. G., Olcott, C. N., Stoney, R. J. Autogenous tissue reconstruction in the management of infected prosthetic grafts. Surgery 1979; 85: 82–92

12. Rob, C. G. Extraperitoneal approach to the abdominal aorta. Surgery 1963; 53: 87–89

13. Inahara, T. Eversion endarterectomy for aortoiliofemoral occlusive disease: a 16 year experience. American Journal of Surgery 1979; 138: 196

14. Moore, W. S., Cafferata, H. T., Hall, A. D., Blaisdell, F. W. In defense of grafts across the inguinal ligament: an evaluation of early and late results of aorto-femoral bypass grafts. Annals of Surgery 1968; 168: 207–214

15. DeWeese, M. S., Fry, W. J. Small bowel erosion following aortic resection. Journal of the American Medical Association 1962; 179: 882–886

16. Hobson, R. W., II, Wright, C. B., O'Donnell, J. A., Zamil, Z., Lamberth, W. C., Najem, Z. Determination of intestinal viability by doppler ultrasound. Archives of Surgery 1979; 114: 165–168

17. Ricotta, J. J., Williams, G. M. Endarterectomy of the upper abdominal aorta and visceral arteries through an extraperitoneal approach. Annals of Surgery 1980; 192: 633–638

18. Queral, L. A., Whitehouse, W. M., Flinn, W. R., Zarins, C. K., Bergan, J. J., Yao, J. S. T. Pelvic hemodynamics after aorto-iliac reconstruction. Surgery 1979; 86: 799–809

Illustrations by Carol Pienta

Reconstruction of the mesenteric and coeliac arteries

Nicholas Ogburn MD
Instructor in Surgery, East Carolina University School of Medicine, Greenville, North Carolina, USA

Walter J. Pories MD, FACS
Professor and Chairman, Department of Surgery, East Carolina University
School of Medicine, Greenville, North Carolina, USA

Introduction

Ischaemia of the viscera may present acutely or as a chronic process. Acute ischaemia is usually due to arterial obstruction from emboli or thrombosis, but may develop in the presence of patent vessels during cardiac failure[1,2].

1a & b

Acute intestinal ischaemia, especially of the colon, is also a preventable complication of surgery and has been reported as a consequence of (a) division of a dominant inferior mesenteric artery during the resection of an aortic abdominal aneurysm, or (b) injury to the artery of Drummond during resection of the colon in a patient with a blocked or previously ligated inferior mesenteric artery[3,4].

Chronic symptoms usually result from arterial stenosis or occlusion caused by aneurysm formation, atherosclerosis, arteritis, retroperitoneal fibrosis and external compression.

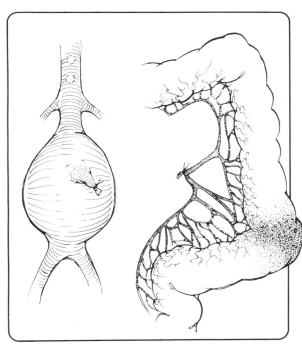

1a

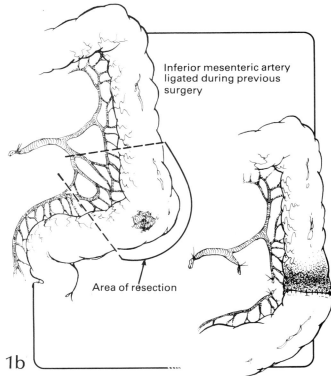

Inferior mesenteric artery
ligated during previous
surgery

Area of resection

1b

ACUTE SUPERIOR MESENTERIC ARTERY OCCLUSION

Acute intestinal ischaemia is associated with a high mortality rate (65–80 per cent) because of the following factors:

1. Difficulty in making the diagnosis before intestinal gangrene is present.
2. Difficulty in distinguishing superior mesenteric artery occlusion from low flow states.
3. Progression of bowel gangrene despite definitive therapy.
4. The poor condition of these patients.

Patients with abdominal pain at risk of a superior mesenteric artery embolus should undergo immediate arteriography of the abdominal aorta and mesenteric vessels. Angiography is extremely important. It is used to differentiate occlusive and non-occlusive ischaemia; to determine the site of the embolus or emboli and the

degree of mesenteric occlusion; to serve as a method of intra-arterial infusion of vasodilators and thrombolytic agents; to evaluate the distal vascular flow; to identify and select patients who might be treated better without an operation (i.e. those with low flow states); and to evaluate the results of therapy.

Risk factors for superior mesenteric artery emboli include significant cardiac disease, particularly recent myocardial infarction or arrhythmias and a history of previous embolic episodes. The source of emboli should be sought without delay and promptly treated[2,3].

Acute thrombosis of the superior mesenteric artery usually occurs at the origin of the vessel and is almost always associated with atherosclerosis. In contrast, emboli usually lodge between the middle colic artery and ileocolic artery and for that reason usually do not cause the degree of ischaemia seen in acute thrombosis[5].

The operation

In spite of the fact that many patients have significant cardiac disease, superior mesenteric artery occlusion from either thrombus or embolus is a surgical emergency and requires operation as soon as the patient's condition permits. Heparin is usually started as soon as the diagnosis is secure to prevent further propagation of thrombosis. Broad-spectrum antibiotics are administered and a Swan-Ganz catheter is inserted for continuous monitoring. Blood and other intravenous fluids must be available and large lines through which to administer them. These patients are frequently unstable and tolerate losses poorly. Digitalis and vasopressors should be withheld if possible as these cause vasospasm of the mesenteric circulation[6].

Incision and exploration

2

A midline incision from the xiphoid to just below the umbilicus usually gives adequate exposure.

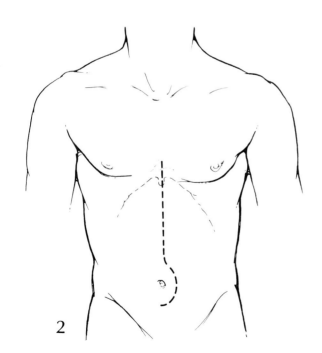

2

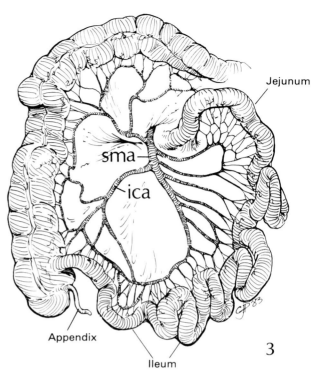

3

Jejunum

sma

ica

Appendix

Ileum

3

sma = superior mesenteric artery; ica = ileocolic artery

3

The abdominal contents are carefully explored with special attention to the jejunum, ileum, appendix and colon to the splenic flexure because these sections of the gut are supplied by the superior mesenteric artery.

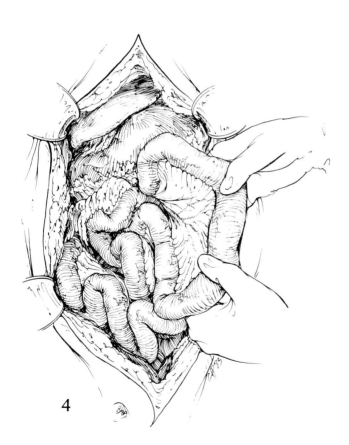

4

4

The bowel is evaluated for colour, motility and gangrene and the mesenteric vessels for the presence and force of the arterial pulsations. The intestinal vessels may be difficult to evaluate, especially in obese patients. Helpful techniques include transillumination of the mesentery, exposure of a mesenteric vessel and observing its pulsation by the reflection of a focused point of light and the use of the Doppler instrument. The injection and distribution of intra-arterial fluorescein as seen with a Wood's lamp has also been described. Arterial pulsations and blood flow should (but do not always) correlate with previous angiography.

For acute intestinal ischaemia, the superior mesenteric artery may be explored near its origin or in a retrograde manner through the ileocolic artery. In the obese patient, where exposure may be difficult, or for the surgeon who operates infrequently on mesenteric vessels, the retrograde ileocolic artery approach is usually easier[7].

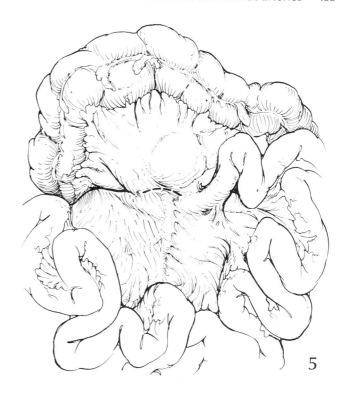

SUPERIOR MESENTERIC ARTERY EMBOLECTOMY (PROXIMAL APPROACH)

5

The transverse colon is retracted upwards and an incision is made in the peritoneum at the base of the transverse mesocolon to expose the lower border of the pancreas and superior mesenteric artery. The artery should be exposed for at least 3–4 cm.

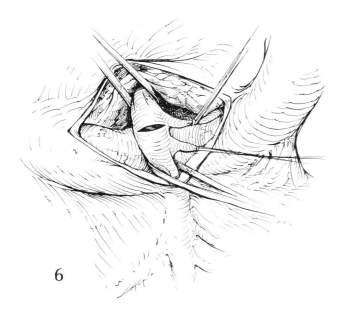

6

The jejunal branches should be carefully controlled with vessel loops; they should not be ligated because they are important collaterals.

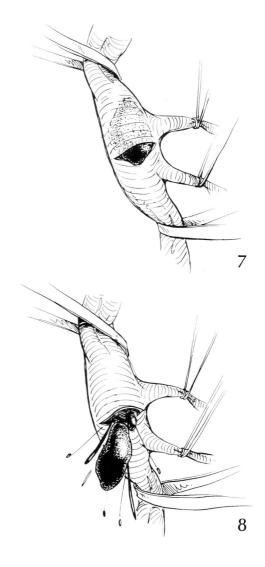

7

7, 8 & 9

Vascular tapes are used to control the vessels and an appropriate vascular clamp is set aside for quick application on the proximal superior mesenteric artery when good flow has been achieved. A transverse arteriotomy is made approximately one-half the circumference of the superior mesenteric artery distal to the embolus and the embolus is allowed to extrude with arterial pressure and gentle traction on the embolus. If good 'back bleeding' from the distal end and good flow from the proximal stump are achieved, the arterial clamp is applied and the arteriotomy closed with a running or interrupted 5/0 or 6/0 Prolene suture.

8

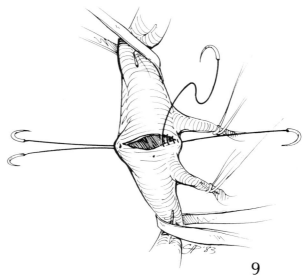

9

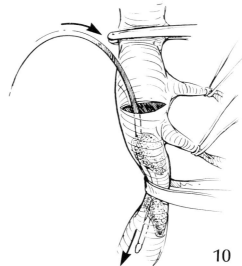

10, 11 & 12

If good flow is not obtained, a balloon embolectomy catheter should be passed gently proximally and distally to remove any remaining clots as necessary. Unfortunately, if the embolus has been present for some time, it may be impossible to remove all thrombi from the smaller distal branches.

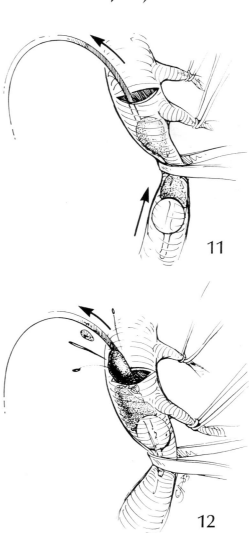

SUPERIOR MESENTERIC ARTERY EMBOLECTOMY (DISTAL APPROACH)

13 & 14

The distal approach to the superior mesenteric artery is technically easier, especially in obese patients, but it has the disadvantage that chunks of the embolus may be forced into the orifices of the distal intestinal vessels during the extraction. With the approach from above it is not uncommon to be able to pull out a thrombus which is a cast of the superior mesenteric artery and several of its branches. When the thrombus is withdrawn from below these extensions of the clot break off, often occluding these vital side branch vessels.

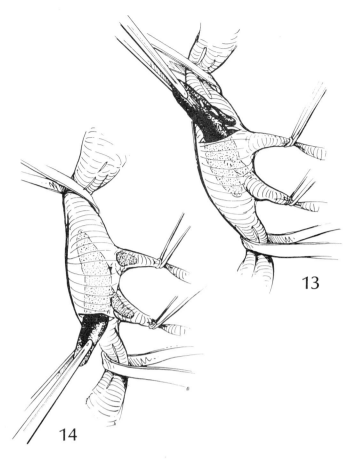

15

In the distal approach the superior mesenteric artery is evacuated through its most distal branch, the ileocolic artery. The caecum is reflected medially and traction on the ileocolic junction reveals the firm cord which contains the ileocolic vessels. The ileocolic artery is dissected proximally through this posterior approach until a diameter of 3–4 mm is reached. Control is achieved with tapes or vessel loops. The vessel is opened and an embolectomy catheter is gently passed to withdraw the clots.

Several passes may be required and the balloon should only be inflated enough to brush gently against the sides of the vessel so that damage to the endothelium (and risk of rethrombosis) is minimized. Milking the various mesenteric branches may also help in clearing these of embolic detritus. If good flow is obtained, the arteriotomy can be closed with fine Prolene.

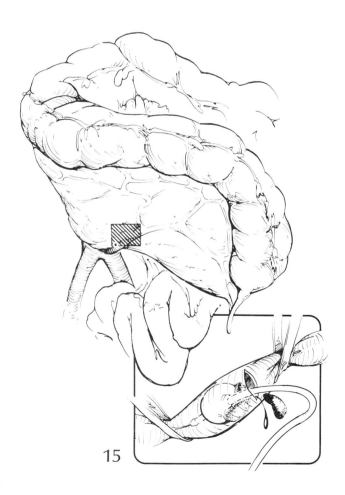

16

If the bowel remains ischaemic because antegrade flow cannot be re-established, retrograde flow can be provided by joining the arteriotomy in the ileocolic artery to an opening in the right common iliac artery. The common iliac artery is isolated at a site where the ileocolic artery can be approximated easily. Control is established either with circumferential tapes, or, preferably, with a partially occluding Satinsky clamp. The side-to-side anastomosis is made with 5/0 or 6/0 Prolene to create as large a lumen as possible.

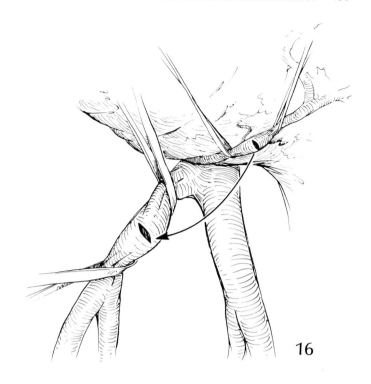

16

SPECIAL CONSIDERATIONS

Whichever approach is used, the anaesthetist should be warned that the blood pressure may drop precipitously when flow has been re-established to the intestine, perhaps through the release of toxic substances. Rapid infusion of fluids may be required to maintain the vital signs.

Areas of intestine which appear non-viable prior to embolectomy may improve to a surprising degree once blood flow is re-established. Operative Doppler measurements, evaluation with fluoroscein dye and intraoperative arteriograms may be helpful in assessing intestinal blood flow.

At least 10-15 min should be allowed to observe the changes in the colour of the intestine before a decision is made as to its viability. All frankly gangrenous and heavily discoloured intestine should be resected. The lines of resection should be made through the intestine with a good pink colour, ready capillary filling and good contraction when stimulated. Small dark spots, 3–5 mm in size, are frequently seen in viable bowel which has been revascularized successfully and can usually be ignored because they almost never represent full thickness loss.

The abdomen is closed with a single running layer of heavy non-absorbable suture because this type of closure is rapid and can be reopened easily if a second-look procedure is needed. If gangrenous bowel is resected the skin and subcutaneous tissues are usually left open; otherwise the wound is closed with widely spaced sutures or skin staples.

If there is concern about the viability of the intestine following revascularization, a second-look operation should be considered between 12 and 24 hours following the initial procedure. It is a difficult decision which must be guided by the patient's condition and prognosis, the extent of questionable discoloration of the bowel left behind, and, most of all, by the experience of the surgeon[5].

A considerable number of patients have gangrene, which will be discovered at surgery to extend from the duodenum to the transverse colon. Little can or should be done in such cases except to close the abdomen and keep the patient and the family as comforted as possible.

CHRONIC OCCLUSION OF THE COELIAC AND MESENTERIC ARTERIES

Patients with chronic occlusion of the coeliac and mesenteric arteries frequently present with a triad of obscure abdominal pain, weight loss and diarrhoea. This symptom complex is also known as the 'small meal syndrome' because eating is soon followed by ischaemic intestinal pain (intestinal claudication), preventing further food intake.

The definitive diagnosis depends upon abdominal arteriography. In general, stenosis or thrombosis of two of the three visceral arteries supplying the alimentary tract is required before symptoms develop, but the syndrome may also result from involvement of only one artery if the collateral circulation is inadequate. It is, however, possible to have a complete thrombosis of the coeliac and both the superior and inferior mesenteric vessels without any symptoms referable to the gastrointestinal tract[1].

Patients with chronic intestinal ischaemia are at great risk from sudden thrombosis of the stenotic superior mesenteric or coeliac arteries and massive gangrene involving the entire small bowel and right colon. In one series of 140 cases of mesenteric infarction[8], almost half the patients (43 per cent) had the premonitory symptoms of anorexia, nausea, diarrhoea and rectal bleeding which waxed and waned for weeks to months before the final illness. The situation is, therefore, comparable to stenosis of the carotid artery with transient ischaemic attacks warning of an impending stroke.

Multiple procedures have been described in the past for management of these patients but most of these have been abandoned because the newer approaches have proved more effective. Dilatations and local endarterec-tomies of the vascular orifices do not last and are soon followed by re-stenosis or occlusion of the vessel. Similarly, reimplantation of the visceral arteries has been abandoned because it is often difficult to re-anastomose a fragile visceral vessel to the thick-walled, diseased abdominal aorta[9].

Three procedures are recommended today. The first is the intra-abdominal placement of an aorta-to-visceral-vessel bypass, usually with a Dacron graft. The other two procedures involve a thoracoabdominal incision with a retroperitoneal approach to the abdominal aorta with an intra-aortic endarterectomy[4] or the implantation of a Carrell patch with the visceral vessels into an aortic Dacron bypass graft[6]. Prophylactic mesenteric revascularization should be performed in asymptomatic patients with documented significant visceral artery disease when other intra-abdominal operations such as renal artery bypass or aortoiliac reconstructive procedures are performed.

Because mesenteric atherosclerosis often involves all three visceral arteries, most surgeons revascularize at least two out of three major vessels and many routinely revascularize all three. The recurrence rate of symptoms is directly dependent upon the completeness of the revascularization at the initial operation. Graft occlusion is not uncommon and, unfortunately, it often results in bowel infarction in the early post-operative period, probably because of changes in visceral haemodynamics following revascularization[10]. Multiple anastomoses seem to minimize this hazard.

The operations

AORTA TO SUPERIOR MESENTERIC AND COELIAC ARTERY BYPASS

17

A standard midline incision is made from xiphoid to below the umbilicus. The abdominal contents are thoroughly explored to rule out other pathology, because malignancies, especially carcinomas of the pancreas and colon, are occasionally the real cause of the symptoms.

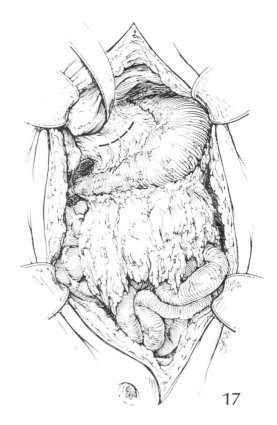

17

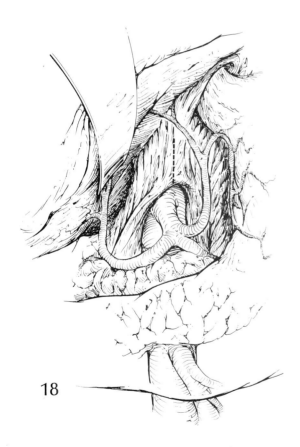

18

18

An opening is made in the gastrohepatic ligament to expose the crural fibres of the diaphragm, and the crura are separated to expose the supracoeliac aorta.

19

A partial occlusion clamp is then placed carefully in this portion of the aorta and an oval of the aortic wall is excised to produce an ample stoma.

20

A bifurcated Dacron graft of appropriate size is then bevelled at its larger end and sewn end-to-side on the supracoeliac portion of the abdominal aorta with continuous 3/0 or 4/0 Prolene sutures. The coeliac artery and its proximal branches and the superior mesenteric artery are then dissected free and controlled with tapes or small vascular clamps. One limb of the graft is then cut to the appropriate length and attached to one of the major divisions of the coeliac artery end-to-side with 4/0 or 5/0 continuous Prolene. The other limb is then run anterior to the pancreas and cut to an appropriate length to lie easily against the exposed superior mesenteric artery. This anastomosis is also accomplished in an end-to-side manner with Prolene. Similarly, a single segment graft can be placed if only one vessel needs to be bypassed.

This antegrade approach, i.e., using the proximal aorta for the proximal vascular anastomosis, does require a more difficult exposure than a retrograde procedure in which the graft is attached to the distal aorta. It is also a more dangerous approach because the aorta may be difficult to control if the clamp slips or cuts the aorta or if the aorta-to-graft anastomosis leaks badly. It has the advantage, however, of permitting clamping and sewing in a generally soft and less diseased area of the aorta and is much less likely to be occluded by advancing disease. If, on the other hand, the distal aorta appears to be pliable and spared from disease, this segment can, of course, be used.

In either approach, the aortic anastomosis should be carried out first. The flow and the security of the aortic suture line should be tested before proceeding with the visceral vessel anastomoses. The flow must be brisk and bleeding well controlled.

Excellent pulses should be palpable in the reconstructed visceral vessels. If these cannot be felt, the repair should be assessed with intraoperative angiography or with a flow meter. If there is any doubt about the adequacy of the anastomoses, these can be readily explored through transverse incisions in the limbs of the grafts.

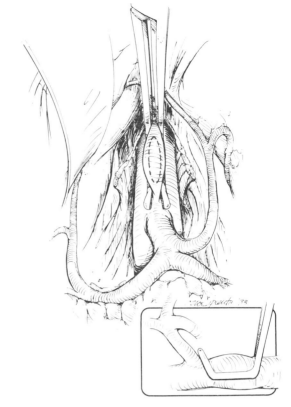

19

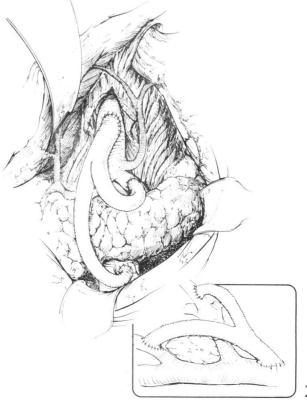

20

THE THORACOABDOMINAL RETROPERITONEAL APPROACH TO THE AORTA

Transaortic endarterectomy

21

The thoracoabdominal retroperitoneal approach involves a much more extensive dissection but gives excellent access to the aorta and its visceral and renal branches. The thoracic portion of the exposure is developed through the fifth or sixth intercostal space and the incision is extended obliquely across the abdomen beyond the midline. A common error is to make the intercostal incision too low; the fifth interspace provides far better exposure than the seventh or eighth.

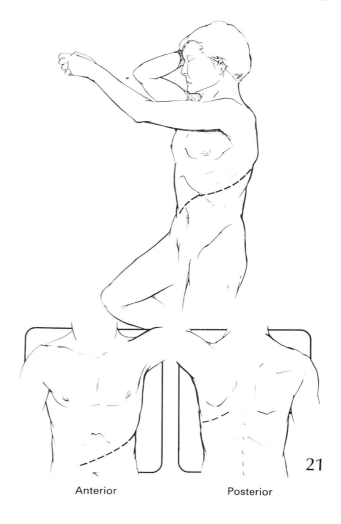

Anterior   Posterior   **21**

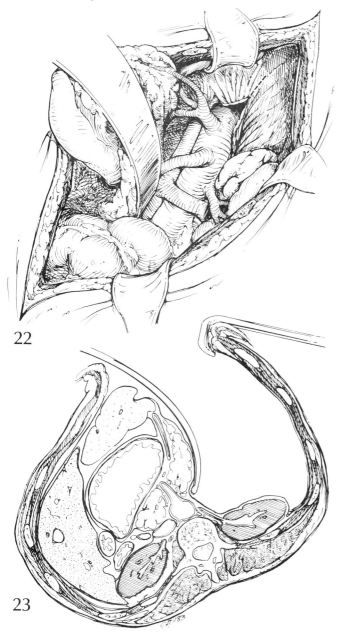

22

23

22 & 23

The retroperitoneal dissection retracts the spleen and the tail and the body of the pancreas to the patient's right. The left crus and the posterolateral and anterior fibres of the left hemidiaphragm are transected circumferentially adjacent to the chest wall to avoid denervation of the diaphragm. Careful resection and forward mobilization of the lymph nodes and vessels exposes the origin of the coeliac axis as it emerges from beneath the median arcuate ligament. Keeping close to the wall of the aorta, a plane of dissection can be developed, leading directly downwards to the origin of the superior mesenteric artery, which usually lies 1–2 cm below the origin of the coeliac axis. When the visceral vessels are exposed, haemodynamic measurements can be made if desired. Vascular clamps are then placed on the aorta above and below the segment which will undergo endarterectomy. If the distal aorta is heavily diseased a vascular clamp should be used with caution because it can break and cut the brittle vascular wall. In such cases, the distal aorta can be controlled more safely with an intraluminal balloon catheter.

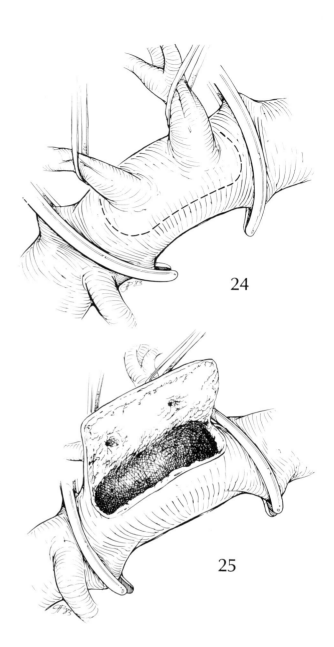

24

24 & 25

An incision is made in the aorta to the left of the coeliac and/or the superior mesenteric artery orifices with a hockey stick extension at each end of the aortotomy. This creates a trapdoor which can be swung back, carrying with it the orifices of the stenotic or occluded arteries.

25

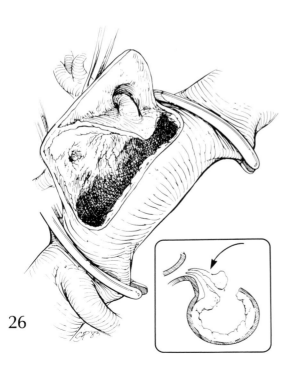

26

26

The intima on the underside of the trapdoor is dissected first from the media of the aortic wall, saving the visceral artery endarterectomy until last. Simultaneous traction on the aortic specimen and instrumental separation of the intima from the media in the branch causes the endarterectomized portion of the visceral artery to prolapse into the aortic lumen. With continuing traction and dissection, the atheromatous intima usually separates smoothly from the inner wall of the visceral arteries. The endpoint of the dissection should, however, be carefully inspected[15] and any residual fragments must be removed. If the intima of the posterior aorta is grossly thickened, it is also removed.

27

The aortotomy is closed with a running suture of 4/0 Prolene. The kidney may benefit from intravenous mannitol administration. Most surgeons prefer to work with the protection of systemic heparinization, but some report good results without anticoagulation. Because the time of occlusion is usually less then 25 min, few renal and spinal cord problems have been reported with this procedure.

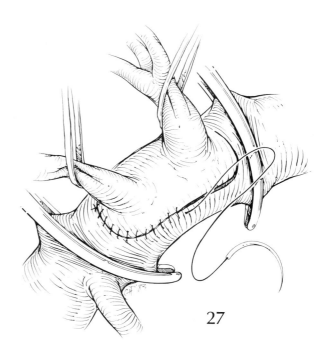

27

Reimplantation of visceral vessels to aortic bypass grafts

Often pronounced visceral artery stenosis is associated with advanced aortoiliac disease and extensive aortic aneurysms. In this setting the aortic graft is put in position in the usual fashion and the visceral vessels are then either reimplanted individually or as a multivessel Carrell patch. Stenotic visceral vessels can also be bypassed with Dacron limbs off the aortic graft to open areas in these arteries.

The intestinal viability and the effectiveness of the intestinal flow should be carefully checked at the end of the procedure. If the pulses are not strong, and if there is any question about the vigorous viability of the intestine, an intraoperative arteriogram should be done. Defects in the vascular repair should be repaired then and there. The association of gangrenous bowel and a Dacron graft leads to disastrous results and must be avoided.

These extensive procedures, in which a long segment of the aorta and a number of its branches are replaced, are difficult and are usually associated with extensive blood loss. These procedures are not to be undertaken lightly and are best left to the experienced vascular surgeon with maximum institutional support.

References

1. Rodgers, D. M., Thompson, J. E., Garrett, W. V., Talkington, C. M., Patman, R. D. Mesenteric vascular problems: a 26 year experience. Annals of Surgery 1982; 195: 554–565

2. Boley, S. J., Sprayregan, S., Siegelman, S. S., Veith, F. J. Initial results from an aggressive roentgenological and surgical approach to acute mesenteric ischemia. Surgery 1977; 82: 848–855

3. Boley, S. J., Feinstein, F. R., Sammartano, R., Brandt, L. J., Sprayregen, S. New concepts in the management of emboli of the superior mesenteric artery. Surgery, Gynecology and Obstetrics 1981; 153: 561–569

4. Stoney, R. J., Wylie, E. J. Surgical management of arterial lesions of the thoracoabdominal aorta. American Journal of Surgery 1973; 126: 157–164

5. Ottinger, L. W. The surgical management of acute occlusion of the superior mesenteric artery. Annals of Surgery 1978; 188: 721–731

6. Crawford, E. S., Morris, G. C., Myhre, H. O., Roehm, J. O. F. Celiac axis, superior mesenteric artery, and inferior mesenteric artery occlusion; surgical considerations. Surgery 1977; 82: 856–866

7. Marston, A. Revascularization of the gut. In: Rob and Smith's operative surgery; alimentary tract and abdominal wall. Pt 1 (4th ed) Dudley, H. (ed). London: Butterworths 1983

8. Pierce, G. E., Brockenbrough, E. C. The spectrum of mesenteric infarction. American Journal of Surgery 1970; 119: 233–239

9. Stoney, R. J., Ehrenfeld, W. K., Wylie, E. J. Revascularization methods in chronic visceral ischemia caused by atherosclerosis. Annals of Surgery 1977; 186: 468–476

10. Hollier, L. H., Bernatz, P. E., Pairolero, P. C., Payne, W. S., Osmundson, P. J.. Surgical management of chronic intestinal ischemia: a reappraisal. Surgery 1981; 90: 940–946

Illustrations by Gillian Oliver

Renal artery reconstruction

Michael E. Snell   MA, MChir, FRCS
Consultant Urologist, St Mary's Hospital, London, UK

Introduction

The refinement in angiographic techniques which took place in the early 1950s resulted in accurate diagnosis of renal arterial lesions, and reports of successful renal artery reconstruction followed soon afterwards.

The principal indication for renal artery reconstruction is hypertension due to renal artery stenosis but other indications include renal artery dissection, aneurysm and trauma. Recently the importance of renal artery reconstruction in conserving or improving renal function has been demonstrated[1].

Where hypertension is associated with renal artery stenosis it is essential to prove that the stenosis is responsible for the hypertension and not merely coincidental[2]. Divided renal function studies performed by catheterization of the ureters have been shown to be an effective means of identifying surgically curable hypertension[3] but most surgeons now rely upon renin estimations[4] because of the lower morbidity associated with the latter technique.

Selection of cases for reconstruction

The natural history of renal artery stenosis is an important consideration in deciding between medical and surgical treatment for renovascular hypertension. In atheromatous cases progression of stenoses resulting in deterioration of renal function was observed in 41 per cent of cases[5]. Similar tightening of stenoses or development of new lesions, sometimes in the contralateral renal artery, were noted in 34.5 per cent of fibromuscular lesions[6]. These findings indicate that reconstruction is the treatment of choice if conservation of renal function and mass is to be achieved. Unfortunately, however, not all cases are suitable for reconstruction. Whilst the excellent results obtained in fibromuscular disease[7] indicate that reconstruction is the best treatment, careful evaluation of each case is required in atheromatous lesions. Where the lesion is confined to the renal artery the results of reconstruction approximate to those achieved in fibromuscular disease and are distinctly superior to those in

whom there is generalized atherosclerosis[8]. In the latter group surgical relief of significant coronary artery and carotid stenosis prior to renal artery reconstruction reduces the postoperative mortality from myocardial infarction and stroke which are two of the major causes of death[9]. In older patients with severe generalized atherosclerosis in whom life expectation is limited, arterial reconstruction should be reserved for those with uncontrolled hypertension or failing renal function in view of the relatively high operative mortality.

Preoperative assessment and care

Significant coronary or carotid artery disease should be sought and treated if found. Cerebral angiography is indicated when there has been a previous subarachnoid haemorrhage. Cardiac failure must be corrected. Antihypertensive medication can often be reduced on admission to hospital but in some cases of severe hypertension intravenous nitroprusside infusion with continuous intra-arterial blood pressure monitoring is required.

Intraoperative care

The aim throughout the procedure is to maintain the blood pressure and urine output at an acceptable level and to minimize ischaemic injury to the kidney during arterial reconstruction. The former is achieved by the judicious use of antihypertensive drugs and fluid replacement.

The kidney is protected against ischaemic injury by the initiation of diuresis with an intravenous infusion of mannitol 20–25 g during the dissection of the renal artery, and inosine 25 mg/kg and heparin 1.5 mg/kg are given intravenously 15 minutes before any occlusion clamps are applied.

In most cases continuous monitoring of the electrocardiogram and intra-arterial and central venous pressure is adequate. In some instances when the patient has been in cardiac failure pulmonary wedge pressure may need to be measured.

Operative techniques

1a & b

The incision

For most reconstructive procedures a transverse upper abdominal incision which divides the muscles or a midline longitudinal incision provides the necessary exposure. The transverse incision is only applicable where there is a broad subcostal arch. The incision employed must allow generous exposure as the distal end of the renal artery reconstruction, which can be difficult, is often deep within the abdomen in adults. A ring retractor is employed with the addition of extra blades for the retraction of viscera as the exposure proceeds. Upon entering the peritoneal cavity a routine exploratory laparotomy is performed including palpation of the adrenal glands.

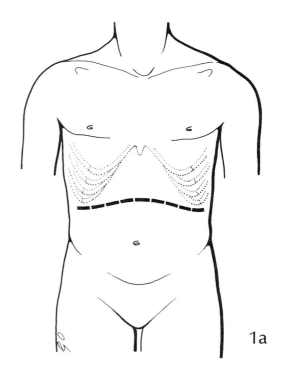

1a

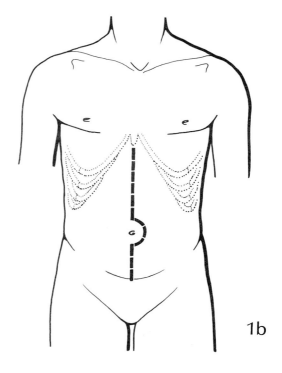

1b

2

Exposure of the right renal artery

The ascending colon is reflected medially and parietal peritoneum is incised along its medial border up to the hepatic flexure after which it becomes possible to retract the ascending colon medially exposing the kidney and duodenum. The duodenum is mobilized in turn and retracted medially until the inferior vena cava and aorta are displayed. At this stage it may be necessary to divide the right gonadal vein.

  The renal artery will normally be found lying behind the renal vein and is exposed by passing silicone slings around the renal vein and inferior vena cava so that these structures may be retracted. The periarterial lymphatics and nervous tissue are cleared from the artery by gentle dissection, taking care not to injure the collateral arteries as they play an important role in maintaining perfusion of the kidney during reconstruction. Throughout the dissection meticulous haemostasis is essential if subsequent retroperitoneal haematoma is to be avoided. Dissection of the artery is continued medially behind the inferior vena cava as far as is necessary to allow subsequent ligation of the artery proximal to the stenosis. If the stenosis is close to the aorta it will be necessary to divide one or two lumbar veins and retract the vena cava laterally to provide access.

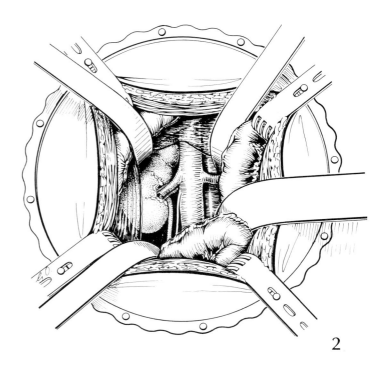

2

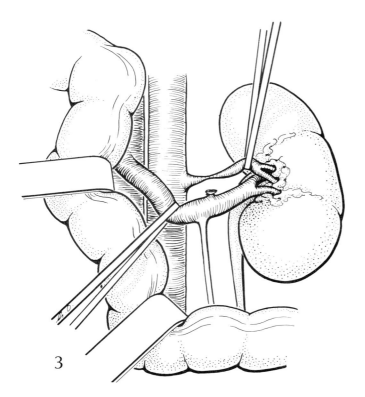

3

3

Exposure of the left renal artery

The descending colon and small bowel are displaced medially. An incision is made in the parietal peritoneum lateral to the colon, commencing just above the pelvic brim and extending upwards and medially around the splenic flexure until it is possible to retract the colon and its mesentery far enough medially to expose the aorta and inferior vena cava. It is often necessary to divide either the adrenal or gonadal vein in order to allow sufficient displacement of the renal vein to expose the renal artery adequately.

MAIN ARTERY STENOSIS

Aortorenal artery graft

The commonest method of renal artery reconstruction is by means of a graft from the aorta to the renal artery. The choice of material is between saphenous vein, internal iliac artery and synthetic material.

Autogenous saphenous vein, in spite of its tendency to dilate[10] is the most widely used material but internal iliac artery is particularly useful when there are two or more branches of the renal artery to reconstruct, and Dacron or polytetrafluorethylene tubes are easier to suture to the aorta when it is atheromatous.

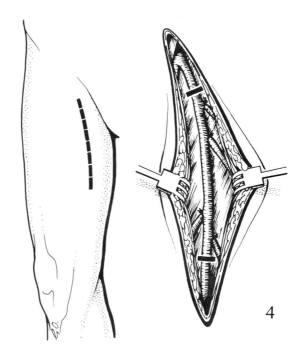

4

4 & 5

Dissection of the saphenous vein

An incision is made in the thigh over the course of the saphenous vein. The vein is exposed and the branches are ligated with fine silk, taking care not to narrow the main trunk by incorporating excess adventitia into the knot. When sufficient length for the reconstruction has been mobilized the vein is divided and lifted from its bed. It is advisable to mark the vein to indicate the direction of flow for the subsequent graft insertion. The lower end of the vein may be dilated to allow insertion of a cannula for perfusion with heparinized blood or Hartmann's solution to look for leakage from any missed branches and to note the position of valves which are undesirable at the anastomotic site.

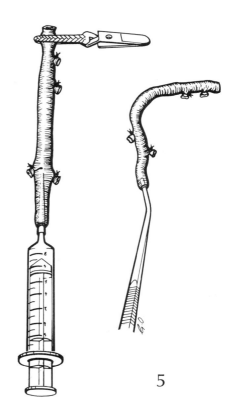

5

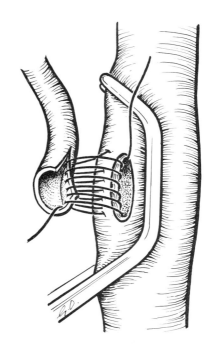

6

6 & 7

Aortic anastomosis

The aorta is cleared of all periaortic tissue from the level of the left renal vein down to the inferior mesenteric artery. It is frequently necessary to divide one or more lumbar arteries on the side on which the anastomosis is to be performed in order to allow sufficient mobilization of the aorta so that a lateral clamp can be placed at the chosen anastomotic site, which should be a relatively disease-free portion of the aorta. An aortic punch is used to make an oval window and the saphenous vein is spatulated. The anastomosis is made with 6/0 Prolene on 13 mm needles, stitching into the lumen of the aorta. The stitches are initially left loose to allow accurate suture placement at the upper end of the anastomosis where it is easy to narrow the saphenous vein by inaccurate stitching.

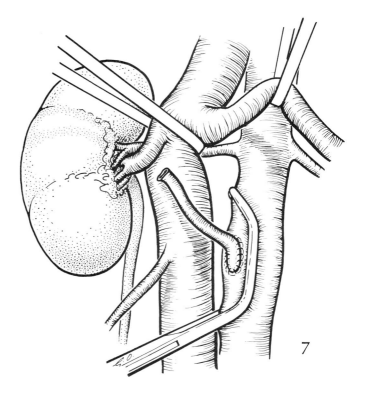

7

8, 9 & 10

Renal anastomosis – end-to-end

The renal artery is ligated proximal to the stenosis and a bulldog clamp is placed on the distal renal artery which is then divided and brought anterior to the renal vein. If the distal stump of the renal artery is short there is a tendency for it to slip through the bulldog clamp and retract into the hilar fat. This can be prevented by encircling the main divisions of the renal artery with silicone slings which are used to lift the artery forwards and compress the branches sufficiently so that the clamp on the renal artery can be dispensed with, allowing greater flexibility during the anastomosis. The renal arterial wall may be very thin if there is significant poststenotic dilatation and it may be necessary to spatulate the saphenous vein to achieve compatibility. If both vessels are small both require spatulation to provide a satisfactory bore. The saphenous vein is brought anterior to the aorta and excess vein is cut off after deciding upon the optimum length. Sometimes the relationship of the renal artery and vein is such that it is more appropriate to pass the vein behind the inferior vena cave, dividing lumbar veins if necessary, to make it lie properly.

The anastomosis is begun by inserting 6/0 Prolene sutures on 10 mm needles at the upper and lower borders of the vessels to be joined. The vessels are then rotated through 180° and the back of the vessels are apposed with a continuous suture. The vessels are then derotated and the anastomosis completed with interrupted sutures, taking care to flush both vessels before inserting the final sutures. The renal artery clamp is released first and then the aortic clamp is partially released. Although the aorta has not been cross-clamped the clamp should be released gradually so as to avoid severe hypotension.

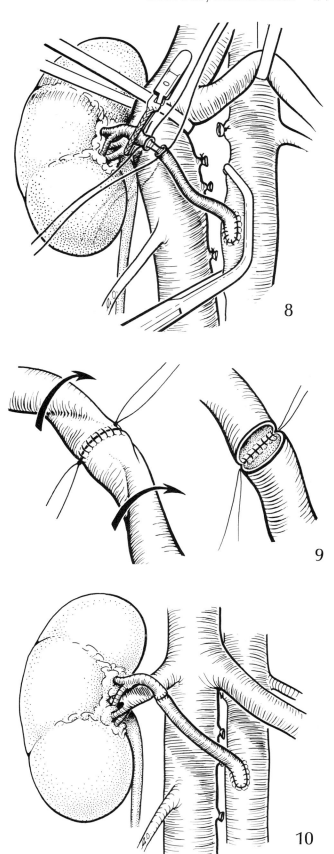

11

Renal anastomosis – end-to-side

Some surgeons prefer an end-to-side anastomosis. This type of anastomosis is required if the stenosis extends down one of the primary branches of the renal artery and it is also easier to perform when a Dacron graft is employed. The aortic anastomosis is performed in the manner described for the saphenous vein. Bulldog clamps are applied to the renal artery or either side of the anastomotic site and an incision 1.2–1.5 cm long is made in the renal artery. If Dacron is used a 6/0 Prolene on a 13 mm needle will be required. The anastomosis is completed with a continuous suture commencing posteriorly. If access to the renal artery is poor it is advantageous to perform the renal artery anastomosis first as this allows the graft to be manipulated freely during suturing. On completion the renal artery clamps are removed, and after flushing the graft is occluded by a bulldog clamp adjacent to the anastomosis. The aortic anastomosis is then constructed.

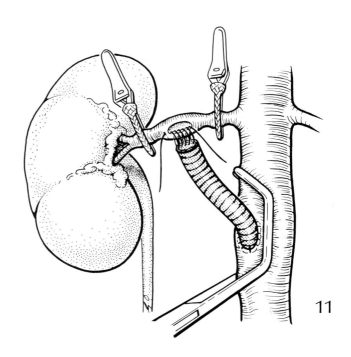

11

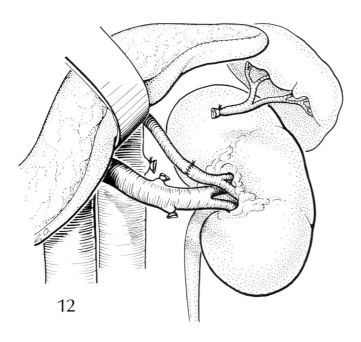

12

ALTERNATIVE PROCEDURES

12

Splenorenal anastomosis

If the coeliac axis and splenic artery are normal this type of anastomosis is often the procedure of choice on the left. The renal artery is mobilized in the usual manner. The pancreas is retracted upwards and the lower border is rotated forwards so as to display the splenic artery. A silicone sling is passed around the artery and it is dissected off the pancreas, dividing the small pancreatic branches. The splenic artery must be handled with great care as it has a marked tendency to spasm and the pancreatic branches are easily torn. When sufficient length has been mobilized the artery is divided between a clamp and a distal ligature and an end-to-end anastomosis is performed. The spleen is left *in situ*.

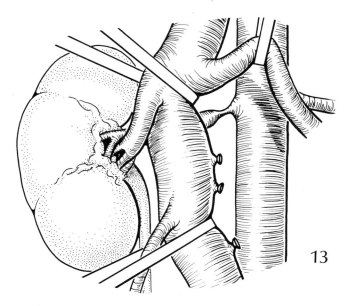

13

13 & 14

Reimplantation of the renal artery

In certain situations, such as an atheromatous stenosis confined to the proximal renal artery or fibromuscular disease in children, there is sufficient length of renal artery to allow reimplantation farther down the aorta. If the stenosis is on the right side the great vessels are exposed as usual and in order to provide adequate exposure of the renal artery at least one lumbar vein is divided to allow retraction of the inferior vena cava and left renal vein. The aorta is prepared and the renal artery is then divided and swung down to be sutured to the aorta in the manner described for aortorenal grafts.

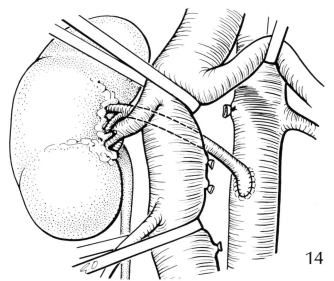

14

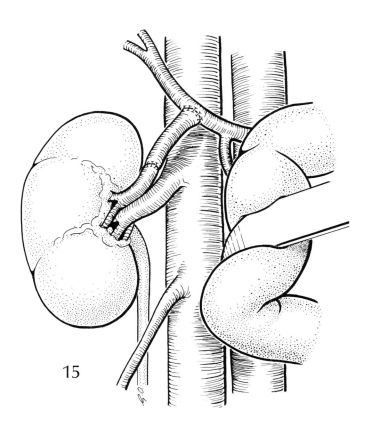

15

15

Hepatorenal graft

If there is gross aortic disease a saphenous vein graft from the hepatic to the right renal artery has considerable merit especially in poor risk patients such as those who are uraemic. The right renal vessels are exposed and the artery is mobilized. The hepatic artery is identified in the lesser omentum as it lies medial to the common bile duct and anterior to the portal vein. It is mobilized and a segment of saphenous vein is anastomosed to it end-to-side. After ensuring that there is adequate flow down the vein the renal artery is ligated and divided and an end-to-end anastomosis made.

SEGMENTAL ARTERY STENOSIS

It is usually possible to reconstruct segmental stenoses *in situ* which has the advantage of maintaining the collateral circulation. Bench surgery is rarely indicated.

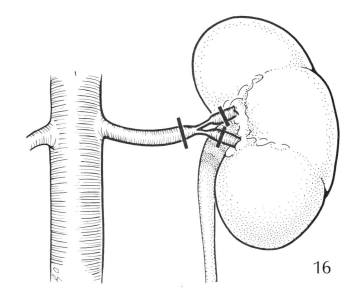

16

16 & 17

Two branches

The simplest technique is to join the two arteries as in a pair of trousers and then anastomose the conjoined arteries to a saphenous vein graft. The latter is anastomosed to the aorta first after which the bifurcation of the renal artery is excised and the adjacent borders of the segmental arteries are spatulated. Beginning at the free border of the arteries a 6/0 Prolene suture is run up to the apex of the anastomosis and back to the opposite free border. The united arteries are then sutured end-to-end to the already established vein graft.

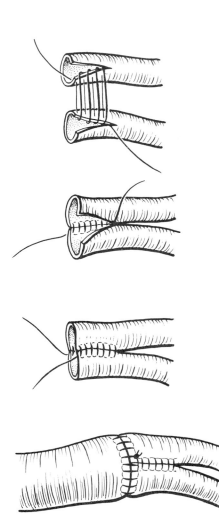

17

Three or more branches

18, 19 & 20

In this situation the iliac internal artery is divided distal to its two major divisions and transected close to its origin. A 1 cm long incision is made in the distal artery to which a segment of saphenous vein is anastomosed with 6/0 or 7/0 Prolene. The internal iliac artery is then anastomosed to the aorta in the usual manner. In order to minimize the ischaemic period the main renal artery is not divided at this stage. The branches are ligated in turn as the previous anastomosis is completed so that there is never more than one segment of the kidney ischaemic at a given time. The main renal artery is ligated on commencement of the final anastomosis.

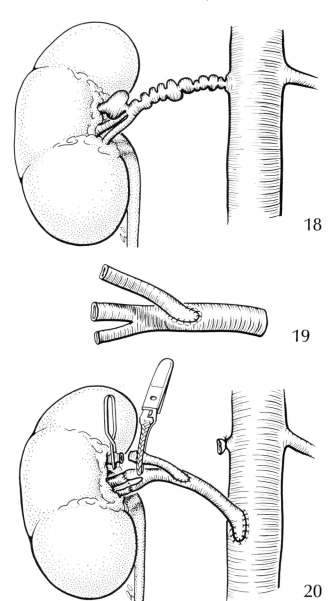

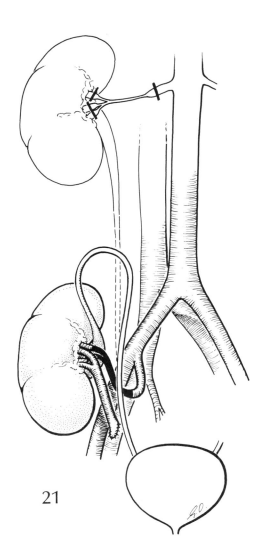

21

On the rare occasion that it is impossible to reconstruct the renal arteries *in situ* the kidney and ureter are mobilized and the renal artery and vein are ligated and divided. The kidney is lifted up to the surface of the wound and the artery is flushed with Collins solution at 5°C from a height of 1 m. The kidney is kept cool between packs soaked in cold saline solution while the branches are reconstructed using segments of saphenous vein which are sutured to one main trunk. The kidney is then replaced extraperitoneally in the iliac fossa. The vein is anastomosed end-to-side to the external iliac vein and the saphenous vein is sutured to the internal iliac artery after it has been transected and turned up towards the kidney.

BILATERAL STENOSES

The mortality from simultaneous bilateral reconstruction, particularly when combined with aortic replacement, is appreciably higher than for unilateral reconstruction[11]. It is often prudent to repair the more ischaemic kidney first and observe the effect on the blood pressure for a few weeks before making a decision about the other kidney.

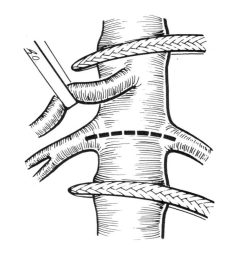

22

Renal endarterectomy

22, 23 & 24

The aorta is exposed as in the exposure of the left renal vessels but the dissection of the aorta continues in a cranial direction until it is possible to place an occlusion clamp across it above the superior mesenteric artery. In order to achieve this it may be necessary to divide the left crus of the diaphragm. Once the dissection of the aorta and both renal arteries is complete occlusion clamps are placed on the aorta above the superior mesenteric and below the renal arteries. Bulldog clamps are used to occlude the distal renal arteries and the superior mesenteric artery. A transverse aortotomy extending a few millimetres into each artery is made. Contrary to general belief the stenosis often commences in the renal artery a few milimetres distal to the ostium and it is therefore not necessary to perform an extensive aortic endarterectomy. A disc approximately 1 cm in diameter is cut in the intima around the renal artery ostium after which the plane of cleavage is entered on the anterior aspect of the artery and developed round the circumference to free the disc. The tube of atheroma is then developed distally by blunt dissection until it ends in a tail and is pulled out. The procedure is repeated on the other side after which both renal arteries are backwashed by temporarily releasing their occluding clamps. A Dacron patch is then tailored to the incision and stitched in with 5/0 Prolene.

If there is extensive aortic disease more radical procedures such as aortic endarterectomy[12] or Dacron substitution of the aorta may be required[13].

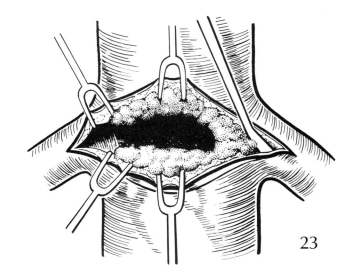

23

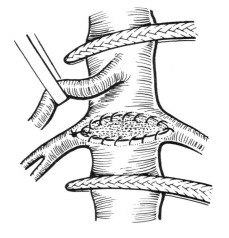

24

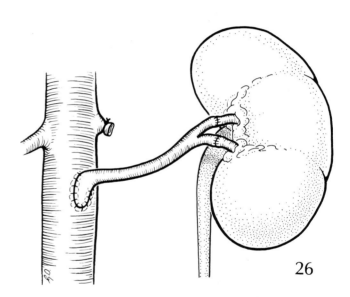

25 & 26

RENAL ARTERY ANEURYSM

The majority of renal artery aneurysms are associated with renal artery stenosis and the principles of reconstruction do not differ from those utilized in renal artery stenosis. Aneurysms greater than 2 cm in diameter require resection in their own right; others only require removal if they are associated with renovascular hypertension.

In the example illustrated the renal vessels are isolated in the usual manner. As both segmental branches are stenosed at their origin they are divided and the internal iliac artery with its two primary divisions is used to replace the renal artery.

Postoperative care

The patient is nursed in an intensive care unit for the first 24–48 hours as the blood pressure often climbs steeply in the first few hours after operation and careful monitoring with active management of the blood pressure and urine output is required. Paralytic ileus is treated by nasogastric aspiration, and routine prophylaxis against thromboembolic disease such as subcutaneous heparin and compression leg stockings is employed.

Persistent severe hypertension is suggestive of graft occlusion and should be investigated by early angiography and isotope renography as it may be possible to salvage the kidney by a second procedure.

Results

The results of surgical treatment of the different categories of patients from selected series are shown in *Tables 1 and 2* and indicate that with careful case selection approximately 90 per cent of patients with fibro-muscular disease and focal atherosclerosis benefit from surgery whilst the figure is lower in patients with generalized atherosclerosis in whom the operative mortality is in the region of 5 per cent.

Table 1 Results of surgical treatment of fibromuscular stenosis

Author	Total number	Cured	Improved	Failure	Operative death
Lawrie et al.[8]	113	43	24	33	0
Stanley and Fry[7]	159	100	53	6	0

Table 2 Results of surgical treatment in atherosclerotic stenosis

Author	Total number	Cured	Improved	Failure	Operative death
Generalized atherosclerosis					
Novick et al.[9]	61	18	36	7	2
Stanley and Fry[7]	51	13	24	14	3
Focal atherosclerosis					
Novick et al.[9]	17	13	4	0	0
Stanley and Fry[7]	54	17	32	5	0

References

1. Dean, R. H., Lawson, J. D., Hollifield, J. W., Shack, B., Polterauer, P., Rhamy, R. K. Revascularisation of the poorly functioning kidney. Surgery 1979; 85: 44–52

2. Eyler, W. R., Clark, M. D., Garman, J. E., Rian, R. L., Meininger, D. E. Angiography of renal areas including comparative study of renal arterial stenoses in patients with and without hypertension. Radiology 1962; 78: 879–892

3. Stamey, T. A., Nudelman, I. J., Good, P. H., Schwentker, F. N., Hendricks, F. Functional characteristics of renovascular hypertension. Medicine 1961; 40: 347–394

4. Vaughan, E. D., Jr. Identifying surgically curable renovascular hypertension. Cardiovascular Medicine 1976; 1: 195–205

5. Dean, R. H., Kieffer, R. W., Smith, B. M. et al. Renovascular hypertension: anatomic and renal function changes during drug therapy. Archives of Surgery 1981; 116: 1408–1415

6. Sheps, S. G., Kincaid, O. W., Hunt, J. C. Serial renal function and angiographic observations in idiopathic fibrous and fibromuscular stenoses of the renal arteries. American Journal of Cardiology 1972; 30: 55–60

7. Stanley, J. C., Fry, W. J. Surgical treatment of renovascular hypertension. Archives of Surgery 1977; 112: 1291–1297

8. Lawrie, G. M., Morris, G. C., Jr, Soussou, I. D., et al. Late results of reconstructive surgery for renovascular disease. Annals of Surgery 1980: 191: 528–533

9. Novick, A. C., Straffon, R. A., Stewart, B. H., Gifford, R. W., Vidt, D. Diminished operative morbidity and mortality in renal revascularisation. Journal of the American Medical Association 1981; 246: 749–753

10. Ernst, C. B., Stanley, J. C., Marshall, F. F., Fry, W. J. Autogenous saphenous vein aortorenal grafts. Archives of Surgery 1972; 105: 855–864

11. Franklin, S. S., Young, J. D., Jr, Maxwell, M. H. et al. Operative Morbidity and Mortality in Renovascular disease. Journal of the American Medical Association 1975; 231: 1148–1153

12. Wylie, E. J. Endarterectomy and autogenous arterial grafts in the surgical treatment of stenosing lesions of the renal artery. Urological Clinics of North America 1975; 2: 351–363

13. Shahian, D. M., Najafi, H., Javid, H., et al. Simultaneous aortic and renal artery reconstruction. Archives of Surgery 1980; 115: 1491–1497

Axillofemoral and femorofemoral bypass grafts

Allyn G. May MD, FACS
Professor of Surgery, University of Rochester Medical Center, Rochester, New York, USA

James A. DeWeese MD, FACS
Professor and Chairman, Division of Cardiothoracic Surgery,
University of Rochester Medical Center, Rochester, New York, USA

Some patients who require an operation for aortic or iliac obstruction cannot safely undergo deep abdominal surgery. In these patients the axillofemoral or femorofemoral bypass graft offers a technique for successful treatment[1,2,3].

AXILLOFEMORAL BYPASS GRAFTS

The particular indications for the axillofemoral bypass graft are: an urgent need to bypass aortoiliac obstruction in the presence of generalized peritonitis or of retroperitoneal infection; as part of the treatment for infection of an aortic prosthesis; or an urgent need to bypass aortoiliac obstruction in the poor-risk patient who cannot tolerate deep abdominal surgery or general anaesthesia[4,5,6].

Frequently a unilateral axillofemoral bypass will suffice even for bilateral severe lower extremity ischaemia. Thus it is wise to drape the patient so that both feet can be observed for colour change and for venous filling (i.e. in sterile transparent plastic bags), and to revascularize the contralateral side only if necessary[7]. If significant contralateral ischaemia persists after axillofemoral bypass grafting, the procedure may be extended by adding a femorofemoral bypass graft. There is some evidence that the long-term patency is better after a femorofemoral graft is added to an axillofemoral graft. The flow appears to be greater through an axillofemoral graft if it supplies both lower limbs[8].

1

The femoral incision

The axillofemoral bypass is constructed with the patient in the supine position and under general or local anaesthesia. A wide area of skin is prepared over the shoulder, base of the neck, anterior and lateral side of the chest, groin and thigh. The femoral artery is exposed first. The skin incision begins at the level of the inguinal ligament about 4 cm lateral to the pubic tubercle and passes medially and inferiorly in a gentle curve. The greater saphenous vein may be seen and should be preserved. The incision is deepened lateral to the saphenous vein and widened by retraction. The pulseless femoral artery can be felt as it is approached and it will be found to lie immediately lateral to the femoral vein and to the termination of the greater saphenous vein. In mobilizing the femoral artery the posterior origin of the deep femoral artery should be remembered, for it is prone to injury in its unobtrusive position. All branches of the femoral arteries should be preserved. Eventually tapes are passed about the common, superficial and deep femoral arteries. These arteries are palpated for evidence of patency and to detect areas, relatively free of atheroma, which can satisfactorily take the graft.

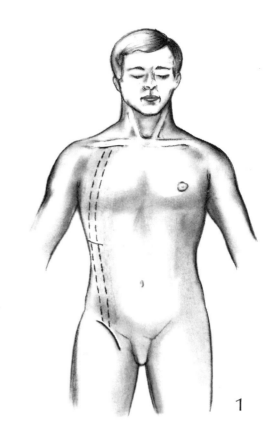

1

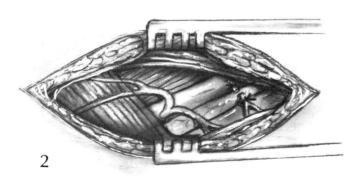

2

2

The axillary incision

The incision to expose the axillary artery is then made. It is 8 cm long, parallel to and one fingerbreadth below the clavicle with its centre at the junction of the medial and middle portions of the clavicle. The two portions of the pectoralis major muscle are retracted and the coracoclavicular fascia is incised. The axillary vessels are uncovered in the space beneath this membrane. Venous branches and the supreme thoracic artery should be tied and divided to allow adequate mobilization of the axillary artery. It is usually possible to preserve the acromiothoracic trunk of the artery. The axillofemoral tunnel is constructed between the pectoralis major and minor muscles, along the midaxillary line in the deep subcutaneous space, passing towards the femoral triangle immediately above the inguinal ligament. It is made with an arterial tunneller. It is usually possible to pass the tunneller from axilla to groin or from groin to axilla without a counter incision.

3

The axillary anastomosis

The upper anastomosis is done first. Heparin sodium 5000 u is given intravenously. A preclotted knitted Dacron prosthesis 8–10 mm in diameter is recommended. The artery is controlled with vascular clamps and a longitudinal incision is made on the inferior aspect of the vessel. An end-to-side anastomosis is made using 5/0 prosthetic arterial suture. After completion of the anastomosis, the vascular clamp is removed briefly at intervals to ensure graft haemostasis. Excess clot is sucked or milked out of the graft and the vascular clamp is repositioned on the proximal graft to restore blood flow to the upper limb.

The prosthesis is placed in the tunnel without twisting and trimmed to reach the site prepared for femoral anastomosis. The femoral clamp is applied, an anterior arteriotomy made and the end-to-side anastomosis made with the same suture material. On completion of the anastomosis, the proximal clamp is removed and the blood allowed to fill the prothesis in order to exhaust air through the distal suture line. As soon as air-bubbles cease to appear, the femoral artery is declamped. The patient is given protamine 50 mg intravenously. Not until all bleeding has been controlled and excess clot expressed from the tunnel are the incisions closed.

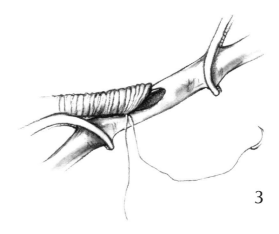

3

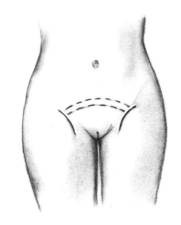

4

FEMOROFEMORAL BYPASS GRAFTS

This cross-leg bypass is useful in the poor-risk patient when unilateral iliac arterial obstruction is significantly the cause of ischaemia; when there is good arterial blood flow to the contralateral lower extremity; and there is a need to avoid deep abdominal surgery. It is possible and sometimes desirable to combine this procedure with the axillofemoral bypass graft[9].

4

Technique

Many aspects of this procedure are the same as those for the axillofemoral bypass graft. The patient is supine and the anaesthesia may be general or local. The lower abdomen, groin and upper thighs are prepared and draped to provide for bilateral femoral and suprapubic exposure. The femoral arteries on the ischaemic side are first exposed to permit evaluation of patency. Operative angiography may be helpful at this time if prior aortography failed to show patency of the femoral arteries. Frequently, revascularization of a patent deep femoral artery alone will suffice to heal a serious lesion of the foot. The patent segment is mobilized so that vascular clamps can be applied. The contralateral femoral artery is exposed and prepared for clamping. A subcutaneous tunnel is developed with the fingers cephalad from one femoral incision passing superior to the mons pubis and descending symmetrically to the contralateral femoral incision.

5

The anastomosis

The upstream anastomosis is completed first. The arteriotomy should be longitudinal and on the anteromedial aspect of the femoral artery. When the anastomosis is finished, the position of the vascular clamp is transferred to the prosthesis at the suture line and the prosthesis, if knitted Dracon, is preclotted by intermittent declamping. Excess clot is removed from the graft, which is then passed through the tunnel without twisting in a gentle curve from one femoral artery to the other. Next the downstream anastomosis is completed. The upstream clamp is removed and the graft freed of entrapped air before downstream declamping is done.

When haemostasis is secured the wounds are closed in layers and provided with simple dry dressings.

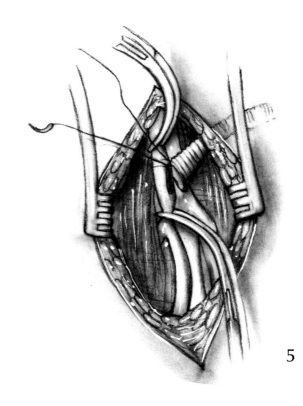

5

Postoperative care

The patients receive preoperative and postoperative antibiotics for 5 days. Early or late thrombosis can usually be successfully treated by thrombectomy of the graft under local anaesthetic over the midportion of the axillary and/or femorofemoral graft[5].

References

1. Blaisdell, F. W., Hall, A. D. Axillary-femoral artery bypass for lower extremity ischemia. Surgery 1963; 54: 563–568

2. Mannick, J. A., Williams, L. E., Nabseth, D. C. The late results of axillofemoral grafts. Surgery 1970; 68: 1038–1043

3. Moore, W. S., Hall, A. D., Blaisdell, F. W. Late results of axillary-femoral bypass grafting. American Journal of Surgery 1971; 122: 148–154

4. Jamieson, C. G., DeWeese, J. A., Rob, C. G. Infected arterial grafts. Annals of Surgery 1975; 181: 850–852

5. Oblath, R. W., Green, R. M., DeWeese, J. A., Rob, C. G. Extra-anatomic bypass of the abdominal aorta: management of postoperative thrombosis. Annals of Surgery 1978; 187: 647–652

6. Plecha, F. R., Pories, W. J. Extra-anatomic bypasses for aortoiliac disease in high-risk patients. Surgery 1976; 80: 480–487

7. Plume, S. K., DeWeese, J. A., Slomczewski, C. M. Intraoperative assessment of peripheral revascularization procedures. Surgery, Gynecology and Obstetrics 1976; 142: 83

8. LoGerfo, F. W., Johnson, W. C., Corson, J. D. et al. A comparison of the late patency rates of axillobilateral femoral and axillobilateral femoral grafts. Surgery 1977; 81: 33–40

9. Vetto, R. M. The femorofemoral shunt: an appraisal. American Journal of Surgery 1966; 112: 162–165

Illustrations by Anita Matthews and Robert Wabnitz

Arterial reconstruction below the inguinal ligament

Richard M. Green MD, FACS
Clinical Assistant Professor of Surgery,
University of Rochester Medical Center, Rochester, New York, USA

James A. DeWeese MD, FACS
Professor and Chairman, Division of Cardiothoracic Surgery,
University of Rochester Medical Center, Rochester, New York, USA

Introduction

Atherosclerotic occlusions of the arterial circulation below the inguinal ligament usually occur in the lower thigh where the artery passes beneath the rigid adductor magnus tendon to become the popliteal artery. The occlusion may extend both proximally and distally from this level, but the common femoral artery in the groin and the popliteal artery in the region of the knee usually remain patent. As the occlusion involves the distal popliteal artery and beyond, the degree of ischaemia increases.

The symptoms associated with chronic femoropopliteal occlusive disease are intermittent claudication, athero-embolic phenomena, rest pain, painful ulcerations or gangrene. Progression from milder forms of arterial ischaemia to more severe forms is often related to associated problems such as diabetes mellitus and continuation of cigarette smoking. The long-term prognosis of these patients is poor. In a long-term analysis of patients with symptomatic femoropopliteal occlusive disease, DeWeese and Rob[1] found that as many as 48 per cent and 73 per cent died most frequently of cardiac causes at 5 and 10 years respectively.

Preoperative

Preoperative evaluation

A general medical evaluation will often disclose diabetes or segmental atherosclerosis in other organ systems such as the extracranial cerebral vessels, and coronary or renal arteries. Priorities of treatment must be made based on the threat to the patient's well-being. When the superficial femoral artery is occluded the femoral pulses are present, but usually no pulses are felt at the popliteal or pedal level. There are some patients with superficial femoral artery occlusion who have weak pedal pulses, but these pulses will disappear with exercise. At the bedside, oscillometric examination and performance of an elevation-dependency test are helpful in determining the severity of the arterial insufficiency. In the vascular laboratory decreased calf and ankle systolic pressures at rest which further decrease after treadmill exercise are important in eliminating other causes of exercise-induced leg pain. Aortofemoral arteriography remains the most definitive of the preoperative studies.

Indications for operation

Patients with limb-threatening rest pain, ulcerations or gangrene are advised to undergo arterial reconstruction if there are patent proximal femoral and distal popliteal or tibial arteries visible on an arteriogram. In severely ischaemic extremities, particularly after acute thromboses, exploration of the run-off vessel with the strongest Doppler signal in the foot and operative arteriography may be necessary. An intact pedal arch in continuity with the run-off vessel is essential for maintaining long-term patency of the more distal bypasses below the popliteal trifurcation. Patients with significant claudication are also offered an arterial reconstruction if there are no serious medical contraindications and if the distal anastomosis is proximal to the knee joint. In some patients with disabling symptoms and a usable saphenous vein, a below-knee operation can be offered. We do not feel that prosthetic grafts should be placed below the knee for the symptom of claudication.

Choice of procedure

The choice of operation is dependent upon the extent of the obstruction as determined by the arteriogram and the status of the greater saphenous vein. Every effort is made to use autogenous tissue by performing a saphenous vein bypass (SVBP), either reversed or *in situ*, thromboendarterectomy (TE) or a combination of these two procedures. Profundoplasties should be considered when there is a haemodynamically significant stenosis or occlusion of the profunda femoris artery. This is not a common occurrence. Percutaneous transluminal dilatation (PTD) can be used in selected cases. When the greater saphenous vein is not available, another method of reconstruction may be required if a TE is also impossible.

We believe that a poor quality autogenous graft (< 4 mm) is not as good as a prosthetic graft. Our current preference for above-knee reconstruction is the PTFE graft. Life table analysis of the patency rates of above-knee PTFE grafts at 24–36 months compares favourably with autogenous vein[2]. These excellent results do not hold for below-knee grafts to the popliteal artery (PTFE grafts) or crural arteries. Our preference, therefore, for below-knee popliteal and crural reconstruction is the human umbilical vein graft[3].

Preoperative preparation

Patients are given aspirin 325 mg and dipyridamole 75 mg three times a day the day before operation unless there is a history of ulcer disease[4]. Either general, spinal or continuous epidural anaesthesia is required. The lower abdomen, groin, and entire leg and foot are prepared and draped. The foot is placed in an intestinal bag to allow its inspection during the course of the operation. The leg is externally rotated and the knee flexed and held in that position with padding beneath the knee joint.

Autogenous venous bypass procedures

Skin incisions

1

(A) For exposure of the common femoral artery and saphenous vein at the fossa ovalis. This should extend above the anterior superior iliac spine to be certain that the artery can be mobilized at the level of the inguinal ligament for optimal flow.

(B) For exposure of the proximal popliteal artery and distal saphenous vein. This incision is placed two fingerbreadths behind the medial femoral condyle.

(C) For exposure of the distal popliteal artery and distal saphenous vein. This incision is placed just behind the edge of the tibia.

(D) For exposure of the posterior tibial artery. The incision is also just behind the tibia.

For exposure of the anterior tibial and peroneal artery *see Illustration 39.*

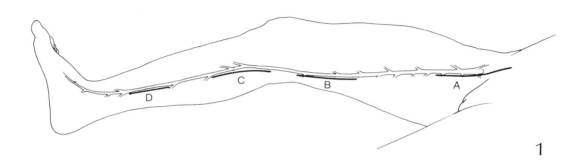

1

OBTAINING AND PREPARING THE SAPHENOUS VEIN FOR REVERSED BYPASS

2

Groin dissection

After making the appropriate incision (*see Illustration 1a*) the saphenous vein is mobilized at the fossa ovalis. The saphenous bulb can be found one fingerbreadth below and one fingerbreadth lateral to the pubic tubercle. It is essential that the dissection of the vein does not create unnecessary skin flaps which may lead to serious postoperative wound complications and jeopardize the reconstruction.

All branches are suture-ligatured with fine silk 1–2 mm from the main vein. Small Hemoclips may be used on the vein remaining in place to save operating time. There is usually a branch of the femoral artery crossing below the bulb here which needs division.

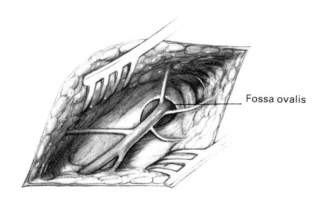

Fossa ovalis

2

3

Leg dissection

The course of the vein is determined and short incisions are made along the medial thigh to mobilize the vein completely. If the identity of the vein opposed to a large branch is in question, the saphenous nerve which runs with the main vein should be followed. An umbilical tape passed around the vein is useful during the dissection for putting gentle traction on the vein. An extra few centimetres of length can be obtained by mobilizing and clamping the common femoral vein, taking a segment of its anterior wall and then repairing the vein with fine Prolene.

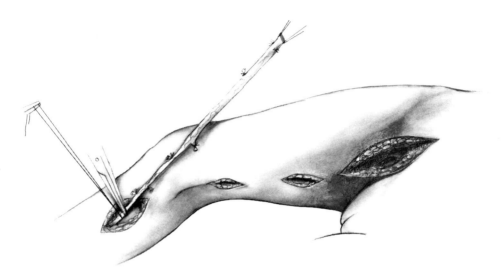

3

4

Distension of the vein

A blunt cannula attached to a 50 ml syringe containing iced, heparinized saline and blood is inserted into the distal end of the resected vein. Alternatively a buffered balanced electrolyte solution containing heparin and papaverine may be used. The proximal end of the vein is occluded by an assistant's fingers. The vein is then gently distended and untwisted by instilling the solution. Unligated branches are secured with 4/0 silk and tears are repaired with 6/0 Prolene, taking care not to narrow the vein by incorporating distant adventitia with the suture. Ocular magnification (2.5×) is useful in preparing the vein. The vein is then placed in the solution of choice and stored until the arteries are prepared for anastomosis.

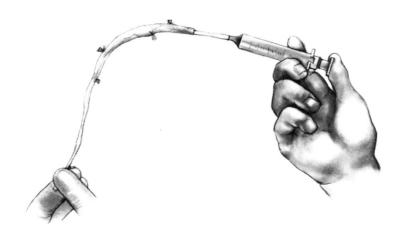

4

EXPOSURE OF THE ARTERIES

5

Exposure of the common femoral artery in the groin

The incision made for exposure of the groin vessels must be above the anterior superior iliac spine to be certain that the common femoral artery can be exposed. The inguinal ligament is identified. The proximal tape should be placed at the level of the superficial iliac circumflex and superficial external pudendal arteries. The best inflow can usually be obtained at this level and whenever possible this should be the level of the proximal anastomosis.

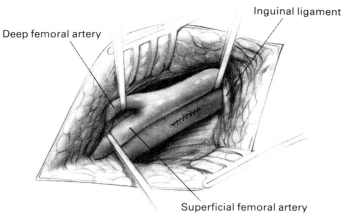

Deep femoral artery

Inguinal ligament

Superficial femoral artery

5

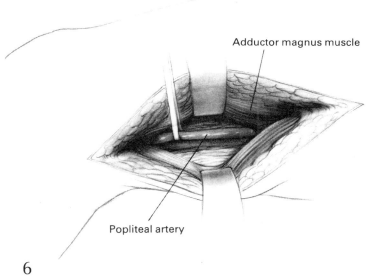

Adductor magnus muscle

Popliteal artery

6

6

Exposure of popliteal artery proximal to knee joint

This incision has already been made for vein harvest. It is two fingerbreadths behind the medial femoral condyle and carried proximally for a distance of 15 cm. The deep fascia anterior to the sartorius muscle is incised. The popliteal artery can be found just beyond the tendon of the adductor magnus muscle. A venous plexus often surrounds the artery which requires ligation. The artery is then mobilized to the level of the knee, preserving all major branches.

When an incision has not been made for vein harvest the suprapatellar popliteal artery can be mobilized with less dissection by making the skin incision immediately over the sartorius muscle.

7

Exposure of popliteal artery distal to knee joint

The skin incision is made over the posterior border of the tibia from the level of the knee joint distally for 15 cm. The crural fascia and semitendinosus tendon is divided. The gastrocnemius muscle is retracted posteriorly to expose the fatty popliteal fossa and neurovascular bundle. Occasionally the medial tendons of the gastrocnemius muscle will have to be divided to provide exposure to a deeply situated artery. The popliteal artery can now be mobilized to the level of its trifurcation.

To expose the tibioperoneal trunk the soleus muscle and the crossing veins must be divided over the distal popliteal artery. Careful dissection is required as these veins are fragile and easily torn. Control should be obtained with suture ligatures. Hemoclips should be avoided in this area. Once the veins are divided the take-off of the anterior tibial artery can be seen and the tibioperoneal trunk can be mobilized.

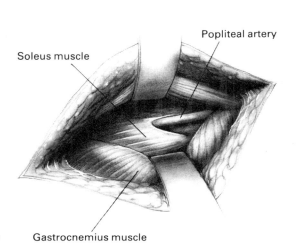

Soleus muscle

Popliteal artery

Gastrocnemius muscle

7

8

Exposure of the tibial arteries

The posterior tibial artery can be exposed by an incision behind the posteromedial border of the tibia. The soleus muscle is retracted posteriorly. As with all tibial artery dissections the artery must be freed from a surrounding venous plexus and its pair of accompanying veins. The anterior tibial and peroneal arteries are best exposed laterally (*see accompanying illustration*).

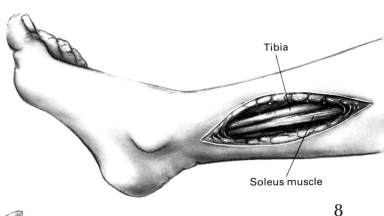

Tibia

Soleus muscle

8

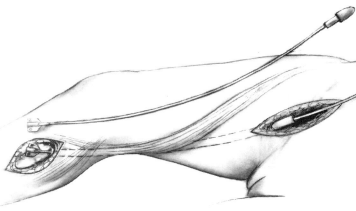

9

TUNNELLING OF THE VEIN

9

Passing the tunneller

The vein graft can be placed in the tunnel vacated by the saphenous vein or in the anatomical tunnel of the superficial femoral artery. We prefer the latter. The tunneller we use is a two-part 50 cm long, slightly curved hollow steel tube with a rod which has one coned end and one flattened end containing two suture holes. It is passed from the popliteal space beneath the sartorius muscle into the groin along the course of the superficial femoral artery. It is important not to put the tunneller through the adductor magnus muscle along the course of the popliteal artery. It is preferable to pass the tunneller prior to administering systemic heparin.

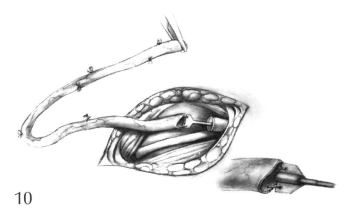

10

10

Passage of vein through tunneller

Insertion of a twisted venous bypass graft will result in early thrombosis. It is important therefore that the vein not twist as it goes through the tunneller. The vein should be distended and untwisted and reorientated to be absolutely certain that the valves are reversed. The groin (inflow) end is then sewn to the two holes in the flattened end of the tunnel rod and the vein is pulled through the metal tube into the groin. The tunneller is now withdrawn over the rod and vein. Heparinized saline is flushed through the vein to check once again for twists.

ANASTOMOSES

Before performing the arterial anastomoses 100 u/kg of heparin sodium are given intravenously.

11

Preparation of the vein for anastomosis

The adventitia on the top of the vein is grasped with a fine clamp. It is important to remove excess adventitia to prevent stenosis of the anastomosis caused by inadvertent gathering of excess distant adventitia. A longitudinal cut 1.5 times the vein diameter is made in the opposite wall of the vein with fine scissors.

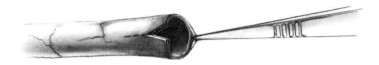

11

12

Arteriotomy and beginning the anastomosis

We begin the distal anastomosis first so that the graft can be manipulated easily. A longitudinal arteriotomy twice the diameter of the vein to be used is made. If the host vessel is thick walled traction sutures in the middle of each side are sometimes helpful. A vascular forceps is inserted into the vein and opened. This allows precise suturing of the heel of the vein graft. A central horizontal mattress stitch is placed which passes from outside to inside vein and inside to outside artery with each needle. We prefer 5/0 or 6/0 double-ended polypropylene. Because this is a monofilament suture several sutures can be taken before the vein and artery are approximated.

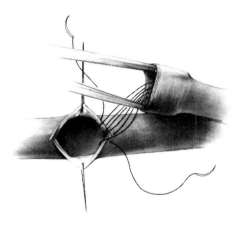

12

13

The distal suture

After the heel suture has been carried midway along the course of the anastomosis a toe suture is placed which approximates the tip of the vein to the distal end of the arteriotomy. This suture is placed from outside to inside vein and inside to outside artery.

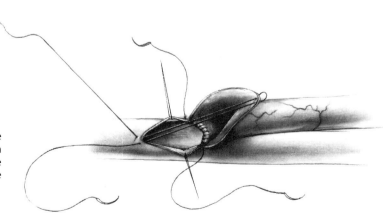

13

Completion of anastomosis

14

The heel suture is then continued toward the toe of the anastomosis as a simple over-and-over stitch. It is important to incorporate all layers of both vein and artery with the suture. The assistant plays an important role as his forceps grasp the adventitia to hold the vein edge away from the arterial edge. This allows the operator to visualize the needle as it passes through the intima of vein and artery and prevents gathering of distant adventitia in the anastomosis.

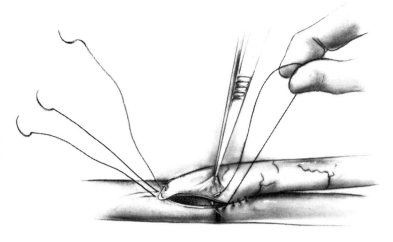

14

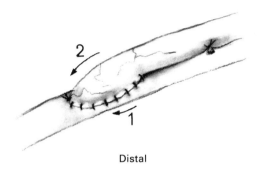

Distal

15

The suturing of the anastomosis always begins at the end of the arteriotomy closest to the centre of the bypass graft. The distal anastomosis begins at the proximal end of the arteriotomy and the proximal anastomosis begins at the distal end of the arteriotomy. This allows for accurate placement of sutures in the critical corners of the anastomosis where the diameter of the entrance to and exit from the graft is determined.

Distal clamps are released first to allow air to escape from the graft. When the graft is full of blood large anastomotic leaks can be repaired before unclamping the femoral artery. Finally, all clamps are removed, heparin is reversed with protamine sulphate and gentle pressure is applied over bleeding areas for 5 minutes.

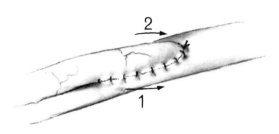

Proximal

15

Completion angiogram and closure

An operative angiogram should be performed if there is any question about the immediate results, e.g. if pulses should be felt and are not, if the foot does not appear revascularized, if the vein appears twisted or if the anastomoses seem stenosed. A 21 gauge butterfly needle is used to inject 20 ml of Angio-Conray into the proximal femoral artery. It is helpful to clamp both proximal to the needle and the deep femoral artery. This ensures that the contrast enters only the vein graft.

After meticulous haemostasis has been achieved closure can be performed. No drains are used. Absorbable synthetic sutures are used for subcutaneous tissue. Staples can be used in the skin.

Prosthetic bypass grafts

Prosthetic bypass grafts can be used for infrainguinal arterial reconstruction but their long-term patency rates do not compare favourably with saphenous vein particularly if the graft crosses the knee joint. When the saphenous vein is not available and arterial reconstruction must be done, two prostheses are currently used most frequently; human umbilical vein and expanded polytetrafluorethylene (PTFE). When the distal anastomo-sis is placed above the knee excellent results can be obtained with both of these grafts. In our experience the human umbilical vein graft works better below the knee but should be reserved for limb salvage. Recent isolated reports of long-term aneurysmal dilatation of the human umbilical vein graft may be a relative contraindication if substantiated in larger series.

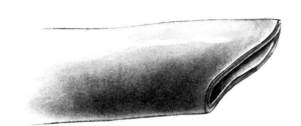

16

16

Use of PTFE

PTFE is an easy graft to handle. Three technical factors merit discussion. First, the length of the graft must be exact. Because no longitudinal expansion is possible redundancy may lead to kinking and occlusion. Second, small vascular needles are important because suture-hole bleeding can be troublesome. If this is a problem, application of microcrystalline collagen is helpful. Third, PTFE should be fashioned as an 'S' for suturing. This eliminates the points at the inflow and outflow of the anastomosis and widens the opening.

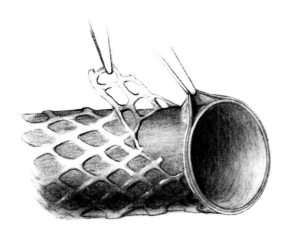

17

17

Use of the human umbilical vein

This graft is more difficult to work with than PTFE. There is a 15 minute soaking process to remove preservative and this is an improvement over previous irrigation procedures recommended by the manufacturer. The most important technical feature in using these grafts is the necessity for partial interrupted suture technique at the heel and toe of the anastomosis. It is important that full-thickness sutures be placed in the graft and to ensure this the needle must pass from inside to outside graft. Because the needle should also be passed from inside to outside the artery interrupted sutures with double-armed needles are essential. Once the anastomosis is set up the sides can be sewn as simple over-and-over sutures. The reason for this technical modification is the tendency of the two layers of the umbilical vein graft to separate and the possibility of creating a graft dissection if flow is allowed in between the separated layers.

Femoropopliteal thromboendarterectomy with patch graft

18

Exposure of distal femoral and proximal popliteal arteries

The longitudinal skin incision is made along the anterior border of the sartorius muscle beginning at the knee joint and carried proximally for 20 cm. The adductor magnus tendon and its proximal membranous extension are divided near their insertions to expose the distal femoral and proximal popliteal artery. Care is taken to preserve the saphenous nerve which accompanies the femoral artery in the adductor canal but pierces the adductor magnus aponeurosis to pass along behind the sartorius muscle. The popliteal artery is then mobilized until it is found to be circumferentially soft.

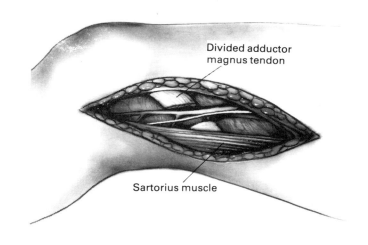

Divided adductor magnus tendon

Sartorius muscle

18

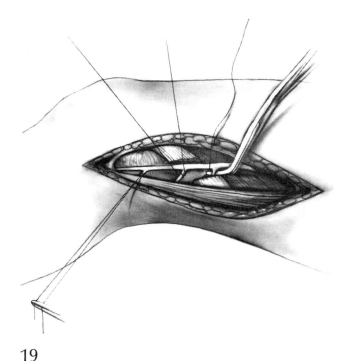

19

19

Control of branches

It is important to obtain control of all the branches of the artery to at least 2 cm beyond the proposed length of the endarterectomy. Otherwise, unnecessary bleeding will occur when the arteriotomy is made or after the atherosclerotic core is removed. Small branches can be controlled by pulling a loop of suture material around the vessel and placing moderate tension on the suture. Atraumatic vascular clamps are used to occlude other vessels.

20

Arteriotomies and developing endarterectomy plane

A superficial longitudinal incision is initially made at the site of the severest disease which is usually at the level of the adductor tendon. The incision is deepened until the yellow atherosclerotic core is identified. This is usually within the media of the artery and the proper plane is reached when the core can be easily bluntly dissected away from the outer wall of the artery. A blunt dissector is used to develop the plane proximally, distally and around the core. The core is divided between two sutures which are gently tied to compress but not cut through the core.

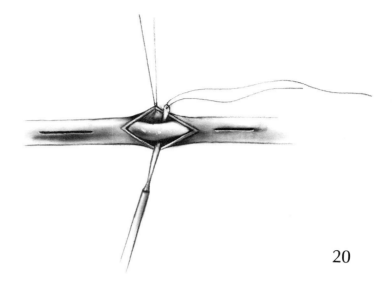

20

21

Distal dissection

The plane of dissection is carried distally to a point where the plaque ends or the core becomes adherent to the outer wall of the artery and is then carefully incised. The endarterectomy should end distally within clear view of the arteriotomy even if it needs to be extended. This allows careful termination of the dissection and incision of the core at a point where it is adherent to the outer wall of the artery.

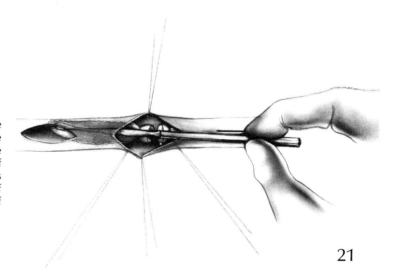

21

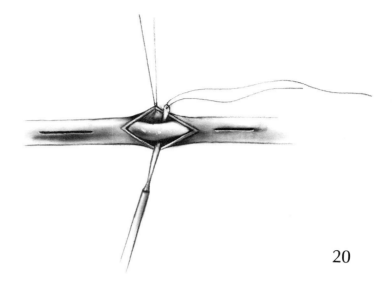

22

22

Tacking of intima distally

It is extremely important that the intima be tightly adherent to the media at the distal end of the endarterectomy to prevent the raising of a flap of tissue which could obstruct the vessel. If there is any question about the adherence, three or four sutures with double-ended needles are used to tack the intima to the arterial wall.

23

Proximal dissection

A ring stripper is then passed around the core and advanced in the plane of cleavage in the media in a proximal direction. It is moved proximally by a combination of rotary and gently pushing movements. Gentle traction can also be applied to the suture attached to the inner core which had been passed through the ring with the endarterectomized specimen. A straight haemostat is used to crush the vessel at the proximal extent of the endarterectomy. The crushing will separate the intima from the atherosclerotic core and the specimen can be easily removed. It is not necessary to tack the intima to the arterial wall proximally. Care must be taken when separating a calcified plaque to prevent adventitial tearing and haemorrhage. Also when using this semiclosed technique it is easy to leave loose flaps of media which can embolize or thrombose the vessel.

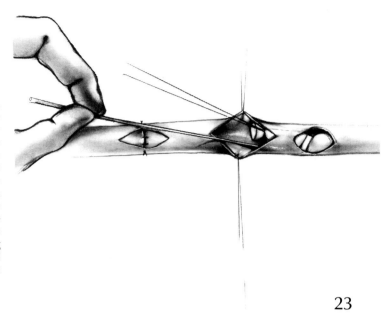

23

24

Patch grafting distal arteriotomy

A patch graft is used to cover the distal arteriotomy to ensure a widely patent outflow from the endarterectomized vessel. A small rectangular piece of vein is obtained, preferably from the arm rather than disturb the saphenous vein. The·width of the vein should be no greater than one-half the diameter of the artery. Mattress sutures are placed in the four tips of the patch and secured. The patch is completed by sewing each corner stitch to another. Securing the corner sutures prevents purse-stringing of the angioplasty.

A continuous everting stitch is run between the stay sutures. A monofilament synthetic suture material is preferred which avoids gathering of the adventitia of the vein.

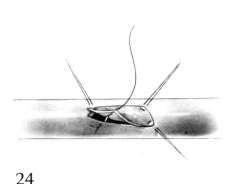

24

25

Completed closures

The middle and proximal arteriotomies are closed with a simple over-and-over stitch between proximal and distal stay sutures. The completed rectangular patch on the distal arteriotomy causes localized enlargement of the arterial lumen and prevents stenosis at the critical distal end of the endarterectomy.

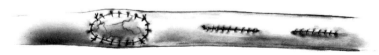

25

Profundoplasty

26

Incision and exposure

There are two varieties of profunda femoris occlusive disease: orifice occlusion, which is due to a large posterior common femoral artery plaque, and disease extending down variable lengths of the profunda femoris artery itself. The treatment of each is different and the exploration must reveal the exact type of occlusion.

A generous groin incision is made to expose the common femoral artery at the inguinal ligament. The superficial femoral artery is also mobilized even if occluded because distal exposure of the profunda femoris artery will require retraction medially of the superficial femoral artery.

If the occlusive disease in the profunda femoris artery extends beyond its orifice the crossing veins must be divided to achieve more distal exposure. The dissection of the profunda femoris artery must proceed until all obvious occlusive disease ends. This often means mobilizing the artery down to its third perforating branch.

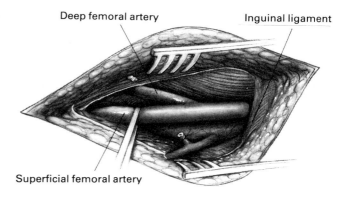

Deep femoral artery   Inguinal ligament

Superficial femoral artery

26

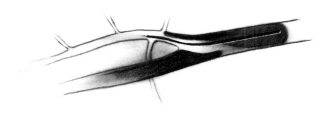

27

27

Arteriotomy for localized lesions

The circumferential or posterior atherosclerotic plaques frequently are localized to the distal common femoral artery and the profunda femoris artery proximal to its medial and lateral circumflex femoral branches. The longitudinal arteriotomy incision is made along the anterior wall of the common femoral artery and carried down the profunda femoris artery to at least 1 cm beyond the palpable plaque.

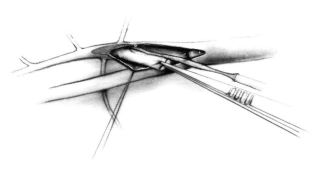

28

28

Endarterectomy of localized lesion

A plane of dissection is established within the media of the vessel and the atherosclerotic core removed under direct vision. Proximally the lesion is separated from the normal artery by the prior application of a straight haemostat. Distally the endarterectomy is ended by sharply incising the intima at a point where it is adherent to the media.

29

Tacking of the intima distally

It is very important that intima at the distal end of the endarterectomy be tightly apposed to the media or a flap can be raised that obstructs the vessel or serves as a nidus for a thrombus. If there is any question about the adherence of the intima and media, double-ended sutures can be passed through the intima and media from within the vessel and tied on the outside of the vessel.

30

Arteriotomy for extensive lesions

The atherosclerotic lesions may extend beyond the circumflex femoral arteries and the first or even second branches of the profunda femoris artery. One short longitudinal incision is made in the common femoral artery and a second incision is made in the profunda femoris artery, making sure to carry it at least 1 cm beyond the palpable plaque.

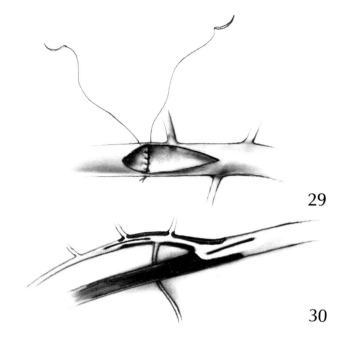

29

30

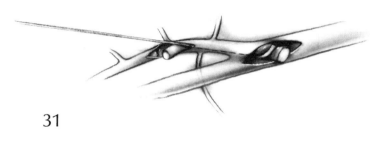

31

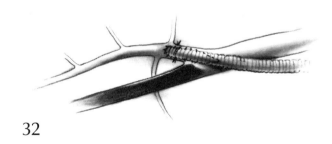

32

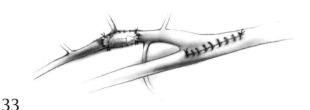

33

31

Endarterectomy of extensive lesion

A plane of dissection is established through the distal arteriotomy in the profunda femoris artery and the endarterectomy ended distally by sharply incising the intima where it becomes adherent. A ring stripper is then used to remove the core to the level of the proximal arteriotomy.

32

Closure of the common femoral arteriotomy incision

The incision in the common femoral artery can be used for the anastomosis of the distal end of an aortofemoral bypass graft or for the proximal anastomosis of a femoropopliteal bypass graft.

33

Closure of profunda femoris vessel

A patch graft, perferably of autogenous vein or disobliterated superficial femoral artery (if occluded), should always be used to cover the incision in the profunda femoris artery to ensure its wide patency (see *Illustration 25*). A patch graft may also be used for covering the incision in the common femoral artery but a simple over-and-over stitch between two stay sutures is usually sufficient.

The distal bypass

IN SITU SAPHENOUS VEIN TECHNIQUE

Our preference for bypasses to the crural vessels is the *in situ* saphenous vein technique[5]. A preoperative phlebogram is useful in locating anomalies and valve sites.

34

Groin incision

A groin incision is made to expose the saphenofemoral junction. The saphenous vein is dissected to expose all branches which are individually ligated with fine silk.

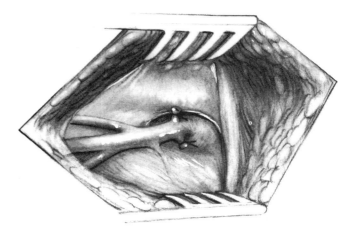

34

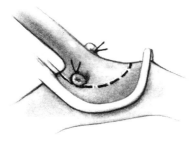

35

35

Division of saphenous femoral junction

After the patient has been heparinized, a vascular clamp is applied to the common femoral vein and the saphenous vein is transected. This manoeuvre provides an extra centimetre of length which allows the saphenous vein to reach the common femoral artery. The common femoral vein is then repaired with fine polypropylene sutures.

Preparation of the vein

36

There are numerous ways to reverse the valves. Early attempts employed a vein stripper forced into the vein from the cut saphenofemoral end. This bluntly disrupted the valves. This method works but is traumatic to the vein and has been replaced by other, more delicate procedures.

The first valve is usually within 5 cm of the saphenofemoral junction. The vein is intussuscepted and the valve leaflets incised under direct vision. A Garrett dilator can be inserted into the vein and this should pass easily down to the first major branch. At this point the vein is prepared for anastomosis.

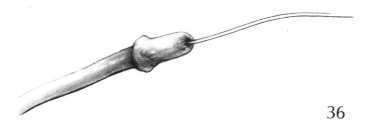

36

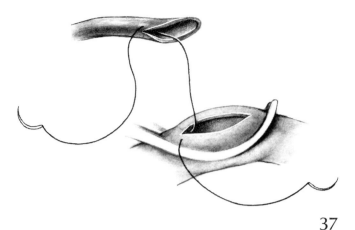

37 & 38

Excess adventitia is trimmed away and the corners of the vein are rounded out. A clamp is placed around the common femoral artery and the anastomosis is constructed as described above.

37

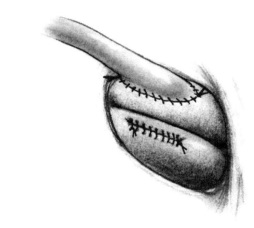

38

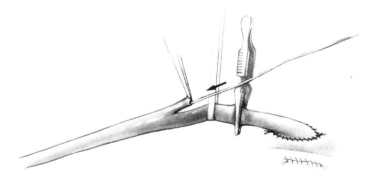

39

39

Clamps are released and the vein is allowed to fill. Pulsatile flow will be felt up to the next competent valve, which will be at a branch. The branch is dissected, the vein clamped and the branch is dilated with Garrett dilators to accommodate the Leather valvulotome available from American V. Mueller. This instrument will cut the valves without damaging the vein. This manoeuvre is repeated until a suitable length of vein is available.

TECHNIQUE FOR GRAFTING TO THE PERONEAL ARTERY

40

Exposure of the peroneal artery

The peroneal artery can be exposed medially through the popliteal space or laterally after resection of the midportion of the fibula. We prefer the latter approach because it gives better, easier exposure and because the artery tends to be less diseased at the midcalf level. The leg is rotated internally and the knee flexed. A 15 cm incision is made directly over the fibula.

41

The musculotendinous attachments to the fibula are incised with electrocautery and, using a large right-angled clamp, an umbilical tape is placed around the bone. The manoeuvre must be done with great care because the peroneal artery and veins can be damaged if one does not stay right on the bone. The umbilical tape can be used to finish the dissection of the fibula by a sawing motion. The bone segment is removed with a Gigli saw.

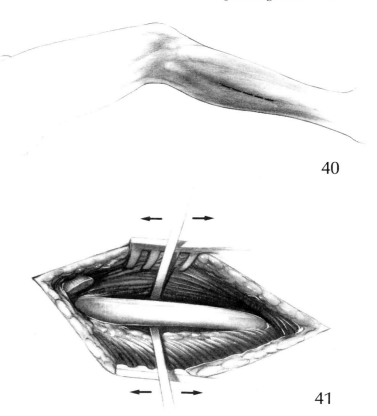

40

41

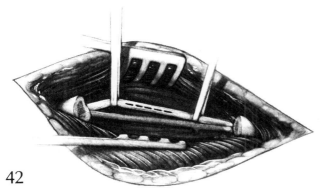

42

42

The peroneal artery is dissected from its surrounding venous plexus with great care. The veins are delicate and should be controlled with fine silk ligatures. Soft vessel loops are placed around the peroneal artery.

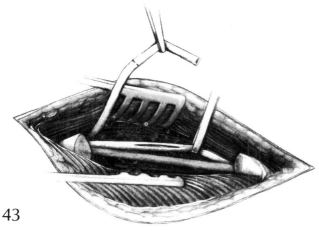

43

43

Making a tunnel

The incision used to expose the saphenous vein below the knee is deepened and the fascia incised to give access to the interosseous membrane. A tunnel is created by finger dissection medially and laterally. A Kelley clamp can be used to pierce the membrane. The vein is brought into the lateral space. The bulldog clip is removed to ensure good inflow.

44

Completion of operation

The anastomosis is constructed with 7/0 polypropylene suture. A completion angiogram is always done. Large arteriovenous communications should be ligated. Heparin is reversed and the wounds closed in layers. A postoperative knee splint is used for 4–5 days.

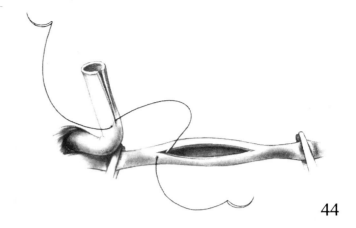

44

Postoperative care

After any arterial procedure on the lower extremity, particularly if the knee joint is crossed, it is important that for a period of 2 weeks the patient should not sit for longer than a few minutes at a time. Patients are allowed to lie down or to be up walking. Elevation of the leg and use of elastic support is prescribed for those patients who develop oedema. Perioperative cephalosporins are given for 3 days. No anticoagulants are used, but antiplatelet therapy is employed in a dose of dipyridamole 75 mg three times a day and aspirin 325 mg three times a day. If prosthetic grafts are used to cross the knee joint we use a posterior splint to prevent knee flexion for the first 5 postoperative days.

References

1. DeWeese, J. A., Rob, C. G. Autogenous venous graft ten years later. Surgery 1977; 82: 775–784

2. Bergan, J. J., Veith, F. J., Bernhard, V. M. et al. Randomization of autogenous vein and polytetrafluoroethylene grafts in femoral-distal reconstruction. Surgery 1982; 92: 921–930

3. Dardik, H., Ibrahim, I. M., Sussman, B. C., Kahn, M., Dardick, I. Glutaraldehyde-tanned human umbilical vein graft. In: Stanley, J. C. et al., eds. Biologic and synthetic vascular prostheses. New York. Grune and Stratton, 1982; 445–465

4. Green, R. M., Roedersheimer, L. R., DeWeese, J. A. Effects of aspirin and dipyridamole on expanded polytetrafluoroethylene graft patency: A randomized, double-blind clinical trial. Surgery 1982; 92: 1016–1026

5. Leather, R. P., Shah, D. M., Karmody, A. M. Intrapopliteal arterial bypass for limb salvage: increased patency and utilization of the saphenous vein used 'in-situ'. Surgery 1981; 90: 1000–1008

Illustrations by Anita Matthews and Robert Wabnitz

Arterial embolectomy

James A. DeWeese MD, FACS
Professor and Chairman, Division of Cardiothoracic Surgery,
University of Rochester Medical Center, Rochester, New York, USA

Preoperative

Indication

With rare exceptions surgical intervention is indicated whenever the diagnosis of arterial embolism to the upper or lower extremity is suspected. At the present time the risk of the operation itself is practically nil and there is an excellent chance of improving distal circulation in all but the most advanced cases. This more aggressive approach to the problem of arterial embolism is warranted owing to two factors: the increased familiarity of surgeons with the mobilization of major arteries and with the making of and proper closure of an arteriotomy; and the availability of the Fogarty balloon catheter, which allows removal of almost all emboli and thrombi from the arteries of the aorta and lower extremity through an arteriotomy in the femoral artery in the groin made under local anaesthesia. The procedure is also indicated in many patients with embolic obstruction of visceral arteries such as the carotid, renal or mesenteric vessels.

Classically, arterial emboli occur in patients with rheumatic heart disease and atrial fibrillation, or in patients with arteriosclerotic heart disease and atrial fibrillation, or in the patient with a recent myocardial infarction. Patients may embolize for other reasons, and any patient with sudden onset of severe limb-threatening ischaemia should not be denied a groin exploration under local anaesthetic because of age, senility or chronic illness. A patient with a viable limb is always happier and easier to manage, even if he is bedridden.

The symptoms of arterial embolus in order of increasing severity include: sudden onset of claudication, numbness, coldness, rest pain and inability to move the extremity. Similarly, the signs in order of increasing severity include: loss of pulse, coldness, pallor, anaesthesia, paralysis, hard and tender muscles and mottled cyanosis.

The time from onset of symptoms should not determine whether or not an operation should be performed. A patient with an embolus without significant propagation of thrombosis and with good collateral circulation may be seen several days after onset of symptoms and still have a localized problem which can be treated successfully with extraction of the embolus.

Preoperative evaluation

A rapid cardiac evaluation should be obtained and appropriate treatment should be started before surgery. The operation should not be delayed, however, for lengthy evaluations and treatment which can be performed following the operation.

A preoperative trial of conservative care is rarely, if ever, indicated today. But heparin may be commenced as soon as the diagnosis has been made.

The operation

1

Preoperative preparation

Both groins and entire legs are prepared and draped. Both feet are enclosed in an intestinal bag to allow direct observation of pulses and appearance of the foot. Local anaesthesia is usually sufficient. Almost all emboli of the lower extremity, including those at the aortic bifurcation can now be removed through an arteriotomy in the common femoral artery with the use of the Fogarty catheter.

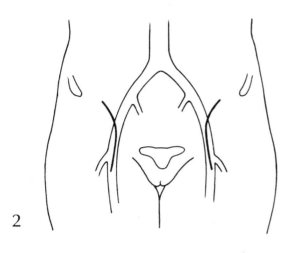

2

3

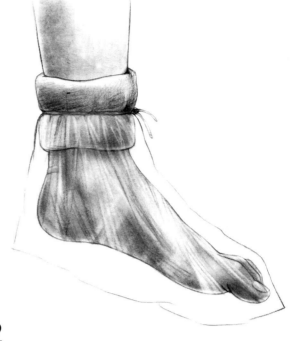

2

1

The incision

The incision begins at the midpoint but one fingerbreadth above the inguinal ligament and is carried medially along the inguinal ligament to a point two fingerbreadths lateral to the pubic tubercle, from which it is extended distally along the course of the femoral artery.

3

Exposure of vessels

The lower edge of the inguinal ligament is identified and dissection carried distally along the femoral artery, which can be found two fingerbreadths lateral to the pubic tubercle. Medially, the saphenous vein is seen but only its superior and lateral branches need be divided and ligated. The common femoral artery is mobilized from just distal to the inguinal ligament to its bifurcation into the deep and superficial femoral artery. Tapes are passed around the common, deep and superficial femoral arteries. The superficial circumflex iliac and external pudendal branches can be controlled with an untied suture which has been thrown twice around the vessel.

COMMON FEMORAL EMBOLUS

The iliac and femoral pulse above the embolus may be bounding, but distal pulses are absent and the temperature and colour changes occur at knee level.

4

Embolectomy

A short arteriotomy is made and stay sutures placed in the edges to avoid repeated handling of the vessel with forceps. The arteriotomy incision should be longitudinal. The embolus may be removed quite easily with forceps and flushing. Completeness of the embolectomy cannot be judged by antegrade bloodflow alone. Non-obstructing thrombi may still be present at the iliac or popliteal level. Fogarty catheters should be passed up the common femoral artery and down both deep and superficial femoral arteries.

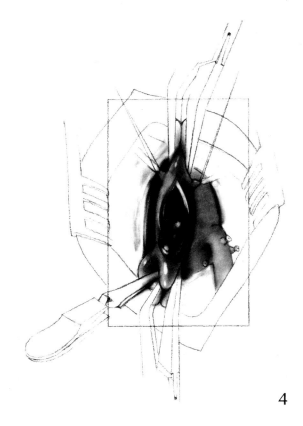

4

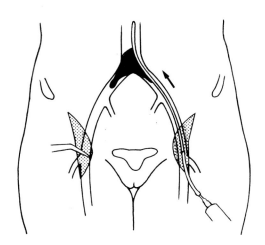

5

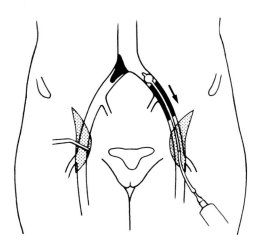

6

AORTIC EMBOLUS

Patients present with no pulses palpable below the aorta. Colour and temperature changes occur in the mid-thigh.

5

Bilateral incisions

It is important to expose the common femoral artery in both groins. Both common femoral arteries are occluded and a Fogarty catheter with the balloon collapsed is passed up one iliac artery.

Aortic embolectomy

6

The balloon is distended and the catheter removed. Usually the saddle embolus will break into smaller pieces during this manoeuvre and becomes extruded through the arteriotomy incision.

7

The catheter is now passed up the opposite iliac artery and further embolus removed. The catheters should be repeatedly passed until no further clot is found. Excessive blood-loss is prevented by occluding the vessel around the catheter with the tape when the catheter is being passed.

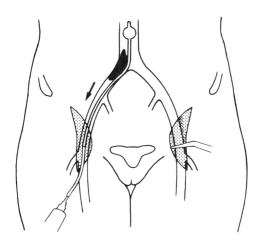

7

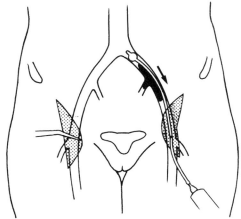

8

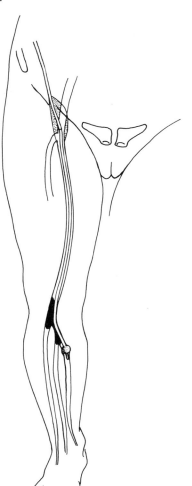

9

ILIAC EMBOLUS

No femoral pulse is present and temperature changes occur at mid-thigh level.

8

Iliac embolectomy

Exposure of the opposite groin is advisable since it is possible to push portions of the embolus into the aorta from whence it could embolize to the opposite leg. The Fogarty catheter is inserted to the common iliac artery, the balloon distended and the catheter removed.

POPLITEAL EMBOLUS

The popliteal pulse may be bounding above the embolus. The temperature changes occur at mid-calf level.

9

Popliteal embolectomy

The Fogarty catheter is passed well down the posterior tibial artery, the balloon distended and the catheter removed. The balloon must not be disturbed too much in smaller vessels since plaques may be cracked or the vessel ruptured. The person blowing up the balloon should be the one to remove the catheter, since he can best judge whether the balloon is under- or over-distended.

TIBIAL-PERONEAL EMBOLI

Although popliteal emboli can usually be satisfactorily removed from the groin it may be necessary to approach the popliteal artery and its trifurcation directly. A general or spinal anaesthesia is required.

10

The incision

It is helpful to have the lower leg flexed 90° and externally rotated. The incision begins one fingerbreadth posterior to the medial malleolus and is extended distally parallel to the posterior border of the tibia.

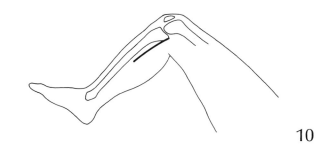

10

11

Exposure

The deep fascia is divided. The gracilis and semitendinosus tendons may be retracted or divided. The medial head of the gastrocnemius muscle is retracted posteriorly.

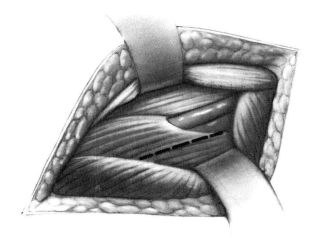

11

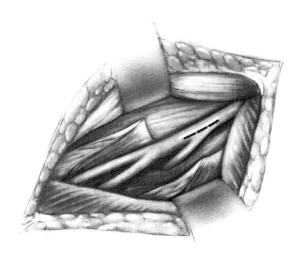

12

Embolectomy

The soleus muscle is incised over the popliteal artery which provides exposure of the anterior tibial as well as the posterior tibial and peroneal arteries. Embolectomy from any of the three vessels can be accomplished through an incision in the distal popliteal artery at the level of the anterior tibial vessel.

12

Intraoperative evaluation

Immediate evaluation of the operative result is possible by visualization of the foot and palpation of the pulses through the intestinal bag. If there is any question as to the patency of the vessels an arteriogram should be obtained (*see* chapter on 'Arteriography', pp. 15–23).

Postoperative care

Anticoagulation with coumarin drugs is begun the day of surgery. There is a significant in-hospital mortality rate for patients requiring embolectomy. The deaths are usually related to the underlying process responsible for the emboli, such as valvular heart disease and myocardial infarctions, and close medical supervision is required.

Further reading

Darling, R. C., Austen, W. G., Linton, R. R. Arterial embolism. Surgery, Gynecology and Obstetrics 1967; 124: 106–114

Fogarty, T. J., Cranley, J. J. Catheter technique for arterial embolectomy. Annals of Surgery 1965; 161: 325–330

Green, R. M., DeWeese, J. A., Rob, C. G. Arterial embolectomy: before and after the Fogarty catheter. Surgery 1975; 77: 24–33

Gupta, S. K., Samson, R. H., Veith, F. J. Embolectomy of the distal part of the popliteal artery. Surgery, Gynaecology and Obstetrics. 1981; 153: 254–256

Illustrations by Anita Matthews

Management of peripheral arterial aneurysms

John J. Ricotta MD
Assistant Professor of Surgery, University of Rochester
School of Medicine and Dentistry, Rochester, New York, USA

Introduction

Although most common in the aortic position, aneurysmal changes can occur throughout the arterial tree and are encountered with some frequency by the vascular surgeon. These aneurysms may lead to thrombosis, distal embolization, rupture or compression of adjacent structures. In most cases, resection is recommended if it is felt that the patient will tolerate operation.

Femoral artery aneurysms

This is the most common site of aneurysmal degeneration after the aortoiliac system. Aneurysms are most often atherosclerotic although they may be mycotic, iatrogenic or anastomotic. Anastomotic aneurysms have been reported following 1–2 per cent of aortofemoral reconstructions. This is a problem that is seen with increasing frequency.

ATHEROSCLEROTIC ANEURYSMS

1

Atherosclerotic aneurysms may involve only the common femoral artery or extend into the superficial and deep femoral arteries as well. These aneurysms present as a pulsatile groin mass and if ignored may go on to thrombosis or be the cause of distal embolization. Rupture of an atherosclerotic femoral aneurysm is rare. The aneurysm is approached through a standard inguinal incision carried high and laterally along the inguinal ligament so that proximal control can be gained at the external iliac artery. Distally control of the superficial and profunda femoris arteries is obtained individually.

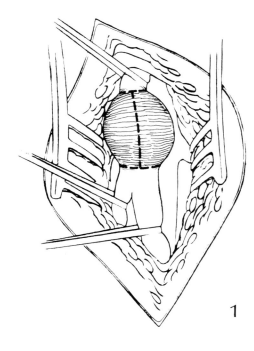

1

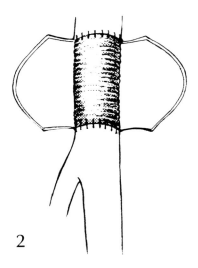

2

2

Graft replacement

After heparinization the aneurysm is opened. The aneurysmal segment is replaced by an interposition graft placed in the bed of the aneurysm. This is usually Dacron since autogenous vein is rarely of sufficient calibre. The proximal anastomosis is performed end-to-end using fine monofilament suture. Distally the anastomosis is performed at the common femoral bifurcation, end-to-end, to include the origin of the superficial femoral artery and all profunda branches.

3

TREATMENT OF EXTENSIVE FEMORAL ARTERY ANEURYSMS

If aneurysmal change extends past the common femoral bifurcation, the superficial and femoral arteries will need to be reimplanted separately. All of the femoral outflow should be preserved. This can be done by attaching the profunda femoris to the side of a straight graft or occasionally by using a small bifurcated graft.

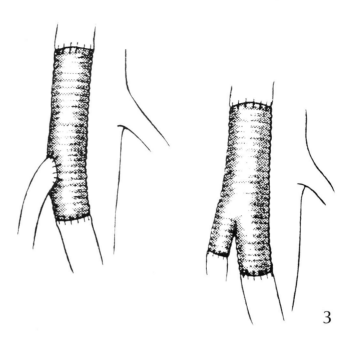

3

EXPOSURE OF ANASTOMOTIC ANEURYSMS

4

Anastomotic aneurysms are most common in the groin and may follow aortofemoral or femoropopliteal grafting. In the absence of infection, these aneurysms are due to defects in suture, graft material or native artery. For the most part these are false aneurysms. They present special problems since there is always scarring present in the area from previous surgery and the outflow is often limited due to a superficial femoral occlusion. These aneurysms are approached through a groin incision. Occasionally proximal control may be obtained extraperitoneally through a separate incision in the iliac fossa. Proximal control of the graft and native vessel is obtained but there is no attempt to secure distal control.

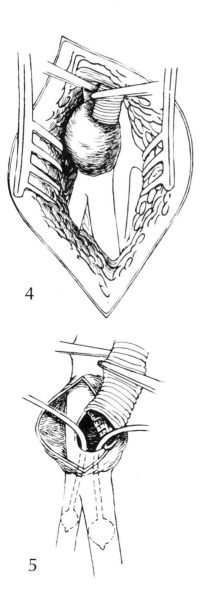

4

5

5

Distal control

After heparinization the aneurysm is opened and distal control is obtained from within the vessel using No. 3 or No. 4 Fogarty catheters. By introducing these catheters to occlude the orifices of the superficial and deep femoral vessels, the chance of damaging these vessels or adherent veins is minimized. Balloons are kept inflated by attaching three-way stopcocks. After control is obtained, the false aneurysm is resected. A new segment of graft is interposed, if necessary, although occasionally the anastomosis may be redone using the original graft segment after some mobilization. Both graft and artery should be debrided back to healthy tissue and the anastomosis must not be under tension. Failure to ensure this may lead to recurrent aneurysm formation.

Popliteal artery aneurysms

These are the second most common peripheral aneurysms. They are often bilateral and quite often associated with aneurysms in other locations (i.e. aorta, femoral). They may be diagnosed by physical examination, angiography or ultrasound (most reliable). Recognition depends on an awareness of their existence by the examining physician. These aneurysms rarely rupture but may cause distal ischaemia by thrombosis, or distal embolization. Large aneurysms may compress the popliteal vein or peroneal nerve. Incidence of amputation may approach 30 per cent in symptomatic popliteal aneurysms and this has led to the dictum that aneurysms greater than 2 cm in diameter should be operated upon in the good risk patient[1,2]. Popliteal aneurysms can be approached posteriorly or by a medial incision.

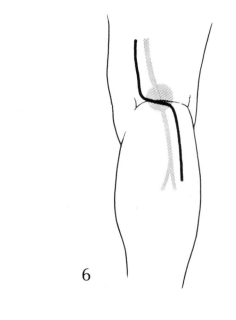

6

6

Posterior approach

The posterior approach avoids transection of any muscle or tendons. The patient is placed prone on the operating table and exposure is achieved through an 'S'-shaped incision, placing the superior limb of the incision medially. The popliteal fascia is opened and the sciatic nerve is retracted. This nerve crosses medial to lateral superficial to the popliteal artery at this level. The proximal popliteal is exposed by retracting the biceps femoris laterally and the hamstring muscles medially; distally the artery is exposed by retracting the head of the gastroenemius muscle. After control is obtained the aneurysm may be resected or bypassed.

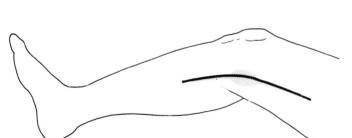

7

7

Medial approach

Although the medial approach may be more traumatic, it is preferred for several reasons. The approach is a familiar one, being identical to that used for femoropopliteal bypass. More important, however, it allows easier exposure of the distal superficial femoral and distal popliteal arteries. Finally, it is better suited for bypass with saphenous vein. The patient is placed supine with the knee in 30° flexion. An incision is made in the lower medial thigh along the anterior border of the sartorius muscle. The popliteal artery is exposed as for femoropopliteal bypass. The tendons of the semimembranosus, semitendinosus, sartorius and gracilis muscles may need to be transected to achieve distal popliteal control.

8

Resection of the aneurysm

Resection or decompression of a popliteal aneurysm is indicated when the aneurysm has caused compression of adjacent nervous and venous structures. Continuity can be restored by mobilization and primary anastomosis, or use of an interposition graft. Resection of the aneurysm may be difficult because of adherence especially to the popliteal vein. We prefer evacuation of the aneurysm with placement of an interposition graft *in situ*. Saphenous vein is preferred since patency is superior to prosthetic materials.

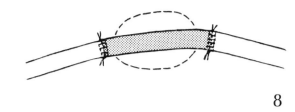

8

9

Exclusion and bypass

We prefer this approach when there are no symptoms of compression, since it avoids extensive dissection of the aneurysm. Proximal and distal control is gained through the medial approach. The artery is ligated immediately proximal and distal to the aneurysm. A bypass of the excluded segment using autogenous vein whenever possible is then performed.

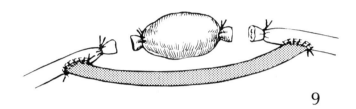

9

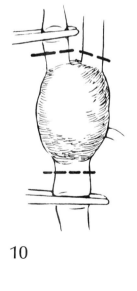

10

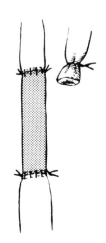

11

Extracranial carotid artery aneurysms

10

These aneurysms are rare and usually present as a mass in the neck or with neurological symptoms due to distal embolization[3]. Whenever possible they should be resected because of their potential for future embolization.

11

Graft replacement

These aneurysms may be treated by resection with primary anastomosis or more commonly an interpositioned saphenous vein graft. The external carotid artery may be sacrificed. A shunt may be employed to maintain flow during grafting as described in the chapter on 'Carotid body tumours' (see pp. 430–434). EEG monitoring is helpful to determine the need for shunt placement. Occasionally, high internal carotid aneurysms may be treated by ligation with or without superficial temporal to middle cerebral bypass.

12

Vertebral artery aneurysms

These aneurysms are rare and usually follow trauma. They are best dealt with by ligation of the proximal vertebral artery or angiographic embolization.

Visceral artery aneurysms

These aneurysms are rare and often asymptomatic. Diagnosis is most commonly made by calcification on a routine abdominal X-ray or at the time of angiography. Treatment varies according to location[4,5,6]. When bypass grafts are used, autogenous saphenous vein is the material of choice.

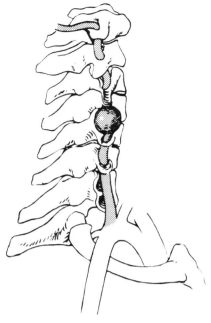

12

13

Splenic artery aneurysms

These are the most commonly reported visceral aneurysms, often noted by crescentic calcification on abdominal films. They are most common in multiparous females. Most of the aneurysms remain asymptomatic. Symptoms are left upper quadrant pain or haemoperitoneum from rupture. Rupture is uncommon except in large aneurysms or in pregnant women. Rupture carries a high mortality and for this reason surgical treatment is recommended for large aneurysms or aneurysms in women of child-bearing age. If the aneurysm is close to the splenic hilum, splenectomy is the procedure of choice. For more proximal aneurysms, exclusion of the aneurysm by ligature is feasible. The spleen may be left *in situ* supplied by the short gastric vessels.

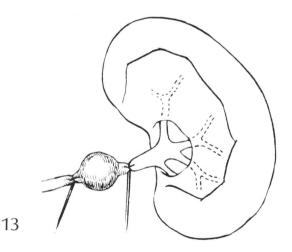

13

14

Hepatic artery aneurysms

These are most frequent in the common hepatic artery but may occur in the intrahepatic location as well. Symptoms include right upper quadrant pain, jaundice due to obstruction by the aneurysms, and haemobilia. Rupture is more common than with splenic aneurysms and has a high mortality. For this reason hepatic artery aneurysms should be resected whenever possible. In the common hepatic artery resection and bypass grafting is the procedure of choice. Intrahepatic aneurysm may be treated by percutaneous embolization.

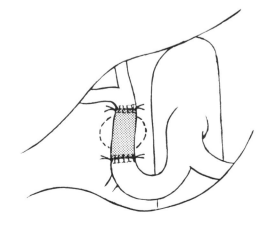

14

15

Renal artery aneurysms

These may be present in the main renal artery, or in the renal hilum. There is little evidence to suggest that renal artery aneurysm in the absence of renal artery stenosis is a significant cause of renovascular disease or hypertension. Nonetheless, occasionally such an aneurysm can be shown to be the source of distal embolization in the kidney. When surgery is indicated, resection and reanastomosis, or aortorenal bypass with exclusion of the aneurysm are the procedures of choice. Distal aneurysms may be dealt with by *ex vivo* bench surgery.

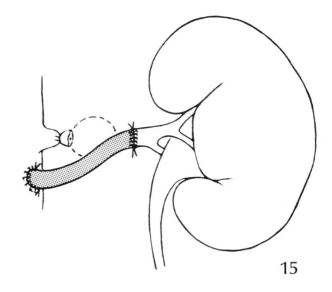

15

16

Coeliac and superior mesenteric artery aneurysms

These aneurysms are rare. When a branch vessel is involved, ligation will often suffice. When the main trunk of the coeliac or superior mesenteric artery is involved, resection with primary anastomosis or interposition grafting is required. Once again, autogenous tissue is the material of choice. Ligation and exclusion of the artery with aortovisceral bypass is also another alternative, and often is technically easier. In this instance, the aortic anastomosis is made end-to-side below the level of the renal artery. It is important that a disease-free segment of the aorta be selected as the site of anastomosis.

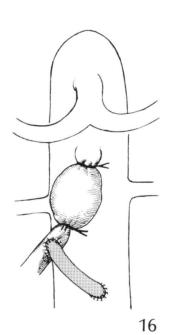

16

References

1. Szilagyi, D. E., Schwartz, R. L., Reddy, D. J. Popliteal arterial aneurysms. Archives of Surgery 1981; 116: 724–728

2. Vermilion, B. D., Kimmins, S. A., Pace, W. G., Evans, W. E. A review of one hundred and forty-seven popliteal aneurysms with long-term follow-up. Surgery 1981; 90: 1009–1014

3. McCollum, C. H., Wheeler, W. G., Noon, G. P., DeBakey, M. E. Aneurysms of the extracranial carotid artery: twenty-one years' experience. The American Journal of Surgery 1979; 137: 196–200

4. Graham, J. M., McCollum, C. H., DeBakey, M. E. Aneurysms of the splanchnic arteries. The American Journal of Surgery 1980; 140: 797–801

5. Busuttil, R. W., Brin, B. J. The diagnosis and management of visceral artery aneurysms. Surgery 1980; 88: 619–624

6. Stanley, J. E., Thompson, N. W., Fry, W. J. Splanchnic artery aneurysms. Archives of Surgery 1970; 101: 689–697

7. Tham, G., Ekelund, L., Herrlin, K., Lindstedt, E. L., Olin, T., Bergentz, S. Renal artery aneurysms: natural history and prognosis. Annals of Surgery 1983; 197: 348–352

Illustrations by Susan Y. Anderson

Popliteal artery entrapment syndrome

Thomas J. Whelan, Jr MD
Professor and Chairman, Department of Surgery,
University of Hawaii, Honolulu, Hawaii, USA

Introduction

Originally considered a rare lesion[1], entrapment of the popliteal artery (and in 12 per cent of cases, the popliteal vein) beneath a musculofascial structure in the popliteal space has been described with increasing frequency. The musculofascial structure is usually the medial head of the gastrocnemius muscle or an accessory head thereof or popliteus muscle or fascial bands deep to the medial head of the gastrocnemius. More recently, cases in which plantaris or semimembranosus has contributed to the entrapment have been reported[2].

Clinical features

The age group in which the lesion becomes symptomatic, in 60 per cent of cases, is below 30 years. Hamming[3] emphasized that, in his vascular clinic, 40 per cent of claudicators under 30 years of age were suffering from complications of this anomaly. Males predominate 9:1. The lesion is often bilateral, at least in 40 per cent of cases. Cases have been reported from all countries of the eastern and western world. The incidence probably ranges from 0.16 to 3.5 per cent. This higher recognized incidence is due to a familiarity with the entity and to reports in two recent papers[4,5]. Gibson[5] described finding the anomaly in 3 of 86 cadavers, in 1 of which the anomaly was bilateral. Bouhoutsos[4] studied approximately 20 000 patients in a Greek military hospital over a 50-month period. The study was prospective and a concerted attempt was made to find these cases: 45 anomalies were discovered in 33 patients, 12 being bilateral.

Symptoms produced by the anomaly are calf claudication or coldness and/or paraesthesias of the foot. Although many cases do not become symptomatic until thrombosis of the entrapped portion of the popliteal artery has occurred, stenosis from mural fibrosis of the artery may precede actual thrombosis and produce symptoms. Temporary kinking and narrowing of the artery from the entrapment when the foot is actively plantar flexed may also produce intermittent symptoms. A small minority, usually in an older age group, have presented with post-stenotic aneurysm formation and a rare patient has developed a markedly ischaemic leg following distal embolism from thrombus in the entrapped artery or in a popliteal artery aneurysm.

The diagnosis is not difficult if the entity is considered. Claudication or other circulatory insufficiency symptoms, occurring in a young male, should alert the physician to the diagnosis. Absence of pedal pulses or a decrease or disappearance of pedal pulses with exercise or with active plantar flexion or passive dorsiflexion is highly suggestive. Doppler ankle pressures in the neutral position with reduction on active plantar flexion or passive dorsiflexion may be helpful although false positive results are possible. Definitive diagnosis is made with arteriography and is not complete unless arteriograms are performed in the neutral position, and in plantar and dorsiflexion. The triad, therefore, of medial deviation of the proximal popliteal artery, segmental occlusion of the mid-popliteal artery when the artery is thrombosed (60 per cent of symptomatic cases), and post-stenotic dilatation, originally felt to be diagnostic of the lesion, must be expanded.

When prospective angiographic studies were done on all persons with ischaemic lower limb symptoms who showed decrease of Doppler pressures at the ankle on passive dorsiflexion of the foot or active plantar flexion, 40 per cent had normal arteriograms in the neutral position. The diagnosis became obvious, with medial displacement of the popliteal artery, upon repeating the angiograms with the foot in either of the above-mentioned positions. The differential diagnosis includes adventitial cystic degeneration of the popliteal artery, arterial embolus and arteritis. Arteriography with the popliteal artery veering away from its normal course in the neutral or stressed arteriograms should lead to the proper diagnosis.

Anatomy

Normal anatomy

1

The normal anatomy is shown through a posterior approach to the popliteal space.

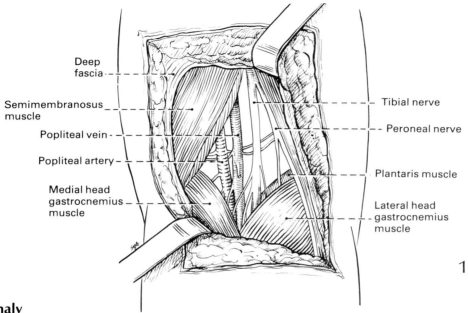

Deep fascia
Semimembranosus muscle
Popliteal vein
Popliteal artery
Medial head gastrocnemius muscle
Tibial nerve
Peroneal nerve
Plantaris muscle
Lateral head gastrocnemius muscle

1

Types of anomaly

The anomaly has been subtyped into four variants, although other types have recently been described[2,4,6].

2 & 3

The most common variants are shown. The main entrapment is beneath a medial head of the gastrocnemius around and medial to which the popliteal artery courses. The only difference between Types 1 and 2 is that in Type 2 the medial head arises more laterally from the back of the femur and the popliteal artery courses straight downwards but still passes medial and beneath the medial head of the gastrocnemius where it is entrapped.

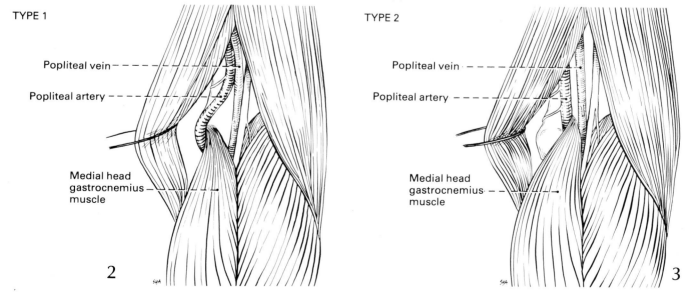

TYPE 1

Popliteal vein
Popliteal artery
Medial head gastrocnemius muscle

2

TYPE 2

Popliteal vein
Popliteal artery
Medial head gastrocnemius muscle

3

4

In Type 3 an accessory slip of the medial head of the gastrocnemius is the entrapping structure.

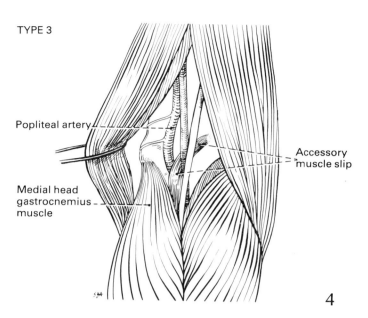

TYPE 3

Popliteal artery

Accessory muscle slip

Medial head gastrocnemius muscle

4

TYPE 4

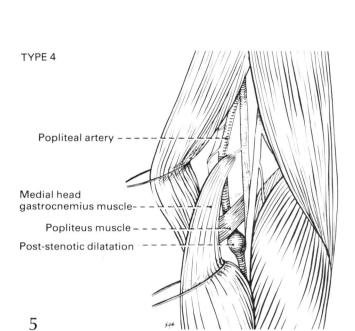

Popliteal artery

Medial head gastrocnemius muscle

Popliteus muscle

Post-stenotic dilatation

5

5

In Type 4 the popliteus or fascial bands entrap the artery. The artery may or may not deviate medially around the medial head of the gastrocnemius but does not appear to be entrapped by this structure. It is in this type that the popliteal vein is most often entrapped.

The plantaris, hypertrophied and displaced caudally and medially, and a combination of semimembranosus, medial head of the gastrocnemius and the plantaris have been shown to cause the entrapment in a few cases recently reported[2].

The operation

6

Incisions

Either the posterior or the medial approach may be used. The posterior approach is preferred[7] as it allows a better definition and identification of the anomaly and lessens the chance of missing it. For most cases, the exposure of the popliteal artery is perfectly adequate. However, if the distal popliteal artery or its trifurcation is involved, there is better exposure via the medial approach. Although saphenous vein harvesting is ideal when the patient is supine for the medial approach, the prone position, necessary for the posterior approach, allows for adequate harvesting either at the ankle or within the medial skin and subcutaneous flap.

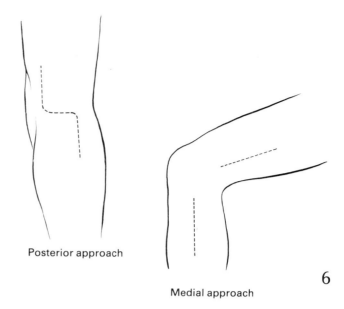

Posterior approach

Medial approach

6

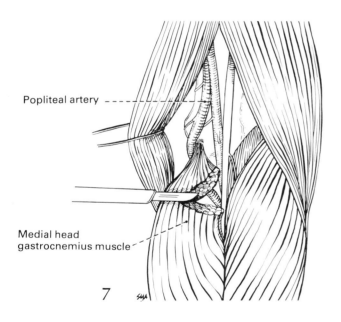

Popliteal artery

Medial head
gastrocnemius muscle

7

7

The entrapment is released by sectioning of the offending muscle(s) or fibrous band.

8

The most common operations performed upon the thrombosed or stenotic popliteal artery are (A) excision and saphenous vein graft replacement[8]; (B) arterial exclusion with vein bypass graft; and (C) thromboendarterectomy with or without vein patch angioplasty.

If symptoms occur prior to structural changes in the entrapped artery, myotomy alone with release of the vessel is sufficient.

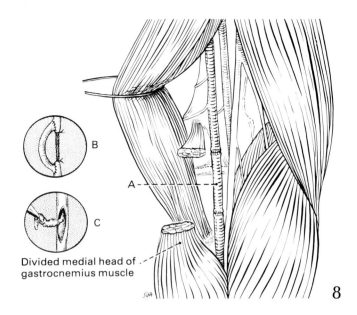

Divided medial head of gastrocnemius muscle

8

Results

Results have been almost uniformly excellent in the over 100 cases which have now been reported.

References

1. Love, J. W., Whelan, T. J. Popliteal artery entrapment syndrome. American Journal of Surgery 1965; 109: 620–624

2. Bouhoutsos, J. Daskalaskis, E. Muscular abnormalities affecting the popliteal vessels. British Journal of Surgery 1981; 68: 501–506

3. Hamming, J. J., Vink, M. Obstruction of the popliteal artery at an early age. Journal of Cardiovascular Surgery 1965; 6: 516–524

4. Bouhoutsos, J. Popliteal artery entrapment syndrome: report of 29 cases. Vascular Surgery 1980; 14: 365–374

5. Gibson, M. H. L., Mills, J. G. Johnson, G. E., Downs, A. R. Popliteal artery entrapment syndrome. Annals of Surgery 1977; 185: 341–348

6. Rich, N. M., Collins, G. J., Jr, McDonald, P. T., Kozloff, L., Clagett, G. P., Collins, J. T. Popliteal vascular entrapment: its increasing interest. Archives of Surgery 1979; 114: 1377–1384

7. Whelan, T. J. Popliteal artery entrapment. In: Rutherford, R. B., ed. Vascular surgery. Philadelphia: Saunders, 1977: 563–568

8. Ferrero, R., Barile, C., Bretto, P., Buzzacchino, A., Ponzio, F. Popliteal artery entrapment syndrome. Report on seven cases. Journal of Cardiovascular Surgery (Torino) 1980; 21: 45–52

Illustrations by Gillian Lee

Management of vascular injuries

Malcolm O. Perry MD
Professor of Surgery, Cornell University Medical College, New York, USA

Aetiology – mechanisms of injury

Although major vascular injuries can be encountered in any civilian setting, the highest incidence is in urban areas where violence is endemic. Penetrating wounds caused by knives and bullets are usually seen, but accidental stab wounds caused by shards of glass or metal also occur. The damage produced by knives or bullets travelling at a low velocity is mainly confined to the wound tract, but high-velocity bullets are associated with blast injury. As the blast cavity collapses, a suction effect is generated which can draw skin, dirt and bits of clothing into the wound. Secondary missiles (bullet fragments or bone splinters) can produce further damage. Such destructive effects may not be suspected from inspection of the skin where, in some cases, rather small wounds are present[1,2].

Motor vehicle accidents are important causes of vascular trauma and victims frequently have multiple injuries. Direct vessel trauma occurs, but often vascular wounds are the result of fractures and dislocations. This is especially likely to occur near joints where the vessels are relatively fixed. Dislocations of the knee, for example, are particularly prone to injure the popliteal artery and similar episodes can damage the brachial or axillary vessels.

Lacerations are seen most often with knife wounds, but contusions, punctures and transections also are encountered. Stretching, angulation and subsequent occlusion are more often seen with fracture dislocations, but the concussive effects of high-velocity missiles can cause such wounds. Immediate vessel disruption and bleeding may not occur, but delayed thrombosis or haemorrhage can lead to ischaemia or false aneurysm formation.

Clinical evaluation

Most arterial injuries can be identified readily because of external haemorrhage or large haematomas. Ischaemia distal to the injury is uncommon with isolated vascular injuries except for wounds of the popliteal and common femoral arteries. Moreover, distal pulses may be intact in up to 20 per cent of patients with acknowledged arterial wounds, although weak or absent distal pulses are important findings[2]. The indications for operative exploration of a suspected vascular wound are summarized as follows:

1. Diminished or absent distal pulse.
2. Persistent arterial bleeding.
3. Large or expanding haematoma.
4. Major haemorrhage with hypotension or shock.
5. Bruit at or distal to suspected site of injury.
6. Injury of anatomically related nerves.

Arteriography can be very useful in the evaluation of potential arterial injuries, especially in patients with multiple pellet wounds, fractures and penetrating injuries of the neck and thoracic outlet. If high-grade, biplane films can be obtained, arteriography presents reliable, although not infallible, evidence regarding the presence or absence of an arterial wound. Moreover, surgical management may be improved by identifying the location and extent of the vascular damage.

Preparation for surgery

Most patients with major vascular wounds require immediate operation, and if haemodynamically unstable they should be taken directly to the operating theatre. If the patient is stable, further diagnostic manoeuvres can be undertaken.

Bleeding is controlled with direct pressure (tourniquets are avoided) and two large-bore intravenous lines secured. Balanced salt solutions are given intravenously while type specific and matched blood is obtained. General anaesthesia is preferred, and special precautions must be taken to avoid extending the damage or dislodging clots in patients with cervical and thoracic wounds. Wide operative fields are prepared since, in patients with wounds in or near the trunk, it may be necessary to enter the abdomen or chest.

General principles

1

Incisions

Vertical incisions are favoured for exposing vascular wounds – they can be extended easily in either direction along the course of the vessel and they are parallel to other neurovascular structures. A vertical incision into the anterior cervical triangle to expose the carotid artery can be extended into a midline sternotomy, for example, or lateral supraclavicular incision as needed. Similarly, a midline abdominal incision can be extended into the sternum or across the costal margin to enter the chest.

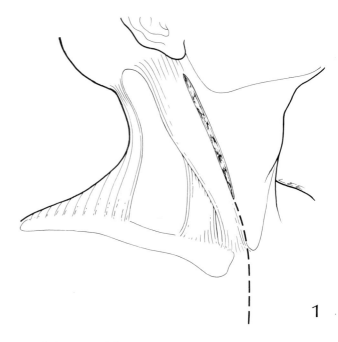

1

Exposure

If the haematoma is large, it is often best to expose the vessels proximally and gain control where the artery is clearly seen. Latex tubing or soft vascular tapes are passed around the vessels and vascular clamps selected. Usually the vascular wound can then be approached safely and the bleeding controlled with direct digital pressure. With multiple injuries, and especially if large veins are involved, temporary proximal and distal vascular occlusion and vigorous suction may be required.

Graft interposition

Resection and end-to-end anastomosis is usually required, but if this cannot be done without tension, graft interposition is indicated. Autogenous grafts (saphenous vein from the ankle, cephalic vein, autogenous artery) are preferred, but prosthetic grafts have been used successfully, and are required in the large vessels of the aortoiliac system. Dacron has been used more often, but polytetrafluoroethylene is chosen frequently now, and may be more resistant to subsequent infection.

Debridement

Lacerations or punctures of larger vessels can be treated by lateral repair, but it is best not to make a firm decision regarding closure until debridement is concluded. Most civilian wounds are inflicted by knives or low-velocity missiles and wide debridement is unnecessary, but blunt trauma and high-velocity bullets cause more extensive damage.

2 & 3

Anastomoses

Continuous suture techniques are satisfactory in most situations, but small vessels (less than 4 mm diameter) are best joined with fine interrupted sutures. A wider suture line in small arteries can be obtained if an oblique or spatulated anastomosis is constructed.

Anticoagulants

Systemic heparin is often given to patients with isolated vascular wounds, but many trauma surgeons believe that full doses of heparin are contraindicated in patients with multiple injuries, and in those with damage to the central nervous system and eyes. Local irrigation of the damaged vessels with a solution containing 100 units of heparin per 10 ml saline is helpful in removing debris and retarding local thrombosis. No anticoagulants are used postoperatively.

Determining patency

A diligent search for distal clots is mandatory, despite what may appear to be adequate backbleeding. Most surgeons routinely pass a Fogarty catheter in both directions prior to completion of the repair. If distal pulses and normal flow are not readily obtained, arteriography is indicated before the operation is terminated.

To illustrate the application of these principles, the management of three of the more common vascular injuries are described: a penetrating wound of the carotid artery, stab wound of the inferior vena cava and a gunshot wound of the femoral artery.

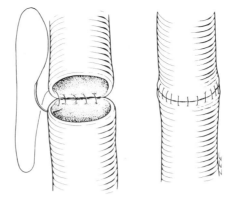

2

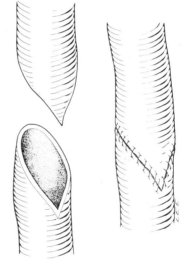

3

Carotid artery injuries

4

Sites of injury

Penetrating cervical wounds which pierce the platysma muscle usually are explored in the operating theatre. The vessels most often injured are the common carotid artery (CCA) and the jugular vein (usually the vein is ligated). The management of carotid artery injuries is assisted by dividing the neck into three zones: Zone I, above the angle of the mandible; Zone II, between the angle of the mandible and 1 cm above the clavicles; and Zone III, below Zone II (includes the thoracic outlet area).

Preoperative arteriography can be helpful in managing any carotid injury, but those patients with wounds in Zones I and III and those with neurological deficits usually require angiograms to plan the operations[3].

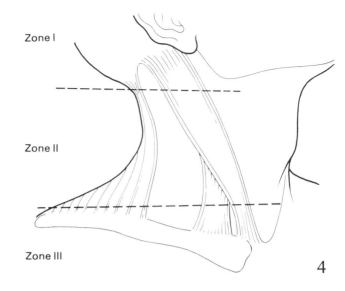

Zone I

Zone II

Zone III

4

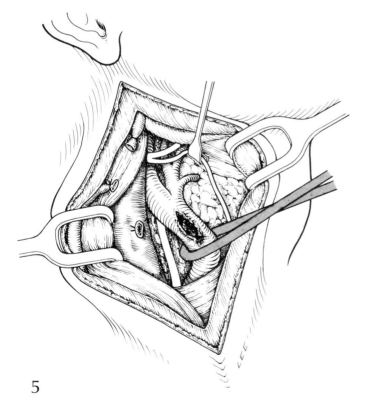

5

5

Zone II injuries (common carotid)

The midcervical carotid artery is exposed through an incision anterior to the sternomastoid muscle. The common carotid artery proximal to the wound is encircled first, then distal control is obtained if feasible. Bleeding initially is controlled with gentle finger pressure, then vascular clamps are applied. If simple suture is impossible, patch graft angioplasty or resection and anastomosis are undertaken.

Zone II injuries (internal carotid)

6

A large proximal wound of the internal carotid artery (ICA) can be repaired by substituting the external carotid. Fine interrupted sutures are used.

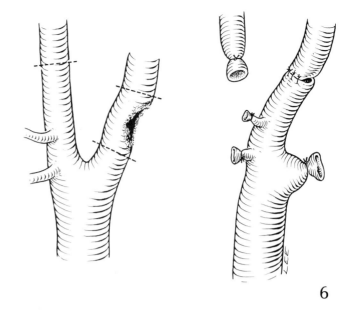

6

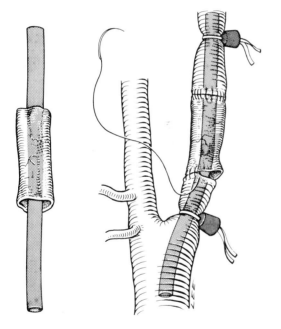

7

7

Graft interposition

If the damage to the ICA is extensive and there is scanty backbleeding from the distal artery, an autogenous saphenous vein graft from the ankle is threaded over a 10 Fr shunt and interposed between the debrided ends of the artery.

Zone III and Zone I injuries

Injuries of the CCA in Zone III may require median sternotomy for control of bleeding before the wound is exposed. ICA wounds at the base of the skull (Zone I) are difficult to expose, and it may be necessary to divide the digastric muscle, excise the styloid process or temporarily dislocate the mandible.

Inferior vena cava injuries

It has been reported that 1 in every 50 gunshot wounds and one in every 300 knife wounds of the abdomen damages the inferior vena cava (IVC). One-third of the victims die before reaching the hospital and half the remainder die during treatment. Multiple wounds of other organs are common – over three-quarters of the patients have damage to other retroperitoneal structures[4].

Most of these patients obviously have a serious injury – usually a bullet wound of the lower chest or abdomen – and shock. There are few laboratory data of diagnostic value and it is best to take unstable patients directly to surgery.

Exposure

The abdomen is opened through a midline incision from xiphoid to pubis, the extent of damage assessed and priorities set. All centrally located retroperitoneal haematomas above the pelvis are explored.

Control of bleeding

8

Initially bleeding is controlled with finger pressure or sponge sticks.

Sometimes small lacerations and punctures can be closed with simple sutures passed beneath an occluding finger or the edges of the IVC can be held together with vascular forceps.

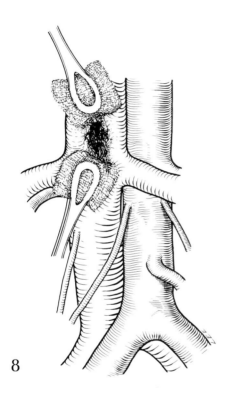

8

9

More often, a partially occluding vascular clamp (Satinsky) is needed to permit accurate repair. Occasionally accurate clamp application may be too difficult and a balloon catheter (Foley or Fogarty) can be inserted to plug the wound and stop the bleeding.

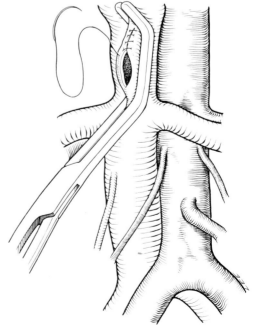

9

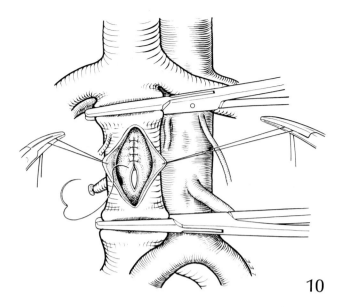

10

10

10

Through-and-through injuries

Wounds which pierce both anterior and posterior walls of the IVC can be closed by lateral repair after mobilizing the cava by ligating and dividing one or two sets of lumbar veins. Alternatively, the anterior wound can be enlarged and the posterior laceration closed from within the IVC. The anterior wall is then repaired.

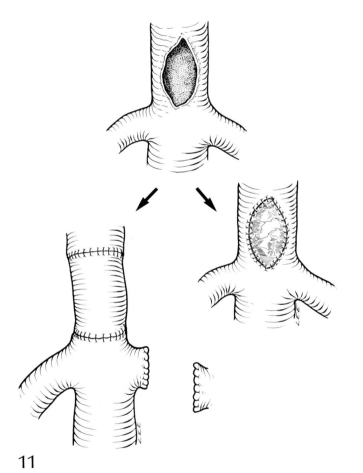

11

Suprarenal cava injuries

11

More extensive suprarenal IVC damage may require a vein graft (the left renal vein or the common iliac vein is preferred) or a patch graft. For the infrarenal cava, especially in unstable patients with multiple injuries, ligation is recommended.

Division of the ligaments and anterior and medial rotation of the right lobe of the liver usually will permit repair of the suprarenal cava and hepatic veins (one major hepatic vein or any small accessory hepatic vein can be ligated safely).

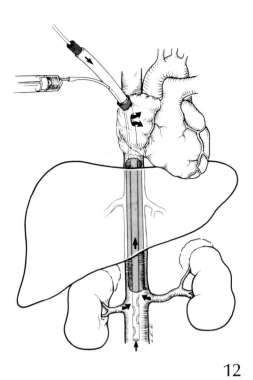

12

12 & 13

If prolonged IVC occlusion is necessary for repair or if bleeding is so brisk as to obscure vision, a transatrial intracaval shunt (Madding-Kennedy) is inserted. The right atrium is reached by extending the abdominal incision into a midline sternotomy. This manoeuvre is not often required, however.

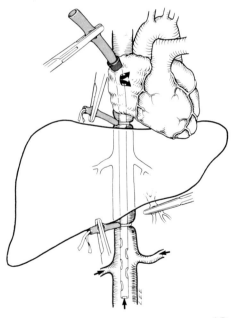

13

Gunshot wound of the femoral artery

Femoral artery wounds comprise approximately 20 per cent of all arterial injuries. These are serious problems. Haemorrhage is often profuse and acute ligation of the common femoral artery results in amputation rates near 50 per cent – only slightly less than that following acute occlusion of the popliteal artery[2].

Most patients with penetrating trauma have severe haemorrhage, or large haematomas: the injury is obvious and immediate surgery is required. If arteriograms are needed to visualize the profunda or popliteal-tibial systems, they can be obtained in theatre.

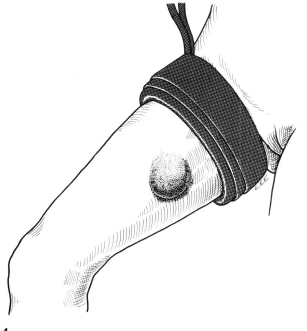

14

14

Compression control

Usually bleeding can be managed at surgery with finger pressure, but if there are multiple wounds, or large haematomas, it is prudent to place an orthopaedic pneumatic cuff proximally before draping the limb. Troublesome bleeding can be arrested quickly by inflating the cuff.

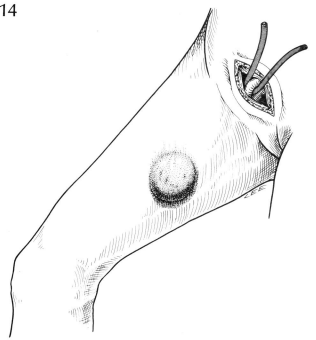

15

15

Proximal control

If there is insufficient room to place a proximal tourniquet, the external iliac artery can be encircled with a vascular tape through a muscle-splitting extraperitoneal incision above the inguinal ligament.

16

Direct control

Once proximal control is secured, the haematoma is evacuated and vascular clamps applied. Although punctures can be repaired with simple sutures, resection and anastomosis is preferred in most situations. If this is not possible without tension a saphenous vein graft is selected.

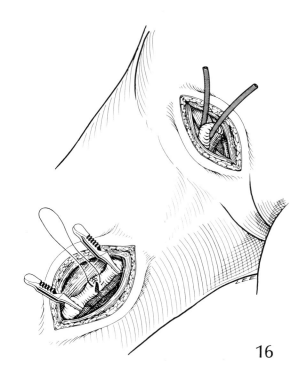

16

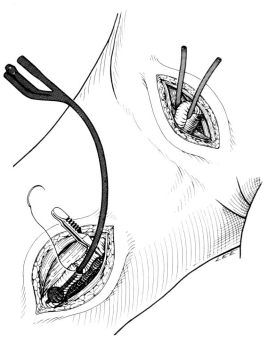

17

17

Determining patency

Prior to completing the repair a Fogarty catheter is passed to ensure a patent system free of clots. Major vein injuries are repaired with simple suture techniques, or resection and anastomosis if this does not prolong the operation unduly. Grafts are needed only on rare occasions (popliteal vein).

Postoperatively the distal pulses and limb blood pressures are followed, but a regular evaluation of neuromuscular function is essential. Any deterioration in the perception of light touch or motor function is a firm indication for further studies – usually arteriography – regardless of skin colour or temperature, distal pulses or limb blood pressure[1].

References

1. Perry, M. O. The Management of acute vascular injuries. Baltimore: Williams and Wilkins, 1980

2. Rich, N. M., Spencer, F. C. Vascular trauma. Philadelphia: W. B. Saunders Co., 1978

3. Thal, E. R., Snyder, W. H., Hays, R. J., Perry, M. O. Management of carotid artery injuries. Surgery 1974; 76: 955–962

4. Perry, M. O. In: Schwartz, S. I., ed. Principles of surgery, 3rd edition. New York: McGraw-Hill, 1979: 273–276

Illustrations by Robert Wabnitz and Anita Matthews

Treatment of iatrogenic vascular injuries

Richard M. Green MD, FACS
Clinical Assistant Professor of Surgery, University of Rochester Medical Center, Rochester, New York, USA

Charles G. Rob MC, MChir, MD, FRCS, FACS
Professor of Surgery, Department of Surgery, Uniformed Services University of the Health Sciences, F. Edward Hébert School of Medicine, Bethesda, Maryland, USA

Introduction

Since the first descriptions of arteriovenous fistulae were made by Hunter in 1757[1] and 1762[2], iatrogenic vascular injuries have been too frequent. The arteriovenous fistulae described by Hunter were between the brachial artery and vein and were caused by barbers performing therapeutic phlebotomy. Today major causes of iatrogenic vascular injuries are surgery, angiography and injections of all types including needle biopsies. As these injuries occur in hospital or in a doctor's office, early diagnosis is both possible and important. This is aided by awareness of the problem and of its frequency. Today arteriography is the most common cause of traumatic arterial thrombosis.

Any artery or vein may be injured by a therapeutic procedure. Vascular injuries may cause haemorrhage, thrombosis or delayed effects such as the formation of a false or dissecting aneurysm or an arteriovenous fistula. Simple ligation of the injured vessel is the simplest form of treatment but should only be considered when the injured vessel is not essential.

Ligation of major arteries carries a predictable risk of ischaemic complications[3] as listed below.

Risk of stroke with ligation of neck arteries:

Common carotid	20%
Internal carotid	40%
Vertebral	8%

Risk of amputation with ligation of upper extremity arteries:

Subclavian	30%
Axillary	43%
Brachial (above elbow)	55%
Brachial (below elbow)	25%
Radial	5%

Risk of amputation with ligation of lower extremity arteries:

Common iliac	53%
External iliac	46%
Common femoral	80%
Superficial femoral	55%
Popliteal	73%

Because of the high complication rates after simple ligation of the injured vessel, repair should be performed whenever possible.

The problems a surgeon faces when treating an iatrogenic vascular injury are numerous and will be illustrated by describing the management of brachial artery thrombosis due to coronary angiography; accidental injury to the femoral artery during a long saphenous ligature and stripping operation; injury to the inferior vena cava during the resection of an abdominal aortic aneurysm; the correction of an arteriovenous fistula between the abdominal aorta and left common iliac vein caused by a lumbar disc operation; and the repair of a false aneurysm of the femoral artery following angiography. These examples illustrate therapeutic procedures which can be applied to all iatrogenic vascular injuries.

The procedures

THROMBOSIS OF THE BRACHIAL ARTERY AFTER CORONARY ANGIOGRAPHY

This problem occurs in roughly 1–2 per cent of coronary angiograms performed via the percutaneous brachial route[4-5]. In most patients the collateral circulation is adequate and the limb is not jeopardized but these patients will usually develop cold intolerance and arm claudication. Ischaemia may be severe, however, and loss of the limb can occur. Thrombectomy followed by arterial reconstruction with a venous patch angioplasty should be done at once if the artery is occluded.

1 & 2

Exposure of the occluded artery

The thrombus begins at the point where the Seldinger catheter enters the artery and at first is localized. A longitudinal incision over the course of the artery is the recommended approach. This incision is medial to the biceps muscle. If the incision crosses the elbow crease it is done so in an 'S' fashion. A 6 cm portion of the artery is exposed and the patient is heparinized. A bulldog clamp is applied proximal to the thrombus but not distally. It is difficult to visualize the intima along the needle path with a transverse arteriotomy in a vessel this size and we therefore open the artery longitudinally through the puncture site.

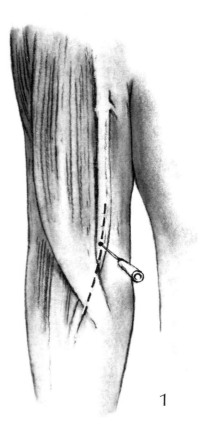

1

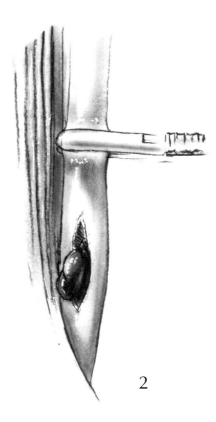

2

3

Removal of the thrombus and any damaged intima

The thrombus often extrudes from the incision and can be removed with suction and irrigation. The distal artery is clamped when retrograde flow develops. The intima is inspected and any loose flaps are excised with fine scissors. A No. 3 Fogarty catheter should always be passed down the distal artery to remove any residual thrombus. If possible, both the radial and ulnar arteries should be catheter thrombectomized. The proximal clamp is removed to flush out thrombus and if necessary the Fogarty catheter can be used to remove residual thrombus.

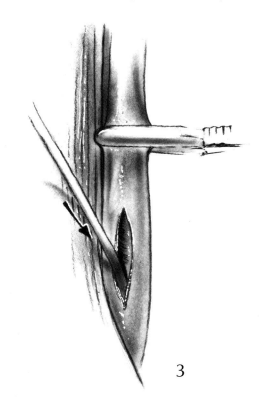

3

4

Closure with a venous patch graft angioplasty

The margin of the artery at the point of insertion of the Seldinger catheter may require excision. The amount of arterial wall removed should be as small as possible. A length of the cephalic vein should now be mobilized and laid open. This piece of vein is then sutured to the margins of the arteriotomy incision with 6/0 Prolene. It is important to use a venous patch graft because stenosis and recurrent thrombosis are likely to follow a simple closure of this arteriotomy. The clamps are now removed and the heparin neutralized with protamine sulphate. If pulses return to the wrist, and the hand becomes pink and warm, all is well. If this does not occur, an intraoperative arteriogram is required to demonstrate the state of the arterial tree. The wound is closed primarily without drainage.

4

ACCIDENTAL INJURY TO COMMON FEMORAL ARTERY DURING LIGATURE OF THE SAPHENOUS VEIN

This unfortunate injury must be recognized at once. It is usually obvious because of the arterial bleeding. It is important not to increase the arterial damage by clamping with haemostats. The correct procedure is to control the bleeding with pressure, dissect out the artery and then deliberately clamp the injured artery with vascular clamps.

Sometimes a far worse situation develops. The surgeon mistakes the superficial femoral artery for the long saphenous vein, carefully dissects the superficial femoral artery and clamps it. A stripper is then introduced into the superficial femoral artery and is passed distally to the ankle. The whole length of the main arterial system of the lower limb is then removed by stripping. The inevitable result is massive gangrene. This error can be avoided by always introducing the stripper into the long saphenous vein at the ankle and passing it proximally by the obvious step of performing an accurate dissection of the saphenofemoral junction in the groin.

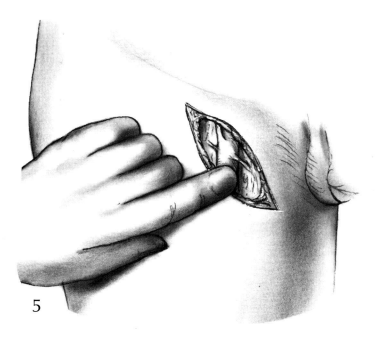

5

5

Control of the arterial haemorrhage

The first step is to apply firm pressure over an area which is gradually reduced in size so that eventually only the actual bleeding point is compressed. The surgeon and his assistant then isolate the artery proximal to the injury. This artery is clamped and the patient is given heparin 50–75 mg by the anaesthetist. Pressure is still applied to the arterial wound and the distal vessel is isolated and clamped. The area is then inspected and if bleeding persists, any unclamped branches are isolated and occluded with bulldog clamps. During this phase of the procedure great care is taken not to injure the femoral vein or femoral nerve.

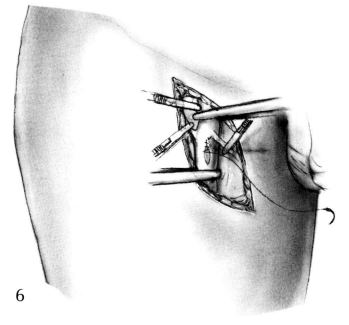

6

6

Repair of the arterial wound

A clean surgical knife wound can be sutured, but if haemostats have been used, the damaged arterial wall must be excised and the defect in the artery can then be repaired with an autogenous venous patch graft. The saphenous vein can be used for this unless the segment is very large and dilated, in which case a small and thick-walled segment of vein, often from the ankle region, may be preferred. The heparin effect is now reversed with protamine sulphate and the arterial clamps are removed.

INJURY TO THE INFERIOR VENA CAVA OR COMMON ILIAC VEINS DURING AN OPERATION UPON THE ABDOMINAL AORTA

This operative complication is best avoided by performing only essential dissection. It is unnecessary to encircle the aorta or iliac arteries routinely during aneurysmectomy and certainly not necessary to remove the aneurysmal sac. The aorta must be completely dissected during aortofemoral grafting but this dissection should be done above the level of the inferior mesenteric artery where adhesions of the aorta to the vena cava are minimal.

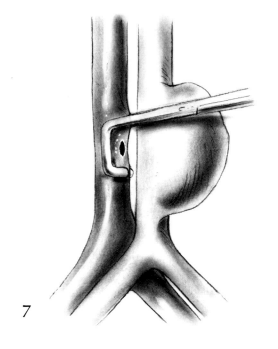

7

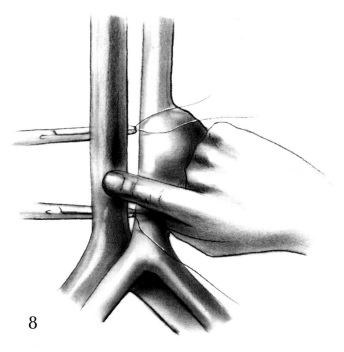

8

Temporary control of the haemorrhage

The injury to the inferior vena cava or common iliac vein is usually small, but it may be enlarged by inefficient attempts to control the bleeding. As a first step, pressure is applied to stop the bleeding. The surgeon then inspects the area and if he can, reduces the pressure point to a small area.

7

If he is successful, the next step is to apply a side clamp after appropriate dissection. It is an error to clamp blindly or to put Hemoclips in the midst of venous hemorrhage. The defect must be seen, isolated and sutured.

The management of a major defect which cannot be controlled with a side clamp

8

If the procedure described above is impossible or fails, the surgeon is presented with a very difficult and possibly disastrous situation. The first step is again to control the bleeding with firm pressure. The surgeon then proceeds in a step-by-step manner. He confirms with the anaesthetist that adequate blood is available for immediate transfusion. He confirms with the operating room nurse that all the instruments he will need are ready and available, including instruments for clamping the vena cava, sutures for repairing the vena cava and ligatures for ligating the vena cava if his attempts at repair fail. He also has prepared and brought to the operating room a machine for autotransfusion if available. The surgeon must be prepared for massive blood loss and its management.

While continuing to control the hemorrhage with firm pressure, the surgeon carefully dissects out the vena cava for a distance of about 2 cm above and below the point of injury. The vena cava is then clamped with vascular clamps above and below the injured segment. If the bleeding persists, any lumbar veins entering the damaged segment of the vena cava must be controlled with bulldog clamps or suture ligatures. During the whole of this phase of the operation, the field is kept clear by pressure on the bleeding point and use of a suction device connected to the autotransfusion system so that the requirement for donor blood is kept to a minimum.

9

Ligature or repair of the inferior vena cava

The surgeon now inspects the injured vena cava. If he can repair the defect, he should do so, but if necessary the inferior vena cava may be ligated. If the effectiveness of the repair is in doubt, a ligature should be placed around the inferior vena cava above and below the point of injury. The surgeon now proceeds to completion of the originally planned aortic operation. Postoperatively the patient's legs are raised and he wears full length elastic stockings.

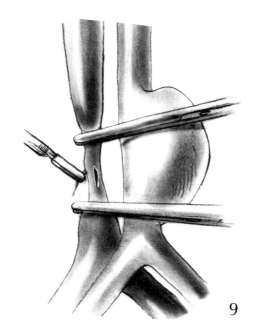

9

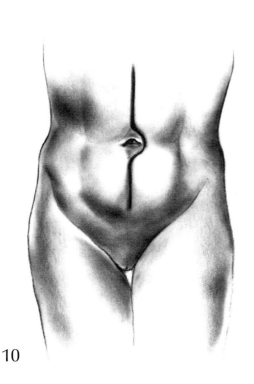

10

CORRECTION OF AN ARTERIOVENOUS FISTULA BETWEEN THE ABDOMINAL AORTA AND THE LEFT COMMON ILIAC VEIN OR INFERIOR VENA CAVA DUE TO LUMBAR DISC OPERATION

This complication was first reported in 1945 by Linton and White[6]. Twenty years later the English language literature contained the reports of at least 27 similar cases[7-8]. The actual incidence is higher because not all cases are reported. Nevertheless, this is a rare but dangerous complication of lumbar disc surgery. It is most likely to occur when the patient is operated upon in the prone position and when the annulus fibrosis is deficient so that the pituitary rongeur used in lumbar disc surgery can slip through the disc space and cause this arteriovenous fistula. A gush of blood follows. This is controlled by packing. Once the diagnosis is confirmed, careful preparation for a major operation is important. This will include the establishment of a reserve of at least 10 u of blood for transfusion. The level of the disc space being operated on determines the site of vascular injury[9]. Most injuries occur through the L4–L5 and L5–S1 interspaces and the common iliac vessels are most frequently involved. Direct aortocaval injury can occur through the L3–L4 interspace.

10

The incision

The abdomen is opened through a midline abdominal incision. After the usual abdominal exploration, as much as possible of the small intestine is removed from the abdomen and placed in a plastic bag. This will expose the aortic bifurcation together with iliac veins and inferior vena cava.

11

Isolation of the abdominal aorta and inferior vena cava proximal to the lesion

If there is time to obtain a preoperative arteriogram the dissection required for vascular control can be limited. At the L3–L4 level, proximal and distal clamps on the aorta and vena cava are all that is necessary. Injuries at the confluence of the iliac vessels at L4–L5 require control of all six major vessels. Unilateral iliac control is adequate for L5–S1. There may be a retroperitoneal haematoma, but this can be surprisingly small. It is important not to approach the actual arteriovenous communication until the major arteries and veins proximal and distal to the lesion have been controlled if the site of the injury is uncertain. The aorta is isolated just distal to the origin of the inferior mesenteric artery and the inferior vena cava, which is also isolated at the same level. Any lumbar arteries or veins immediately distal to this point are clamped with bulldog clamps.

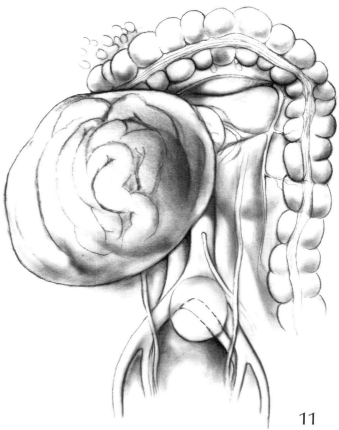

11

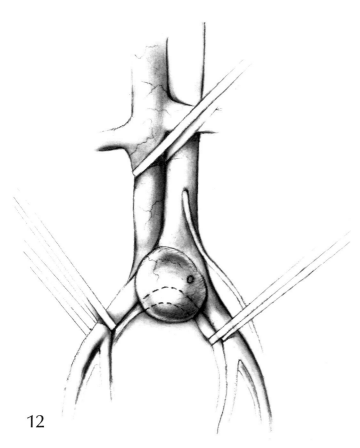

12

12

Isolation of the iliac vessels distal to the lesion

The right and left common iliac arteries and veins are now isolated well away from the lesion and close to the bifurcation of the common iliac artery and the junction of the hypogastric and external iliac veins. The blood flow to the area of the arteriovenous fistula will now be under control except for the middle sacral artery and vein, sometimes a second pair of lumbar arteries and veins closer to the aortic bifurcation and an occasional vessel supplying the ureter. If possible, these vessels are located before opening the vessels and occluded with bulldog clamps, but this step, although desirable, is not essential.

13

Exposure of the arteriovenous fistula

After the anaesthetist has given the patient heparin 50–75 mg, all the vessels are clamped and the distal abdominal aorta is opened opposite the arteriovenous fistula with a longitudinal incision on the anterior aortic wall which may, if necessary, be extended onto one of the common iliac arteries. The surgeon will now see the defect in the posterior wall of the distal aorta. If bleeding still occurs, the orifices of the middle sacral or other small vessels should be oversewn with vascular sutures from within the lumen of the aorta. The defect in the left common iliac vein will be seen behind the arterial injury. If bleeding occurs from a branch of this vein, it should be temporarily controlled with a small pack.

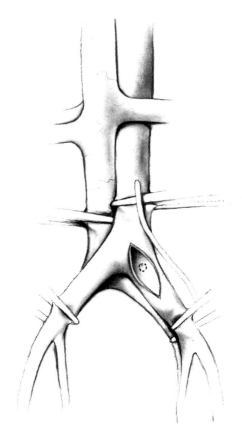

13

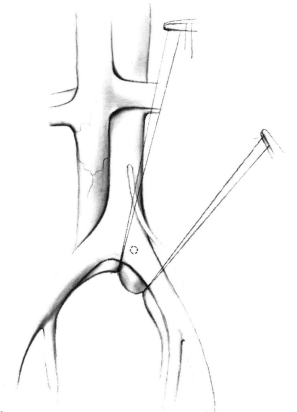

14

14

Ligature of the left common iliac vein

It is a mistake to attempt to repair the left common iliac vein. A ligament or suture is tied around the left common iliac vein proximal and distal to the injury. The fact that this vein has been injured with rongeur or similar forceps means that repair is difficult and ligature is safer and better in most cases. Once this is completed all clamps on the veins involved in the operation are removed.

15

Repair of the arterial injury

The artery is now open on both sides anteriorly because of the surgeon's incision and posteriorly because of the injury which caused the arteriovenous fistula. The posterior defect is closed first. Usually a patch is required. A patch of Dacron velour is sutured to the margins of this defect with a continuous 4/0 Prolene suture from within the lumen of the aorta. The anterior arteriotomy incision is then closed by a simple Prolene suture. However, if it appears that this will constrict the lumen, a second patch of Dacron velour may be used. The clamps are now removed. The heparin effect is reversed with protamine sulphate and the abdominal incision closed in the usual manner. Alternatively, the damaged arterial segment may be replaced by a Dacron prosthesis.

If a Dacron patch or prosthesis has been used, we recommend a 5-day course of antibiotics as a prophylactic measure against infection.

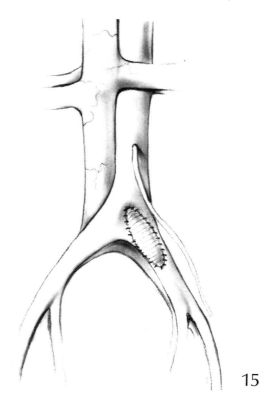

15

REPAIR OF A FALSE ANEURYSM OF THE FEMORAL ARTERY AFTER ARTERIOGRAPHY

Patients may present with a painful, pulsatile mass in the groin, days, weeks or months following retrograde catheterization. The pain may radiate down the leg, mimicking nerve compression. Often there is a history of extensive ecchymosis immediately after the procedure. The diagnosis of a false aneurysm can be made at the bedside. Ultrasonography is useful if there are any doubts. Repair should be undertaken promptly.

16

Incision and control of the artery

A groin incision is made over the femoral artery. Although local anaesthesia may be used for groin explorations dealing with arterial thrombosis, we prefer a general anaesthetic for this operation. A great deal of inflammatory reaction is often present and the area should be sharply incised down to the pulsatile mass. If the mass has been present for some time a fibrous capsule will be present and vascular control can be obtained above and below the aneurysm. Often only a haematoma is encountered, and once this is evacuated brisk arterial bleeding occurs. Fortunately, the arterial opening is usually quite small and a finger can be placed over the bleeding point for temporary control. Proximal dissection of the femoral artery can then be done, heparin given and a vascular clamp applied.

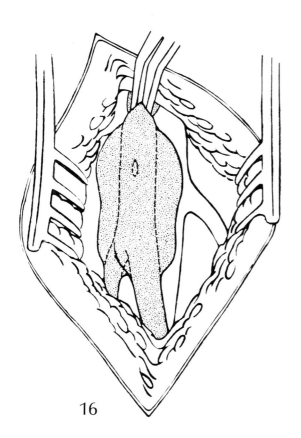

16

17

Repair of the injury

Once proximal control has been obtained and the vessel clamped, the dissection is completed. We have noticed that these injuries are often due to tangential entry into the artery by the catheter, often at the bifurcation of the common femoral artery. Two or three interrupted sutures of 5/0 Prolene are usually sufficient for repair. In a small child, a saphenous vein patch may be required.

Closure

Any remaining haematoma should be evacuated. The heparin is reversed with protamine. A two-layer closure without drainage is performed. Antibiotics are unnecessary unless a prosthetic patch has been used.

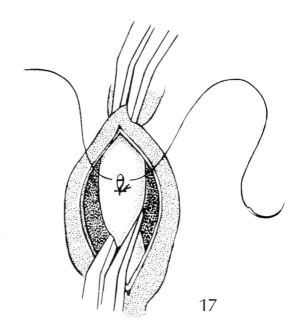

17

References

1. Hunter, W. The history of an aneurysm of the aorta with some remarks on aneurysms in general. *Medical Observations and Inquiries.* 1757; 1: 323–357

2. Hunter, W. Further observations upon a particular species of aneurysm. *Medical Observations and Inquiries.* 1762; 2: 390

3. Ehricks, E. Major vascular ligations. In: Eiseman, B., ed. Prognosis of surgical disease. Philadelphia: W. B. Saunders, 1980: 102–105

4. Adams, D. F., Fraser, D. B., Abrams, H. L. The complications of coronary arteriography. Circulation 1973; 48: 609–618

5. Sones, F. M., Shirley, E. K. Cine coronary arteriography. Modern Concepts of Cardiovascular Disease 1962; 31: 735–738

6. Linton, R. R., White, P. D. Arteriovenous fistula between the right common iliac artery and inferior vena cava. Report of a case of its occurence following an operation for a ruptured intervertebral disc with cure by operation. Archives of Surgery 1945; 50: 6–13

7. Horton, R. E. Arteriovenous fistula following operation for prolapsed intervertebral disc. British Journal of Surgery 1961; 77: 49

8. Harbison, S. P. Major vascular complications of intervertebral disc surgery. Annals of Surgery 1954; 140: 342–348

9. Bernhard, V. M. Aortocaval fistulas. In: Haimovici, H., ed. Vascular emergencies. New York: Appleton-Century-Crofts, 1982: 353–363

Illustrations by Kevin Marks

Treatment of acquired arteriovenous fistulae

H. H. G. Eastcott MS, FRCS
Honorary Consultant Surgeon, St Mary's Hospital, London, UK

A. E. Thompson MS, FRCS
Consultant Surgeon, St Thomas's Hospital, London, UK

Preoperative

Indications

Acquired arteriovenous fistulae are the result of trauma to blood vessels or mycotic aneurysms[1]. Such a connection occasionally occurs as a result of operative trauma or may be surgically created to allow access to the circulation for haemodialysis. Shunting of the blood from the arterial to the venous system produces both general and local effects. The general effects are produced by lowering of the peripheral vascular resistance. If the fistula is large and involves major vessels, progressive increase in the left ventricular output can be followed by ventricular hypertrophy and high output failure[2]. All fistulae will be accompanied by a relative increase in blood volume. Subacute bacterial endocarditis can occur at the site of the fistula or in the heart.

Local effects depend on the site and size of the fistula. Venous insufficiency and peripheral ischaemia are common if the proximal limb vessels are affected, with ulceration of the ankle and calf developing in the lower limbs. These problems are avoided in the arteriovenous fistula for haemodialysis by using a small distal fistula in the arm. In pathological fistulae adjacent structures may be compressed by aneurysmal vessels. Buzzing may greatly distress the patient with a carotid-jugular or cavernous sinus fistula.

Primary repair has been the first-line treatment of choice in accessible pathological fistulae. However, the increasing success of radiographic techniques, particularly in areas inaccessible to surgery, may change this approach[3].

Contraindications

Operation should not be lightly undertaken and the possible radiological alternatives need to be carefully considered. The cure of this condition presents considerable technical difficulty and if the lesser procedure of proximal arterial ligation has to be performed, drainage of the remaining effective circulation back through the fistula may result in gangrene of a limb.

Small aneurysmal varices need nothing more than an elastic support and regular review for cardiac complications. Very occasionally an arteriovenous fistula closes spontaneously by thrombosis.

Preoperative preparation

Preoperative assessment of the patient includes careful examination of the cardiovascular system followed by estimation of the haemoglobin, blood volume and cardiac output. If fever is present, repeated blood cultures are made. Preparation must be made for blood transfusion, but it must be remembered that this condition is normally accompanied by a significant increase in blood volume with overloading of the heart. Although some loss of blood is beneficial, blood replacement must be available if profuse bleeding occurs.

Plain radiographs should be taken to localize any suspected metal fragments in the region of the fistula. Several investigations are helpful in planning the surgical approach. Arteriography will help to define the extent of acquired fistulae of this type[4]. A Doppler ultrasound probe is useful in identifying the site of the fistula. An increase in the volume of a peripheral pulse may follow accurate occlusion of the fistula with digital compression.

Anaesthesia

General or spinal (epidural) anaesthesia is suitable. Hypotensive agents may be necessary to reduce hypertension when flow through the fistula has been arrested.

The operation

A wide exposure is essential. The incision should be centred over the position of the fistula as shown on the arteriogram, at the point where the bruit is loudest, or where local digital pressure will abolish it, rather than over the region of greatest soft tissue swelling, which may be only the partly clotted sac.

Application of tourniquet

1

Pneumatic type

There is much to be said for using a tourniquet: the blood loss is reduced and the preliminary dissection is much simpler. A wide pneumatic type is preferable as it can be released at the stage when the fistula itself is exposed, as a test of whether it has been obliterated.

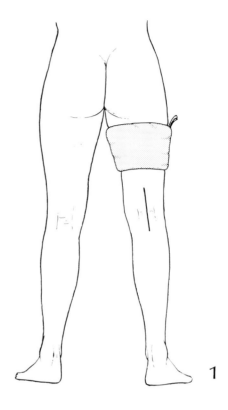

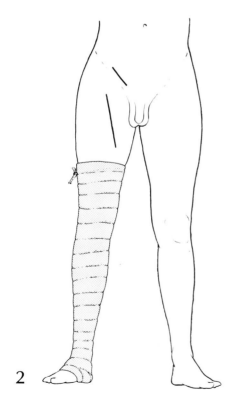

2

Esmarch's bandage

If the fistula is large and lies at the root of the limb, a separate formal exposure of the main vessels is made proximally. The subclavian artery, the common iliac artery or the external iliac artery is temporarily controlled. If necessary the clavicle can be removed or the inguinal ligament divided. The engorged and hypertrophied limb may be emptied by elevation and by the application of an Esmarch's bandage. It is either taken tightly up to the proximal tourniquet and then removed, or, if no proximal tourniquet is used (as on the higher fistula sites), it is applied much more loosely, up to the lower limit of the sterile field, and is left in place, thus serving to diminish venous bleeding.

3

Superficial dissection

Many dilated superficial veins are encountered in making the long incision. Correct application of the tourniquet will have helped to reduce this difficulty, although if the pressure is not correctly adjusted it may only increase the venous bleeding.

The muscle layers

Whenever possible the approach to the deep vessels is by muscle separating or splitting, for many large collaterals course through the bellies.

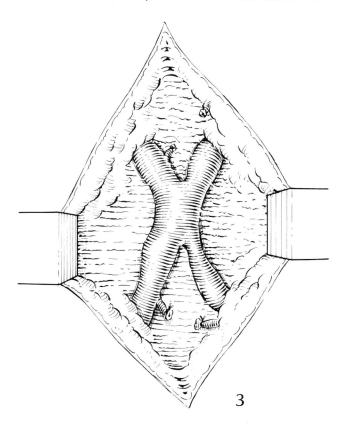

3

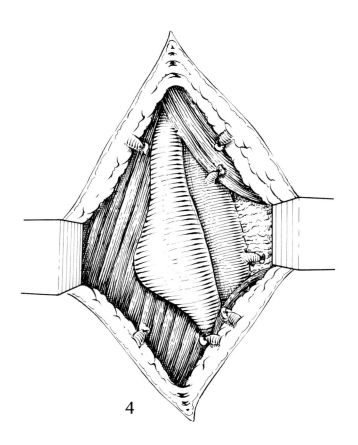

4

4

Deep dissection

The dilated afferent artery must first be located, particularly if other means of controlling the bloodflow have not been adopted, and a temporary tape ligature or arterial clamp applied. Several medium-sized vessels require ligation and division before the main vein can be approached, often along a tributary. Sometimes the sac or fistula itself is the best guide to the main vein which, when found, is temporarily clamped above and below the communication.

5

Exploring the fistula itself

The pulsation and thrill in the communicating region are now abolished by the clamps, and, although the sac may still refill slowly after digital compression, it should be opened. The source of any remaining branch is seen and can be sutured, or the vessel can be located and tied outside the sac, the operator being guided by the position of its opening within the sac. Any foreign body is removed. The site and size of the fistula can then be assessed.

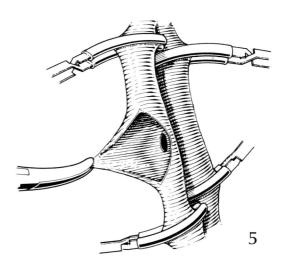

5

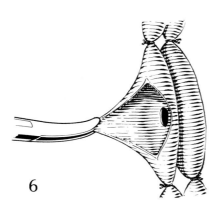

6

6

Quadruple ligation

This simple procedure has been the one most generally used. It carries some risk of producing ischaemia, but it is safer than a complicated repair operation when fibrosis and collateral formation are extensive. The ligatures must be placed between the fistula and the first branch of each vessel, whenever possible, to prevent backward loss through the fistula. More than four ligatures are usually needed. The bruit should be completely abolished at this stage, although a small peripheral pulse may be felt.

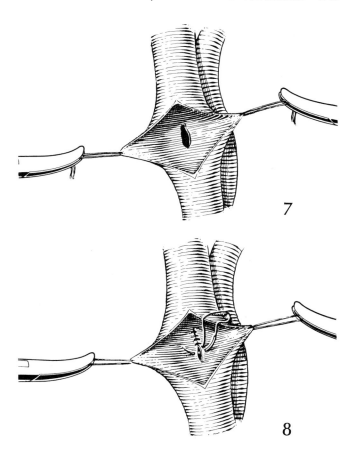

7 & 8

Transvenous repair of fistula

Where the vein is dilated, or forms a sac, the fistula can be explored through it, and repaired with a simple continuous suture. The vein is then repaired. It should not be sacrificed to the repair of the artery unless its condition precludes a separate repair, lest venous insufficiency follow. Transvenous repair is best suited to cases with a wide zone of adherence between the artery and the vein around the fistula[5].

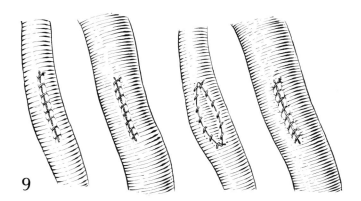

9

Simple repair of artery and vein

There is sometimes sufficient varicose aneurysm formation, or increase in the diameters of the artery and vein themselves, to allow tissues to spare for a longitudinal suture of each, without much narrowing of the lumen. A patch graft may be required for the arterial repair.

10

Repair of artery by excision and anastomosis

The artery wall may be involved in the formation of the sac. Local repair in these circumstances is likely to be followed by recurrence as a simple aneurysm. It is better to excise the damaged segment, which is seldom more than 2.5 cm or so in length, and then to restore the artery by an end-to-end anastomosis. This is the ideal treatment. Tension can be avoided and the gap closed by the use of posture: for example, by raising the shoulder or flexing the knee. The disparity in size between the two ends is overcome by appropriate traction upon the two supporting stitches (*see* p. 65). The vein is sutured first, if clotting is thought to be likely, or if it would be obscured by the repaired artery.

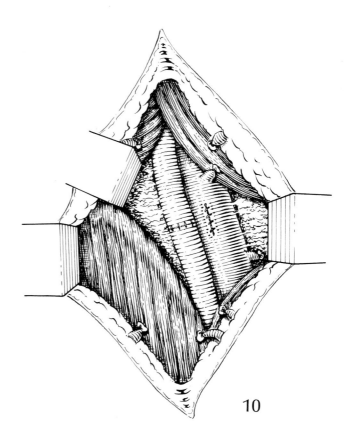

10

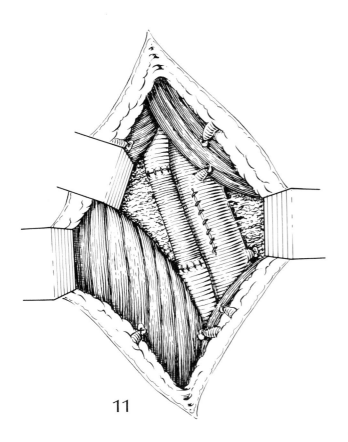

11

11

Repair of artery by excision and grafting

A longer gap in the artery than can be closed by direct anastomosis is an indication for the insertion of an arterial graft. Although only a short length is usually needed it is better not to sacrifice one of the nearby veins for the purpose, for hyperaemia and venous insufficiency are likely sequelae of the reconstruction of the artery. A separate dissection of a vein from another part is permissible, however, and the upper saphenous trunk is very suitable. It must be reversed to avoid obstruction by valves. Alternatively, in the larger arteries a Dacron graft may be used.

Postoperative care and complications

The restoration of a normal circulation with a pre-existing raised blood volume may cause postoperative complications. Monitoring of the central venous pressure by an indwelling catheter is essential. Direct measurement of the circulating volume may also be helpful. The use of diuretics or venesection will reduce the circulating volume.

Complications

Cardiac failure may follow the repair of a large fistula. Postoperative transfusion should be withheld to avoid precipitating this complication in the presence of an already overloaded circulation. The cooperation of a cardiologist both before and after surgery is valuable.

The use of heparin during the operation and the presence of the numerous high-flow collaterals in the operative field maybe complicated by postoperative haemorrhage. Suction-drainage and close observation reveal this complication at an early stage. Ischaemia of the extremity occurs more commonly after the multiple ligation procedure and reconstruction is preferable.

Reconstruction is followed by a phase of reactive hyperaemia in the operated extremity. The foot pulses and temperature must be closely watched. Any sudden deterioration is an indication for re-exploration.

References

1. Ross, J. The surgery of arterial disease and injury. British Medical Journal 1946; 1: 1–4

2. Sako, Y., Varco, R. L. Arteriovenous fistula: results of management of congenital and acquired forms, blood flow measurements, and observations on proximal arterial degeneration. Surgery 1970; 67: 40–61

3. Ricketts, R. R., Finck, E., Yellin, A. E. Management of major arteriovenous fistulas by arteriographic techniques. Archives of Surgery 1978; 113: 1153–1159

4. Bell, D., Cockshutt, W. P. Angiography of traumatic arteriovenous fistulae. Clinical Radiology 1965; 16: 241–247

5. Beall, A. C., Harrington, O. B., Crawford, E. S., DeBakey, M. E. Surgical management of traumatic arteriovenous aneurysms. American Journal of Surgery 1963; 106: 610–618

Further reading

Gomes, M. M. R., Bernatz, P. E. Arteriovenous fistulas: a review and ten year experience at the Mayo Clinic. Mayo Clinical Proceedings 1970; 45: 81–102

Graham, J. M., McCollum, C. H., Crawford, E. S., DeBakey, M. E. Extensive arterial aneurysm formation proximal to ligated arteriovenous fistula. Annals of Surgery 1980; 191: 200–202

Treatment of congenital arteriovenous fistulae

J. Leonel Villavicencio MD, FACS
Professor of Surgery, Uniformed Services University of the Health Sciences,
F. Edward Hébert School of Medicine, Bethesda, Maryland;
Director, Vein and Lymphatic Clinic, Walter Reed Army Medical Center, Washington, DC, USA

Introduction

In dealing with congenital vascular malformations during the past 20 years we have become convinced that one can almost always demonstrate the involvement of both arterial and venous systems.

In some lesions, the active passage of blood from the arteries to the veins results in important haemodynamic manifestations, both local and systemic. Locally, the gradual increase in arteriovenous shunting produces venous stasis, dilatation of veins and ischaemia distal to the fistulae. Systemically there are changes in cardiac haemodynamics which may lead to significant heart failure[1]. This occurs most commonly in arteriovenous angiomas and cirsoid (or racemose) aneurysms which may have a rapid evolution.

There are other congenital vascular malformations which seem to be haemodynamically stable and grow very slowly, if at all. In these types of lesions – usually localized haemangiomas – the predominance of the venous system is quite evident. We have occasionally observed, how-ever, sudden spontaneous or post-traumatic activation of the dormant arteriovenous communications with a tendency to rapid progression[2]. It is fair to mention that we have also observed spontaneous regression of some of these malformations with gradual disappearance of the lesion over some years as has been reported by Rigdon[3] and Sariñana[4]. Because of this behaviour, lesions present at birth should be closely observed for the first 4–5 years of life. Untimely surgical attempts to excise these lesions in small children may result in permanent disfigurement.

Finally there is another type of congenital anomaly in which there are extensive vascular malformations with widespread arteriovenous fistulae involving a whole extremity. In these cases, the surgical challenge is formidable. However, acceptable functional results can be obtained with interruption and/or embolization of all vessels feeding the affected areas. This is followed by segmental excisions carefully planned on the basis of intraoperative angiography. The resection of tissue may include skin, muscle and even bone. Modern plastic surgical techniques provide several means of coverage of relatively large defects.

When all surgical resources have been used (or cannot be employed because of the extensive nature of the malformation), conservative measures should be instituted until gradual deterioration of the extremity demands a major amputation or disarticulation of the diseased limb. The same applies for extensive arteriovenous fistulae of the hand or foot.

Therapeutic alternatives

In localized congenital arteriovenous fistulae, radical surgical excision provides an excellent opportunity for permanent cure. This can be accomplished when the arteriovenous fistulae are sharply circumscribed or in those rare instances where an isolated malformation communicates with a single arterial vessel. In haemangiomas, the whole lesion should be removed *en bloc*. The skin should be closed without undue tension. If this is not possible, free skin grafts or myocutaneous flaps should be used. The collaboration of a competent plastic surgeon should be sought. The great advances in plastic and reconstructive surgery have enabled us to resect large lesions which previously were considered inoperable.

In the generalized types of vascular malformation there is a series of procedures that can be used to diminish the amount of shunting through the lesions. These include: synovectomy to avoid haemarthrosis; epiphyseal stapling to prevent excessive growth of an extremity; interruption of all afferent vessels feeding the malformation; excision of varicose venous trunks in cases of relatively stabilized or moderately active arteriovenous fistulae. The removal of large, dilated veins in one or more staged operations helps a great deal in reducing the flow through the fistulae.

Sclerotherapy has been found very useful, either alone or in the postoperative period. Sessions of sclerotheraphy can be scheduled once or twice a week followed by compression bandages. Elastic stockings should be worn for life.

Roentgentherapy produces excellent results in some lesions, particularly in those with a tendency to rapid growth in which there is a great deal of angioblastic activity in the tissues. A low dose is given at low voltage (2–4 applications of 50–80 rad at 30–40 kV repeated after 4 months if necessary).

Kasabuchi[5] and Zarem[6] report success following the systemic use of corticosteroids in cases of extensive haemangiomas in children. Azzolini[7] reported far better results with the local infiltration of corticosteroids into the lesions using small dosages of triamcinolone acetonide. The results are especially good in predominately subcutaneous haemangiomas of the cheek and parotid region.

Transcatheter vessel embolization has been widely used in the preoperative management of tumours and arteriovenous malformations[8]. We have used it successfully with radiological control at the time of surgery.

Available materials for embolization include autologous tissue, absorbable haemostatics, synthetic particulates and liquid polymers. Each material has advantages and disadvantages as has been carefully reviewed by Greenfield[9]. We will describe our method of embolization with muscle fragments.

Major amputation or disarticulation of an extremity is the only alternative in those cases of extensive vascular malformations with multiple sites of arteriovenous fistulae in which the magnitude of the anomalies leads to deterioration of the extremity and the cardiovascular system.

Preoperative

If it is reasonably certain that the lesion is well localized, radical surgical excision can be accomplished without the need for preoperative angiography. If there is the slightest doubt about the extension of the malformation, angiography must be carried out, including selective serial arteriography of the branches feeding the arteriovenous lesion.

When the lesions are in the extremities, we have found the use of temporary ischaemia with Esmarch bandage and pneumatic tourniquet (300 mmHg for the upper extremity and 400–500 mmHg for the lower extremity) greatly facilitates the surgical procedure. We keep the time of ischaemia to a maximum period of one hour.

Often it is necessary to perform a series of staged operations in order to stabilize a lesion and the patient and relatives should be warned of this possibility.

Anaesthesia

General anaesthesia is preferable in adults with extensive lesions and should always be used in small children. In some adults with small localized lesions, local or regional anaesthesia is satisfactory.

Operations for localized lesions

RESECTION OF CIRSOID ANEURYSM OF THE SCALP

Temporary clamping of external carotid artery and division of facial vein

1

These lesions are often located on the temporal area and can bleed profusely if the main feeding vessels are not controlled before the direct attack on the aneurysm. A 6 cm incision is made at the level of the carotid bifurcation, following the skin folds of the neck. The sternocleidomastoid muscle and the jugular vein are retracted laterally. The facial vein is identified and divided between ligatures.

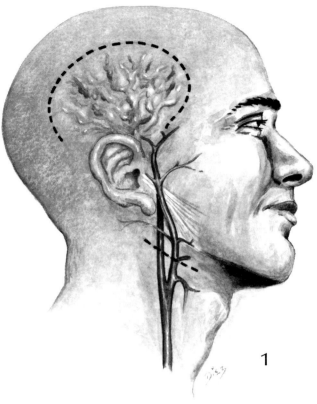

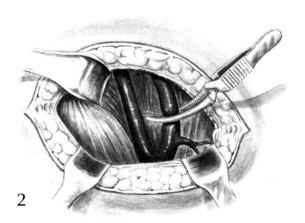

2

The cervical fascia is opened longitudinally. The carotid vessels are gently dissected, trying to avoid unnecessary handling of the carotid bulb. The external carotid artery is identified by its branches and temporarily occluded with a bulldog clamp.

Scalp incision and removal of lesion

3

A deep curved incision is made down to the periosteum. The lesion should be contained in the flap. The dissection is continued in the plane between the lesion and the periosteum, using the electrocoagulation unit. The flap is thus developed, ligating individually the large vessels and coagulating the smaller ones until the large mass of anomalous vessels is completely separated from the periosteum.

The next step is to remove the lesion from the inner aspect of the flap in order to interrupt any significant bloodflow coming from the base. After the lesion has been excised, the clamp is removed from the external carotid artery and any bleeding points are either ligated or coagulated.

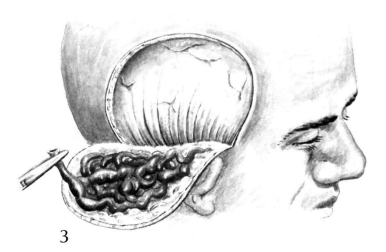

4

Closure of the incisions

The galea aponeurotica is approximated with interrupted 3/0 polyglycolic sutures, leaving suction drainage for 24 hours. The skin is closed with nonabsorbable interrupted stitches. The wound in the neck is closed in layers. Here, we prefer to close the skin with fine monofilament sutures (5/0) or an intradermic running suture of 4/0 polyglycolic material. The wound will heal with an excellent cosmetic appearance.

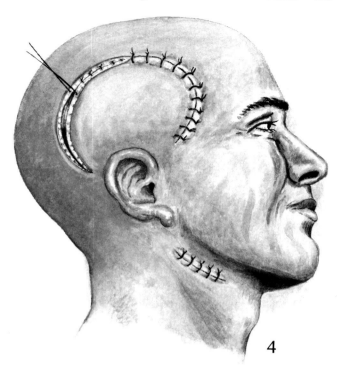

4

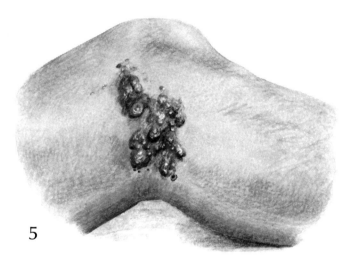

5

EN BLOC EXCISION OF A KNEE HAEMANGIOMA

5

Many haemangiomas can be resected *en bloc*. A cavernous haemangioma in the knee of a 16-year-old boy illustrates the verrucoid aspect of the skin lesions typical of these types of congenital anomalies. The haemangioma has dilated veins and bluish skin crusts which bleed easily either spontaneously or after minor trauma.

6

An incision is made well clear of the lesion, ligating and coagulating all bleeding vessels. The subcutaneous lesions often resemble small blueberries. The dissection should continue towards the deeper tissues until the fascia is identified. Care should be taken to remove all pathological tissues and destroy with cautery or suture-ligatures all suspicious lesions on the edges of the apparently healthy remaining tissue.

It is important to remember that recurrence or worsening of the lesions after surgery usually reflect either an incorrect diagnosis or an incomplete operation. The lesion should be removed completely, leaving a clean area to be covered by a skin graft. The skin graft can be applied immediately after removal of the lesion or 4–5 weeks later, when the wound has been covered with healthy granulation tissue and the defect is almost at the level of the skin. The latter technique produces a better cosmetic appearance.

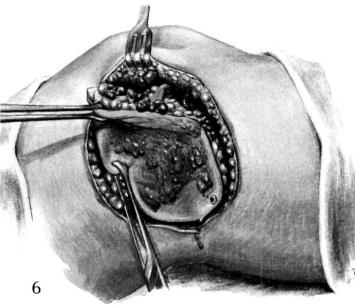

6

Operations for generalized lesions

The aim of surgery here is to reduce bloodflow through the fistulae. Ligature of the main feeding artery proximal to the anomaly usually makes the situation worse. Better results can be obtained with ligation of all the arterial branches feeding the lesion and excision or destruction as complete as possible of all involved tissue. Embolization of the shunting areas through the main feeding vessels has proved to be a therapeutic method which can obliterate a good number of lesions. Both methods are illustrated.

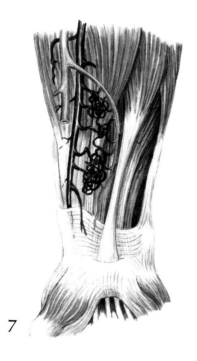

7

LIGATION OF AFFERENT ARTERIES

7

The main artery feeding the lesion should be carefully identified in the angiographic study. An incision as long as is necessary is made parallel to the artery (in this case the radial artery at the anterior aspect of the forearm). The artery and veins leading to and from the lesion are identified and dissected throughout their entire length.

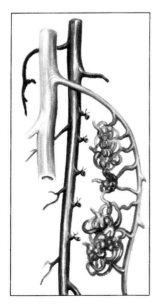

8

8

All the afferent branches leading to the fistulae are divided between ligatures.

An important surgical decision has to be made at this time. If the lesion is considered resectable, it should be removed, excising all the pathological tissue and destroying with diathermy and/or suture-ligation all suspicious non-resectable tissue. If the lesion cannot be excised without impairing the function of the extremity, then embolization should be performed through each one of the distal ends of the divided feeding arteries. After embolization has been completed, an effort should be made to resect as much as possible of the pathological tissues. The wound is closed in layers.

TRANSCATHETER VESSEL EMBOLIZATION

Embolization of the vessels feeding the vascular malformation has been increasingly used to obliterate the shunting areas. It can be done either percutaneously or in the course of a surgical procedure planned to remove a lesion. It can also be done as one of a series of staged procedures in the course of the palliative treatment of extensive arteriovenous communications.

Fistulae involving a lesion in the thigh

9

A vertical incision is made over the femoral vessels in the groin.

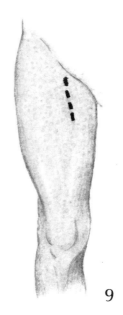

9

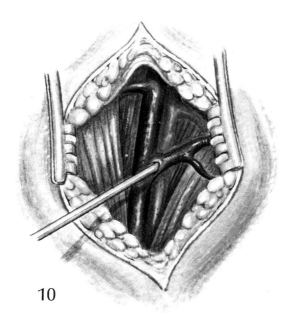

10

10

The femoral artery is dissected and the branches feeding the lesion are identified by angiography. A vessel is shown being injected with contrast material.

11

Muscle embolization is then carried out. Small fragments of muscle which have been taken from the neighbouring tissues, are placed in saline and injected into as many branches as necessary until angiography confirms obliteration of the fistulae. Silicone spheres or surgical gelatin (Gelfoam) have also been successfully used as embolization material[9].

After embolization, it is convenient to try to resect the lesion.

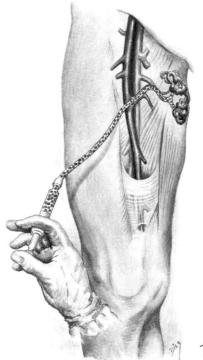

11

Inoperable lesions

12

Here we see an extremity with extensive vascular malformations, large dilated venous trunks, cutaneous necrosis and widespread arteriovenous communications. Intractable oedema and limb hypertrophy with skeletal lesions are commonly seen in these cases. The conservative measures described previously have been used without success and amputation or disarticulation remain the only alternatives.

Postoperative measures

Suction drainage should be used in all cases in which extensive dissection or tissue resection has been done. Pressure bandages with limb elevation are mandatory in all cases in which the pneumatic tourniquet has been employed to perform the operation. The pressure dressings and bandaging should be applied before releasing the tourniquet. Care should be taken to place adequate padding between fingers or toes and over bony prominences.

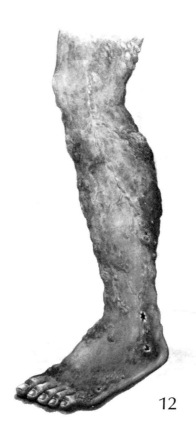

12

References

1. Holman, E. Abnormal arteriovenous communications: peripheral and intracardiac acquired and congenital. 2nd ed. Springfield, Illinois: C. Thomas, 1968

2. Malan, E., Puglionisi, A. Congenital angiodysplasias of the extremities. Journal of Cardiovascular Surgery, 1965; 6: 255–345

3. Rigdon, R. H. Spontaneous regression of hemangiomas: an experimental study in the duck and chicken. Cancer Research 1955; 15: 77–79

4. Sariñana, C., Vargos, L., Mota, F. Manejo de los hemangiomas de la infancia. Boletín médico del Hospital infantil 1962; 19: 6

5. Kasabuchi, Y., Sawade, T., Nakamura, T. Successful treatment of neonatal retroperitoneal hemangioma with corticosteroids. Journal of Pediatric Surgery 1973; 8: 59–62

6. Zarem, H. A., Edgerton, M. T. Induced resolution of cavernous hemangiomas following prednisolone therapy. Plastic and Reconstructive Surgery 1967; 39: 76–83

7. Azzolini, A., Nouvenne, R. Nuove prospettive nella terapia degli angiomi immaturi dell'infanzia. 115 lesioni trattate con infiltrazioni intralesionali di triamcindoneone acetonide. Ateneo Parmense 1970; 41 (Suppl. 1): 51–77

8. Grace, D. M., Pitt, D. F., Gold, R. E. Vascular embolization and occlusion by angiographic techniques as an aid or alternative to operation. Surgery, Gynecology and Obstetrics 1976; 143: 469–482

9. Greenfield, A. J. Transcatheter vessel occlusion: selection of methods and materials. In: Athanasoulis, C. A., Abrams, H. L., Zeitler, E., eds. Therapeutic angiography. Berlin, Heidelberg, New York: Springer-verlag, 1981

Role of the vascular laboratory in the diagnosis of venous disease

Robert W. Hobson II MD
Professor of Surgery and Chief, Section of Vascular Surgery, University of Medicine and Dentistry of New Jersey,
New Jersey Medical School, Newark, New Jersey, USA

Thomas G. Lynch MD
Assistant Professor of Surgery, Section of Vascular Surgery, University of Medicine and Dentistry of New Jersey,
New Jersey Medical School, Newark, New Jersey, USA;
Chief, Vascular Surgical Section, VA Medical Center, East Orange, New Jersey, USA

Joseph A. O'Donnell MCh, FRCSI
Consultant Surgeon, Department of Surgery, UCC Regional Hospital, Cork, Ireland

Introduction

The surgical treatment of acute deep venous thrombosis and its subsequent postphlebitic complications requires accurate techniques for the diagnosis and characterization of the extent of the venous disease. The clinical diagnosis of acute venous obstruction secondary to deep venous thrombosis (DVT) is frequently inaccurate. The symptoms and physical findings associated with DVT tend to be non-specific, and cases of unsuspected DVT may occur in the absence of physical findings. Several authors[1-5] have documented the inaccuracy of clinical evaluation in this diagnosis. Although McLachlin, Richards and Paterson[6] observed that the only reliable physical sign of DVT was the presence of significant unilateral oedema, Cranley, Canus and Sull[7] reported that even oedema was not of great value in discriminating between patients with and without DVT. While most pulmonary emboli originate in the lower extremities, Sevitt[8] reported the absence of clinical signs of venous thrombosis in 60 per cent of autopsy-proven pulmonary emboli arising from DVT. Walker[9] documented that 49 per cent of pulmonary emboli arose from clinically silent lower extremities, while Kakkar et al.[10] similarly reported an absence of clinical signs in about half of their patients.

Since it is apparent that the clinical diagnosis of DVT is accurate in only about 50 per cent of cases, it is important to supplement the clinical examination with a more objective assessment. The purpose of this chapter is to examine our experience, as well as that of others, with the use of impedance plethysmography, phleborheography, Doppler ultrasound, ^{125}I labelled fibrinogen scanning and ambulatory venous pressures in the diagnosis of acute and chronic venous disease.

Plethysmography

The plethysmographic techniques are used to assess venous capacitance and outflow in response to temporary extrinsic venous compression. Various plethysmographic techniques have been utilized, including impedance, air displacement, water displacement and strain gauge. The two most commonly employed methods, however, are impedance plethysmography[11-13] and phleborheography, an air displacement technique introduced by Cranley[14,15].

Impedance plethysmography (IPG) reflects the changes in electrical impedance which accompany changes in blood volume. Based upon Ohm's law, if a fixed current is passed through a biological segment, such as the lower extremity, changes in the measured voltage are a function of impedance and, by extension, of blood volume.

1

Position of patient

With the patient in the supine position, the lower extremities are elevated, externally rotated and comfortably flexed at the hips and knees. The impedance electrodes are applied to the calves bilaterally. Pneumatic cuffs of 30 cm width are used to effect temporary, extrinsic venous occlusion.

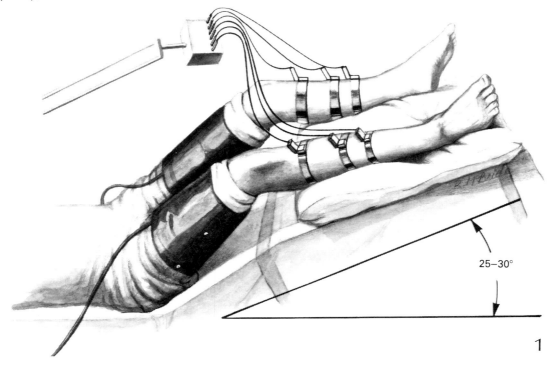

25–30°

1

2

Measuring impedance

The change in impedance 1 min following proximal venous compression reflects the venous capacitance (VC) and is expressed as a percentage change in the impedance (% $\triangle$ I) relative to a standard calibration (C, 0.1% $\triangle$ I/mm). The venous outflow (VO) is measured 3 s following the release of proximal venous compression, and is also expressed as a percentage change in the impedance.

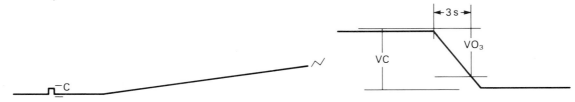

2

3

Acute deep venous thrombosis

In comparison to a normal examination, the presence of an acute deep venous thrombosis is characterized by a decreased capacitance ($<1.85\%\triangle I$) and outflow ($<0.95\%\triangle I$). A representative tracing demonstrates decreased capacitance and outflow in the left lower extremity (below), characteristic of deep venous occlusion. The upper tracing, from the right lower extremity, is normal.

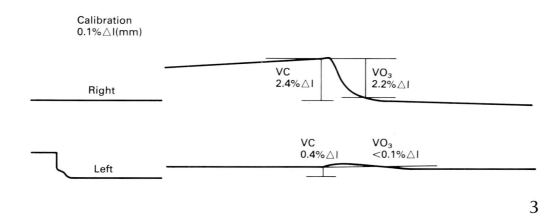

3

Results

The results of IPG in 88 consecutive patients (108 limbs) was reported recently by O'Donnell et al.[16] The overall accuracy of this technique, when compared with venography, was 90 per cent (Table 1). Two false negative results occurred when DVT was confined to the calf. However, the accuracy of IPG in detecting acute DVT in the popliteal or iliofemoral veins was 100 per cent. Five of 9 false positive results occurred in patients with previous DVT in whom abnormal haemodynamics persisted. Of the 4 normal extremities with abnormal haemodynamics, 2 reverted to normal on repeat examination while venous outflow in 2 remained equivocal.

Table 1 Accuracy of IPG compared to venography

		IPG		
Venography		Normal	Abnormal	Accuracy of IPG
Normal	(n = 57)	53	4	93%
DVT	(n = 25)	2	23	92%
Insufficiency	(n = 26)	21	5	81%
				—
				90% Overall

Phleborheography

4

The method

Phleborheography is an air displacement plethysmographic technique employing five cuffs on the extremity as well as a chest cuff to record respiration. The patient is examined in the recumbent position with the lower extremities placed 10–15° below the level of the right atrium and the patient's weight shifted to the side of the examination. Unlike the impedance technique utilized in our institution only one extremity is examined at a time.

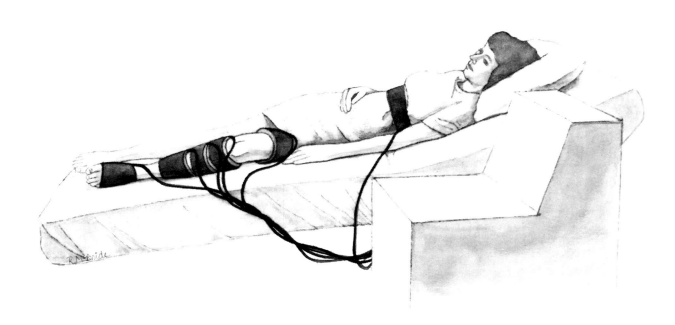

4

5

Results

A six-channel strip chart-recorder is utilized to show the pneumograph and any volume changes in the thigh and calf cuffs. Volume changes in the thigh, calf and ankle are observed coincident with respiration. In addition, volume changes are observed in the more proximal cuffs in response to foot compression (*a*). A decrease in foot volume, is observed following compression of the calf (*c*).

In the presence of obstructive DVT the characteristic tracing may show absence of spontaneous respiratory volume changes (*b* – upper, mid and lower calf), poor emptying of the foot on calf compression (*d*) and increases in the baseline segmental limb volume distal to the thrombosis in response to calf and foot compression (*b*). Cranley[15] has reported an overall accuracy of 97 per cent, with a sensitivity of 92 per cent and a specificity of 100 per cent. Although these data are perhaps somewhat superior to our own results with IPG, we have continued with this technique because of the greater ease of bilateral testing.

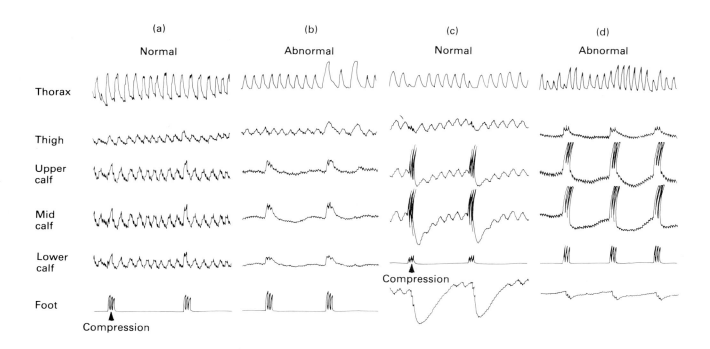

5

Doppler ultrasound

6

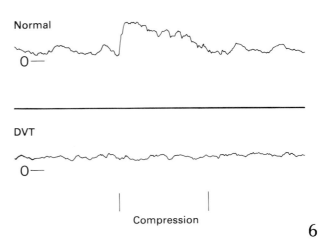

Normal

DVT

Compression

6

The examination

The application of Doppler ultrasound to the diagnosis of deep venous thrombosis is based upon the transcutaneous detection of venous flow patterns. The Doppler flowmeter employs a transducer coupled to the skin with an acoustic gel. One piezoelectric crystal in the transducer emits an ultrasonic signal at a frequency of 5 MHz, while a second receives the reflected signal. There is a shift in the transmitted frequency when that signal is reflected from a moving surface, so that venous (or arterial) flow velocity is proportional to the frequency shift which occurs when the transmitted signal is reflected from the moving red blood cells.

DVT is characterized by the absence of spontaneous venous flow, the presence of a continuous flow velocity pattern without phasic respiratory variation, and/or diminished augmentation on compression.

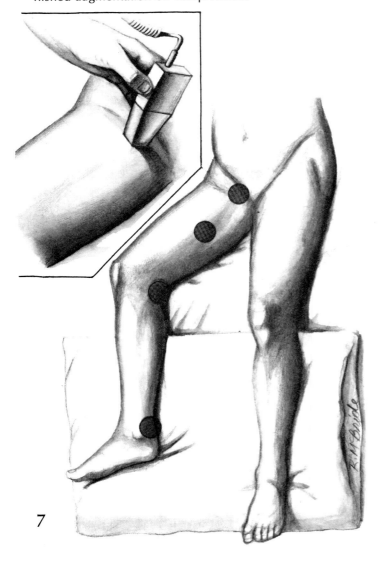

7

7

Position of patient

The Doppler venous examination is performed with the patient in the supine position. The leg to be examined is externally rotated, and the patient's weight is shifted onto the ipsilateral hip. The common femoral, superficial femoral, popliteal, and posterior tibial veins are identified relative to the corresponding artery with the Doppler probe (*inset*). The presence or absence of spontaneity and phasicity of venous flow are then noted at each level, as well as the response to thigh and/or calf compression.

Venous flow in the common femoral, superficial femoral and popliteal veins is spontaneous. Flow velocity in the posterior tibial vein, however, is often below the threshold sensitivity of the instrument, and identification of this vein may require augmentation of flow by compression of the foot. Venous flow is phasic in character, decreasing with inspiration and increasing during expiration. Compression of the thigh, distal to the superficial and common femoral veins, or the calf, distal to the popliteal and femoral veins, should also augment venous flow and confirm patency of these distal veins (*see Illustration 6*). Conversely, compression of the calf interrupts venous flow through the posterior tibial vein in the presence of competent valves, while release of compression augments flow and confirms patency of the tibial venous system.

Results

Strandness and Sumner[17] reported a 93 per cent accuracy with the technique in 51 patients, false negative examinations being most commonly associated with thrombi in the small veins of the calf. Like phleborheography, the technique is more useful in the diagnosis of calf vein thrombosis than impedance plethysmography. Barnes *et al.*[5] reported an 84 per cent accuracy in the diagnosis of calf vein thrombosis in 55 extremities. The majority of inaccurate studies were falsely positive and resulted from subfascial haematoma, cellulitis and muscle paralysis.

^{125}I Fibrinogen scanning

The method

In 1960, Hobbs and Davies[18] reported that fibrinogen tagged with ^{131}I was incorporated within experimental thrombi and could be localized with suitable gamma-counting equipment. Investigations involving humans followed[19]. The use of ^{125}I, a low-energy gamma emitter, by Atkins and Hawkins in 1965[20], allowed use of portable counting equipment and made the technique practical. The patient is given sodium iodide to saturate the thyroid (100 mg per day), after which a dose of 50–100 mCi of ^{125}I tagged human fibrinogen is administered intravenously.

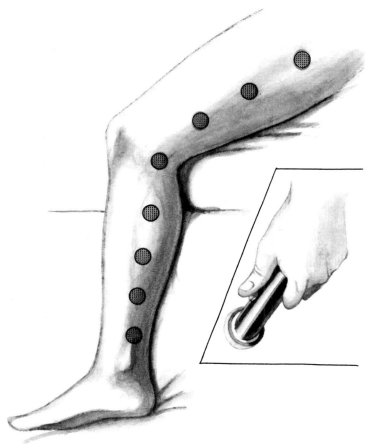

8

Counting sites over the medial thigh and calf are selected and scanned daily for 5 days (*inset* demonstrates the small hand-held probe which is used). These peripheral counts are then expressed as a percentage of the precordial count. An increase of 15 or 20 per cent relative to the precordial count[10, 21] is considered diagnostic of venous thrombosis. Using these criteria, Kakkar *et al.*[22] reported a 92 per cent correlation with phlebography while Browse *et al.*[23] reported an 80 per cent correlation.

Clinical usefulness

A major disadvantage of this technique is the inaccuracy associated with established venous thromboses, as well as the decreased sensitivity to iliofemoral thrombosis. However, ^{125}I labelled fibrinogen is extremely sensitive to the presence of calf vein thrombi. While the clinical significance of these thrombi remains controversial, the technique is useful in evaluating the efficacy of prophylactic techniques in the prevention of postoperative DVT. Because of the time required to complete the test, however, its applicability in the diagnosis of acute DVT has been limited in our clinical practice.

8

Ambulatory venous pressures

The surgical management of patients with chronic venous insufficiency should be based upon precise diagnosis. A reasonable approach to such therapy requires the surgical extirpation of superficial veins in patients with saphenofemoral or saphenopopliteal incompetence, and the control of incompetent perforating veins by sclerotherapy, operative ligation or conservative therapy in patients with deep venous disease. Newer reconstructive procedures in the treatment of deep venous insufficiency include venous bypass and valvular reconstruction or transplant. Clinical evaluation, including the palpation of incompetent perforating veins and use of the Trendelenburg and Perthes tests, has generally been employed in the diagnosis of venous insufficiency. Ambulatory venous pressure measurements have also been advocated to characterize more precisely the aetiology and extent of such insufficiency. In addition, such techniques are essential to evaluate the efficacy of venous reconstructive procedures.

9

The method

Direct venous pressure measurements, recorded at rest as well as during and after ambulation, can be obtained by introducing a butterfly needle into a vein on the dorsum of the foot. The infusion set is connected by disposable plastic tubing to a calibrated pressure transducer. Resting pressures are measured with the patient on the treadmill, following which ambulation is initiated for 20–30 s at 0.5 mile per hour (0.8 km/h). The patient is then asked to stand quietly in place until pressure measurements return to preambulatory levels. Saphenous vein and superficial venous haemodynamics are assessed by repeating the procedure following inflation of a 7.5 cm wide thigh tourniquet so that the resting pressure is increased by at least 5 mmHg. The fall in venous pressure during ambulation is expressed as a percentage of the maximum measured pressure (%P). The time for restitution of pressure to preambulatory values is measured in seconds (RP).

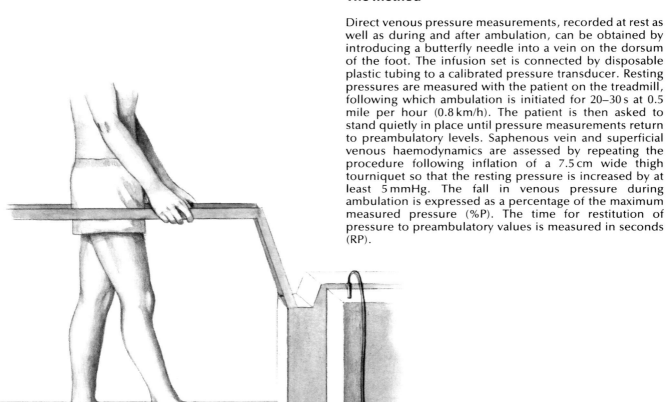

10a, b & c

Results

The resulting pressure in patients with and without venous insufficiency is equivalent to the hydrostatic pressure referable to the right atrium and ranges from 80 to 100 mmHg. Tracings from normal volunteers (a) show a significant fall in venous pressure during ambulation (solid lines indicate period of ambulation), followed by a slow return to preambulatory values. Tracings characteristic of saphenofemoral incompetence and deep venous insufficiency are illustrated in (b) and (c), respectively. RP and %P are significantly lower in all patients with venous insufficiency. Following application of a proximal tourniquet (broken line), RP and %P return to normal in patients with saphenofemoral incompetence and are unimproved in patients with deep venous insufficiency.

Comparable data may also be obtained by the photoplethysmographic technique recently described by Abramowitz et al.[24] Reflux times as determined by the technique correlate closely with RP as determined invasively; however, the additional pressure data available by direct measurement have also been of interest to us in selected groups of patients.

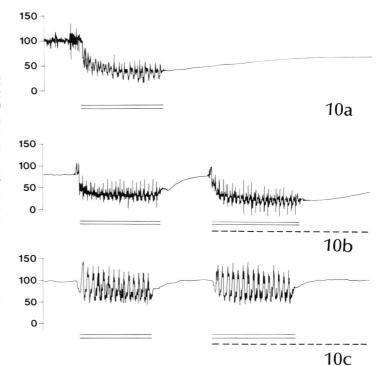

10a

10b

10c

References

1. Evans, D. S. The early diagnosis of deep vein thrombosis by ultrasound. British Journal of Surgery 1970; 57: 726–728

2. Haeger, K. Problems of acute deep venous thrombosis. I. The interpretation of signs and symptoms. Angiology 1969; 20: 219–223

3. Hume, M., Sevitt, S., Thomas, D. P. Venous thrombosis and pulmonary embolism. Cambridge, Massachusetts: Harvard University Press, 1970

4. Alexander, R. H., Folse, R., Pizzorno, J., Conn, R. Thrombophlebitis and thromboembolism: results of a prospective study. Annals of Surgery 1974; 180: 883–887

5. Barnes, R. W., Russell, H. E., Wu, K. K., Hoak, J. C. Accuracy of Doppler ultrasound in clinically suspected venous thrombosis of the calf. Surgery, Gynecology and Obstetrics 1976; 143: 425–428

6. McLachlin, J. A., Richards, T., Paterson, J. C. An evaluation of clinical signs in the diagnosis of venous thrombosis. Archives of Surgery 1962; 85: 738–744

7. Cranley, J. J., Canos, A. J., Sull, W. J. The diagnosis of deep venous thrombosis: fallibility of clinical signs and symptoms. Archives of Surgery 1976; 111: 34–36

8. Sevitt, S. Venous thrombosis and pulmonary embolism. In: Clark, R., Badger, F. G., Sevitt, S., eds. In: Modern trends in accident medicine and surgery. London: Butterworths, 1959 :247–263

9. Walker, M. G. The natural history of venous thromboembolism. British Journal of Surgery 1972; 59: 753–754

10. Kakkar, V. V., Howe, C. T., Nicolaides, A. N., Renney, J. T. G., Clarke, M. B. Deep vein thrombosis of the leg: is there a high risk group? American Journal of Surgery 1970; 120: 527–530

11. Wheeler, H. B., Mullick, S. C. Detection of venous obstruction in the leg by measurement of electrical impedance. Annals of the New York Academy of Science 1970; 170: 804–811

12. Wheeler, H. B., O'Donnell, J. A., Anderson, F. A., Penny, B. C., Perua, R. A., Benedict, C. Jr. Bedside screening for venous thrombosis using occlusive impedance phlebography. Angiology 1975; 26: 199–210

13. Wheeler, H. B., O'Donnell, J. A., Anderson, F. A., Benedict, K. Jr. Occlusive impedance phlebography, a diagnostic procedure for venous thrombosis and pulmonary embolism. Progress in Cardiovascular Diseases 1974; 17: 199–205

14. Cranley, J. J., Gay, A. Y., Grass, A. M., Fiorindo, A. S. Plethysmographic technique for the diagnosis of deep venous thrombosis of the lower extremities. Surgery, Gynecology and Obstetrics 1973; 136: 385–394

15. Cranley, J. J., Canos, A. J., Sull, W. J., Grass, A. M. Phleborheographic technique for diagnosing deep venous thrombosis of the lower extremities. Surgery, Gynecology and Obstetrics 1975; 141: 331–339

16. O'Donnell, J. A., Hobson, R. W., Lynch, T. G., Jamil, Z., Hart, L. Impedance plethysmography: noninvasive diagnosis of deep venous thrombosis and arterial insufficiency. American Surgeon 1983; 49: 26–30

17. Strandness, D. E. Jr, Sumner, D. S. Ultrasonic velocity detector in the diagnosis of thrombophlebitis. Archives of Surgery 1972; 104: 180–183

18. Hobbs, J. T., Davies, J. W. L. Detection of venous thrombosis with ^{131}I labelled fibrinogen in the rabbit. Lancet 1960; 2: 134–135

19. Nanson, E. M., Palkco, P. D., Dick, A. A., Fedoruk, S. Q. Early detection of deep vein thrombosis of the legs with I-131 tagged human fibrinogen: a clinical study. Annals of Surgery 1965; 162: 438–445

20. Atkins, P., Hawkins, L. A. Detection of venous thrombosis in the legs. Lancet 1965; 2: 1217–1219

21. Negus, D., Pinto, D. J., LeQuesne, L. P., Brown, N., Chapman, M. [125]I labelled fibrinogen in the diagnosis of deep vein thrombosis and its correlation with phlebography. British Journal of Surgery 1968; 55: 835–839

22. Kakkar, V. V., Howe, C. T., Flanc, C., Clarke, M. B. Natural history of postoperative deep vein thrombosis. Lancet 1969; 2: 230–233

23. Browse, N. L., Clapham, W. F., Croft, D. N., Jones, D. J., Thomas, M. L., Williams, J. O. Diagnosis of established deep vein thrombosis with the I-125 fibrinogen uptake test. British Medical Journal 1971; 4: 325–328

24. Abramowitz, H. B., Queral, L. A., Flinn, W. R., Nora, et al. The use of photopléthysmography in the assessment of venous insufficiency: a comparison to venous pressure measurement. Surgery 1979; 86: 434–441

Illustrations by Anita Matthews and Robert Wabnitz

Phlebography

James A. DeWeese MD, FACS
Professor and Chairman, Division of Cardiothoracic Surgery,
University of Rochester Medical Center Rochester, New York, USA

Indications

Phlebography remains the most accurate method for evaluation of anatomical variations, congenital abnormalities and pathological changes in the veins of the leg or arm. Phlebography is most useful in establishing the correct diagnosis in patients with suspected deep venous thrombosis of either the upper or lower extremity. Classic physical signs of swelling, tenderness or Homans' sign are frequently absent in patients with deep venous thrombosis and conversely the signs may be present in the absence of venous thrombosis[1]. The pattern or extent of venous thrombosis can be useful in determining rational medical or surgical treatment including venous thrombectomy, interruption of the vena cava, and pulmonary embolectomy[2, 3, 4, 5, 6]. The changes occurring in veins following all treatments of acute venous thrombosis can be demonstrated[7]. A functional evaluation of intermittent compression symptoms of the arm can be obtained[8]. A functional evaluation of venous drainage of the leg can be obtained by the study of phlebograms taken in the semi-erect position before and after exercise[9]. The aetiology of venous ulcers in patients with complicated varicose vein problems can be determined[10].

263

Phlebography of the lower limb

Equipment

Special requirements for the performance of functional ascending phlebography are a tilt table, a 90 cm (36 inch) long cassette holder, and the ability to make serial film changes.

1

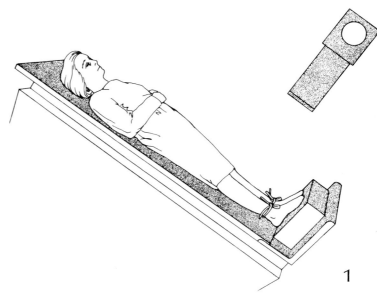

Position of patient

The patient is placed on a table which is tilted 30–45° from the horizontal. Films are best exposed with the patient in the semi-erect position. The radiopaque material is heavier than blood and it is possible to fill more veins more completely in that position and avoid layering artifacts.

A needle is introduced into any superficial vein on the dorsum of the foot. A rubber tourniquet is applied snugly around the ankle.

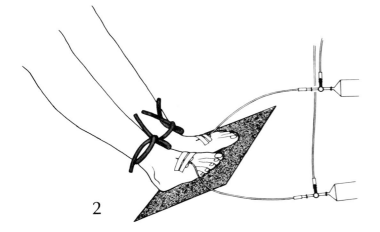

2

Injection

After injection of 40–80 ml of radiopaque contrast material, one or two long films are exposed. The patient is then asked to push himself up on his toes five times. Additional films are then exposed. The extent to which the contrast material will fill the venous system is unpredictable and the use of long films and multiple exposures can decrease the number of injections and amount of contrast material necessary for a satisfactory study. The patient is returned to a horizontal position and 300 ml of saline are infused.

3

Normal phlebogram[11]

Normal veins have smooth parallel walls and sharply demonstrated valve cusps. The anterior tibial, peroneal and posterior tibial veins taper slightly and are usually double. The doubled veins join at varying levels below and above the knee joint to form the popliteal vein. The superficial femoral vein is also doubled over a varying distance in about 25 per cent of normal extremities. The deep femoral vein is frequently visualized because of its distal connection with collateral veins from the popliteal vein, but may not be demonstrated except through reflux at its proximal end.

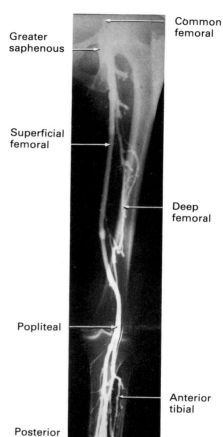

3

4

Calf vein thrombosis[1]

The unequivocal diagnosis of deep venous thrombosis was based on the presence of well defined filling defects and heavily opacified veins and the demonstration of these defects on at least two radiographs. The defects are frequently globular. In some instances they appear serpentine and seem to be waving in the proximal bloodstream. Smaller bubble-like defects are frequently seen distal to a thrombus defect.

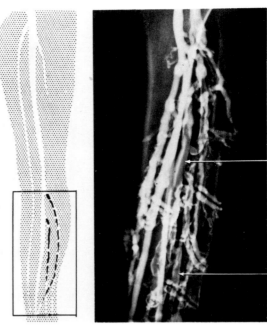

4

(Reproduced from DeWeese, J. A., Rogoff, S. Phlebographic patterns of acute deep venous thrombosis of the leg. Surgery 1963; 53:99)

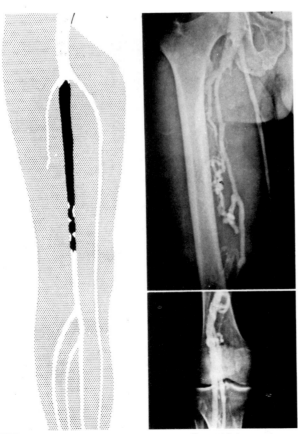

(Reproduced from DeWeese, J. A., Rogoff, S. Phlebographic patterns of acute deep venous thrombosis of the leg. Surgery 1963; 53:99)

5

Femoral vein thrombosis[1]

Femoral vein thrombosis is usually seen in association with proximal or distal occlusion, but on occasion is localized to the femoral vein. Bubble-like defects are demonstrated distal to a non-visualized segment of obstructed femoral vein. Non-visualization of the femoral vein with good opacification of the proximal and distal veins and the presence of collaterals is considered thrombotic obstruction.

6

Iliofemoral venous thrombosis[1]

Thrombotic obstruction of the iliac and femoral vein is usually associated with thrombosis of the calf veins. In those instances only numerous feathery collaterals are visualized in the entire lower leg (a). In most instances there is localized occlusion of the iliac and femoral vein with remarkably normal appearing calf veins and popliteal veins (b). In rare instances, localized iliac vein obstruction with bubble-like defects of thrombi in the femoral vein are seen. The distal femoral, popliteal and calf veins are remarkably normal (c).

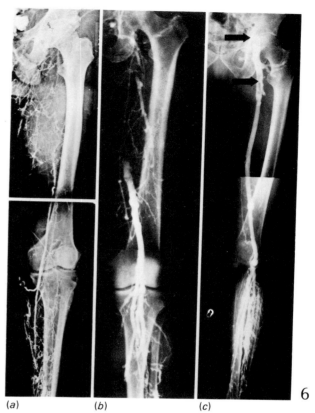

(a)   (b)   (c)   6

(Reproduced from Haimovici, H., ed. Vascular surgery principles and techniques. New York: McGraw-Hill, 1976)

7

Post-thrombotic changes

Veins which have been the site of venous thrombosis usually appear to have irregular walls with lack of valvular structures or remain occluded. In some instances there is little phlebographic evidence of previous thrombosis[7]. These phlebograms were obtained prior to treatment (a), following 2 weeks of heparin therapy (b), and 6 months later (c). Lysis of the thrombus and adherence to the venous wall has occurred at 2 weeks with further healing obvious at 6 months. On the other hand the iliac vein remains occluded and only collateral veins are visualized in the pelvis.

Special studies

It may be possible to visualize the iliac veins and inferior vena cava by injections at the ankles. Better visualization of those structures is best obtained with direct injections into the femoral vein. Retrograde injections of contrast material into the common femoral vein to identify incompetent valves is possible but there is controversy regarding what is normal. Incompetent perforators may be visualized on ascending phlebography and can also be visualized by special cineangiographic techniques.

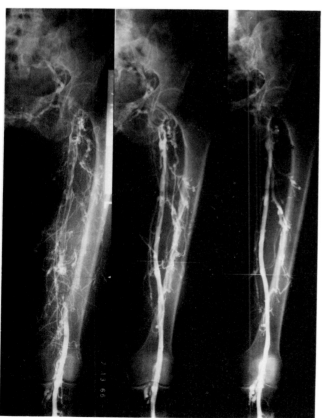

(a)   (b)   (c)

7

Upper extremity phlebography

Position of patient

Satisfactory phlebograms can usually be obtained with the patient supine and the arm in neutral position. To demonstrate the site of obstruction in patients with intermittent venous obstruction other positions are necessary. The obstruction may be identified by hyperabducting the arm of the supine patient. Alternatively the phlebogram can be performed in the upright position in association with venous pressure studies with the shoulders in both neutral and exaggerated military position.

8

Injection

A needle is inserted into the median antecubital vein or median antebrachial vein which communicate directly with the basilic vein, axillary vein and subclavian vein. Injections into the radial side of the arm or cephalic vein do not usually allow visualization of the basilic vein. After injection of 25 ml of radiopaque material multiple films are exposed.

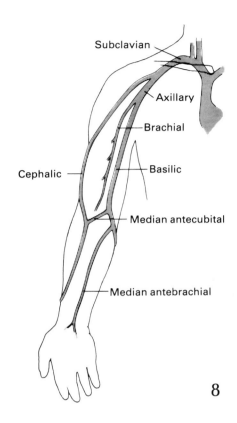

8

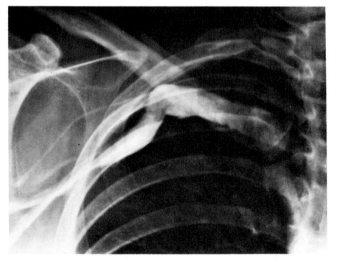

9

9

Normal phlebogram

The basilic vein is occasionally bifid. The cephalic vein and brachial vein are rarely seen. The axillary and subclavian vein are smooth walled. Short segments of other tributaries may be seen. The superior vena cava is rarely visualized well because of the dilution by blood from the internal jugular vein.

10

Intermittent venous obstruction[8]

With the arm in the hyperabducted position or the shoulders in military position, phlebrograms usually demonstrate the column of dye ending as a beak-like deformity at the outer edge of the first rib. Distal distension of the vein is observed and collaterals may be seen. The venous pressure will be at least three times normal.

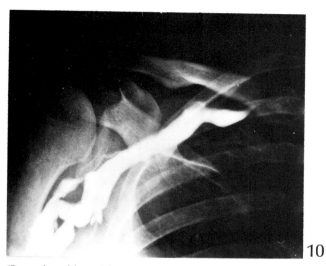

10

(Reproduced from Adams, J. T., DeWeese, J. A., Mahoney, E. B., Rob, C. G. Intermittent subclavian vein obstruction without thrombosis. Surgery 1968; 63:147)

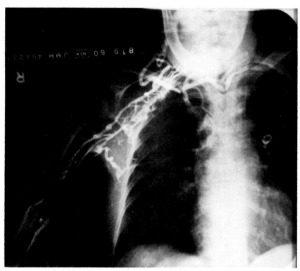

11

(Reproduced from Adams, J. T., DeWeese, J. A. Effort thrombosis of the axillary and subclavian veins. Journal of Trauma 1971; 2:923)

11

Acute venous thrombosis

Phlebograms taken during the acute phase of effort thrombosis usually demonstrate an occlusion of the subclavian vein with small collaterals visible near the jugular vein. Thrombi may be seen in the axillary vein[2].

12

Post-thrombotic

The usual appearance is of continued obstruction of the subclavian vein with the patent axillary vein draining into the jugular vein and superior vena cava through large collaterals which bypass the first rib. These collaterals may be obstructed by elevation of the arm. Secondary collaterals in the chest wall are then seen.

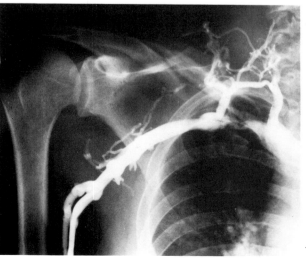

12

Complications

Radiopaque materials may rarely produce allergic reactions consisting of urticaria or even anaphylactic shock. Benadryl or even cortisone may be required for the reaction or for the preparation of patients who have had previous reactions.

The materials may produce acute phlebitis. This has been observed in less than 5 per cent of patients and usually these are patients with postphlebitic varicosities. The flushing of the vein with saline and immediate elevation of the leg may decrease the incidence of this complication.

Skin sloughs may occur following intradermal or subcutaneous injections of the contrast material and great care must be taken with placement of the needles into the vein.

References

1. DeWeese, J. A., Rogoff, S. M. Phelbographic patterns of acute deep venous thrombosis of the leg. Surgery 1963; 53: 99–108

2. Adams, J. T., DeWeese, J. A. 'Effort' thrombosis of the axillary and subclavian veins. Journal of Trauma 1971; 11:923–930

3. DeWeese, J. A. Thrombectomy for acute iliofemoral venous thrombosis. Journal of Cardiovascular Surgery 1964; 5:703–712

4. DeWeese, J. A., Adams, J. T., Gaiser, D. L. Subclavian venous thrombectomy. Circulation 1970; 51 & 52 Suppl. II-158–II-164

5. Adams, J. T., Feingold, B. E., DeWeese, J. A. Comparative evaluation of ligation and partial interruption of the inferior vena cava. Archives of Surgery 1971; 103:272–276

6. DeWeese, J. A. The role of pulmonary embolectomy in venous thromboembolism. Journal of Cardiovascular Surgery 1976; 17:348–353

7. Lipchik, E. O., DeWeese, J. A., Rogoff, S. M. Serial long-term phlebography after documented lower leg thrombosis. Radiology 1976; 120:563–566

8. Adams, J. T., DeWeese, J. A., Mahoney, E. B., Rob, C. G. Intermittent subclavian vein obstruction without thrombosis. Surgery 1968; 63:147–165

9. DeWeese, J. A., Rogoff, S. M. Functional ascending phlebography of the lower extremity by serial long film technique. Evaluation of anatomic and functional detail in 62 extremities. American Journal of Roentgenology 1959; 81:841–854

10. DeWeese, J. A., Rogoff, S. M. Clinical uses of functional ascending phlebography of the lower extremity. Angiology 1958; 9:268–278

11. Rogoff, S. M., DeWeese, J. A. Phlebography of the lower extremity. Journal of the American Medical Association 1960; 172:1599–1606

Illustrations by Robert N. Lane

Operations for varicose veins

John T. Hobbs MD, FRCS
Senior Lecturer in Surgery, University of London;
Consultant Surgeon, St Mary's Hospital, London, UK

CLASSIFICATION OF VARICOSE VEINS

The term 'varicose veins' refers to abnormally prominent veins on the lower limb. These can be classified into distinct types as follows.

Dilated venules, venous 'flares', 'bursts' or 'stars', telangiectases

These small vessels are only of cosmetic importance, being related to skin structure and hormonal effects but may be secondary to varicosis, as with the typical 'ankle flare'.

Athlete's hypertrophic veins

In healthy athletes the veins may be prominent but this dilatation is not abnormal being due to high blood volume and increased flow through muscular limbs.

Arteriovenous fistulae

Arterial pressure transmitted to the venous system directly will result in venous dilatation. This may be associated with congenital disorders such as Klippel-Trenaunay syndrome, where grossly dilated veins may be present which are atypical in distribution. Dilated veins are also seen in association with acquired arteriovenous fistula which may follow gunshot, stab wounds or surgical trauma.

1a & b

Internal iliac vein incompetence

This only occurs in women as a complication of pregnancy or, rarely, following pelvic infection and may be a sequel to thrombosis in the pelvic veins. Varices arise from the posterior vulval region and extend down the medial aspect of the upper thigh and over the back of the thigh or across the adductor tendon to join the long saphenous system. These small veins are particularly painful during the premenstrual period and sometimes following coitus.

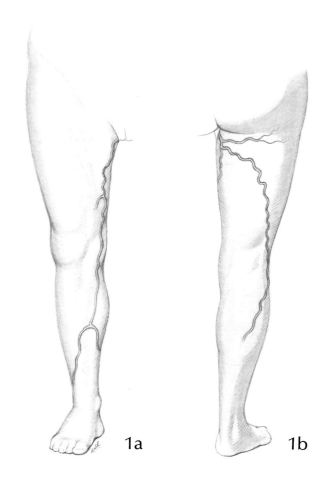

1a   1b

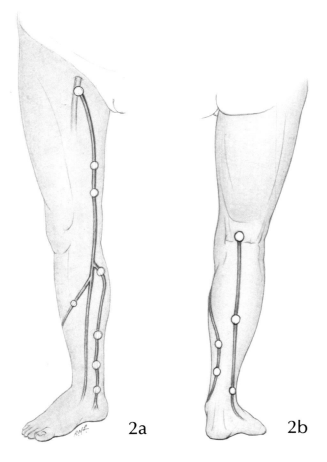

2a   2b

2a & b

Primary varicose veins

This is the most common problem requiring treatment. There is usually a family history and the inherent defect is either a weakness of the vein wall or valvular insufficiency and often a combination of both. The long saphenous system is the most frequently involved vein and the incompetence of the saphenofemoral vein junction may result in dilatation of the long saphenous vein or its anterolateral tributary. Below the knee, the incompetence usually involves the posterior arch tributary, sometimes the anterior tibial vein but rarely the long saphenous vein below the upper third of the calf. Incompetence of the short saphenous system may be associated with incompetence of the long saphenous system or may occur alone. The primary incompetence may also involve the large direct perforating veins.

Secondary varicose veins

The superficial leg veins may become dilated if the venous outflow from the leg is obstructed by extrinsic pressure caused by enlarged lymph nodes, pelvic tumours and bony displacements, or by occlusion of the lumen due to iliac vein thrombosis. Similarly, the superficial veins in the thigh, particularly the long saphenous vein, may become varicose when functioning as collateral pathways to overcome occlusion of the superficial femoral vein in the post-thrombotic syndrome.

In the later stages of the post-thrombotic syndrome with valvular insufficiency of the popliteal vein distal to proximal obstruction or valvular destruction, the perforating veins in the lower leg become grossly incompetent resulting in dilated veins on the lower leg and secondary skin damage. Sometimes the perforating veins become incompetent after local thrombosis without involvement of the deep veins.

Treatment should be confined to eliminating the incompetent perforating veins by sclerotherapy. This protects the skin from the underlying deep vein damage, which cannot be cured.

TREATMENT OF VARICOSE VEINS

It is evident that to treat venous problems effectively each limb must be carefully assessed and an accurate diagnosis established. The correct plan of treatment must then be made and precisely executed. The methods of treatment include reassurance, elastic stockings, sclerotherapy and surgery.

Some patients can be reassured that the veins are not significant and that the symptoms are due to some other cause, such as referred pain from the lumbar spine, arthritis or arterial disease.

Elastic stockings will hide veins and prevent the condition deteriorating but will not cure them.

Venous problems can only be cured by either sclerotherapy or surgery. For sclerotherapy to be effective the vein must be kept occluded after the introduction of a destructive agent until fibrosis is permanent. Therefore injection compression is an effective method whenever the treated veins can be bandaged. The termination of the long and short saphenous veins and the upper thighs cannot be adequately bandaged; therefore venous problems involving these veins and those on the upper thigh are best treated by surgical methods, rather than sclerotherapy.

There is no standard operation for varicose veins–each leg must be carefully assessed, accurately marked and dealt with accordingly. The commonest operations are those on the long saphenous and short saphenous vein systems. Incompetent perforating veins can either be treated surgically whilst dealing with the saphenous systems or they can be treated by sclerotherapy. With the use of effective injection techniques there is now no need for the radical subfascial approach to ligate perforating veins.

Indications for operation

Primary varicosis is progressive and, if untreated, the veins increase in number and size. The condition may often be cured by adequate surgery during the earlier stages. Therefore, progression of the disorder is an indication for active treatment.

The two most common complaints causing patients to seek treatment are aching discomfort in the legs when standing and the cosmetic appearance. Treatment is also indicated for complications, which include superficial thrombophlebitis, acute bleeding, eczema and ulceration.

Operations available

The standard operations are the following.

1. Flush ligation and division of the long saphenous vein at the groin, together with stripping of the main trunks down to the upper calf and removal of the dilated and tortuous tributaries (LSV strip).

2. Flush ligation and division of the short saphenous vein at its termination, which is usually in the popliteal fossa, and stripping of its trunk and major tributaries (SSV strip).

3. Occasional exposure, ligation and division of ankle-perforating veins if they are grossly enlarged and incompetent.

Note: In this context 'flush' refers to ligation and division of the saphenous veins flush with the femoral or popliteal vein, so that the ligature is proximal to all tributaries.

The surgery need not be radical because any residual small tributaries can later be treated by injection if they do not disappear after surgical removal of the proximal incompetent vein. Both legs can be treated together and meticulous care is required to prevent recurrence. Although the operation provides excellent training for the trainee surgeon, supervision is necessary because of the high recurrence rate when the surgery is not accurate.

Preoperative preparation

On admission, a careful physical examination is made and routine investigations include urine examination, chest X-ray, ECG, haemoglobin estimation and other specific tests as indicated. The whole of the leg and adjacent pubic area is shaved.

3a & b

The patient then stands in a good light and the legs are carefully examined to check the venous pathology which is reassessed and compared with the outpatient assessment, previously detailed on the record card.

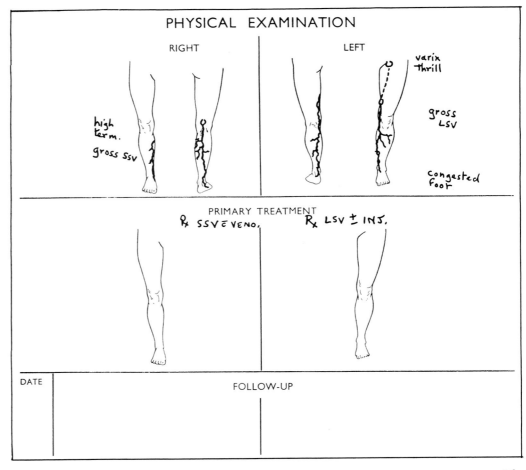

3a

3b

4

The accurate marking of the veins by the surgeon who is to operate is a most important step, because when the legs are elevated many of the veins will no longer be apparent. The superficial veins are outlined between parallel lines which indicate the size of the veins and this is best done with a felt-tipped indelible marker (Pentel, N50).

After the veins have been fully and carefully outlined, the sliding finger method is used to find the points of control from which various sections of vein refill after being emptied, and these points are intended to include the incompetent perforating veins. In the lower leg, in association with incompetence of the long and short saphenous veins there will be a definite perforating vein where the refluxing blood re-enters the deep system but because of gross dilatation this will also show reversed flow during some stages of the walking cycle. There may be further primary and secondary perforating veins which are identified and marked by a circle. Tourniquet tests and examination with Doppler are not necessary at this time.

Anaesthesia

General anaesthesia is used and endotracheal intubation is only necessary if there is difficulty in maintaining an adequate airway. If general anaesthesia is contraindicated because of cardiac or pulmonary disease the operation may be carried out under lumbar epidural anaesthesia.

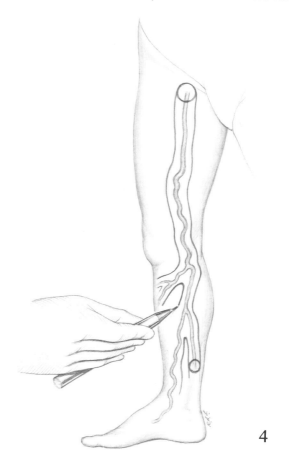

4

Equipment

The following equipment should be available.

Instruments

2 Sponge holders
5 Towel clips
1 Suture scissors
1 Size 3 scalpel handle with No. 10 blade
1 Size 3 scalpel handle with No. 15 blade
1 McIndoe dissecting scissors
1 McIndoe dissecting forceps
2 Small retractors
1 Needle holder
6 Crile artery forceps, 5½ inch, straight
3 Crile artery forceps, 5½ inch, curved
3 Mosquito forceps, 5 inch, straight
3 Mosquito forceps, 5 inch, curved
4 Stripper cables, Bowden with threaded ends
2 Cylindrical stripper tips
2 Olive stripper tips
4 Stripper heads, 9 mm
2 Stripper heads, 12 mm
2 Stripper heads, 6 mm

Sutures

2/0 Plain CGS (W103) for ligature
 0 Chromic CGS (W114) for large vessel ligature
3/0 Plain on 25 mm round body curved needle (W438) or 2/0 (W439)
5/0 Ethilon on fine straight skin needle (W624)

Position of patient

5

For operations on the long saphenous vein and front of the legs the patient is placed in the supine position with feet apart but a spreading board or table is not necessary.

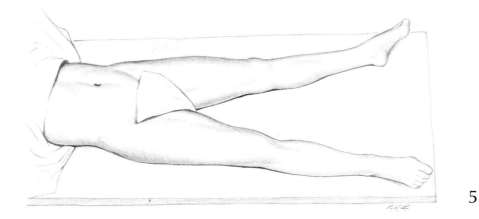

5

6

For operations on the short saphenous vein the patient is placed in the lateral position with the lower leg flexed.

After the proximal part of the operation is complete the table is tilted head down to an angle of more than 10°. This reduces venous pressure to zero and minimizes bleeding. Excessive tilt for a long period may result in oedema of the face, especially the eyelids, and introduces the risk of air entering the circulation if a vein is opened.

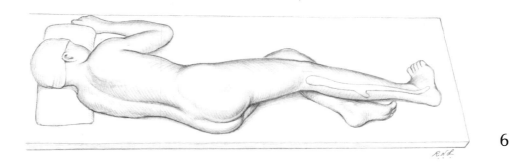

6

Operation for long saphenous vein incompetence

7

The incision

The hip is abducted and the knees slightly flexed so that the tension lines in the upper thigh are parallel to the inguinal ligament.

The saphenofemoral junction is approximately 3 cm below and 4 cm lateral to the pubic tubercle and is located as a slight filling deficiency medial to the femoral artery pulse. A 5 cm incision is centred on this point and made in the line of the skin creases. In case of difficulty the incision should be lengthened. Diathermy is not used.

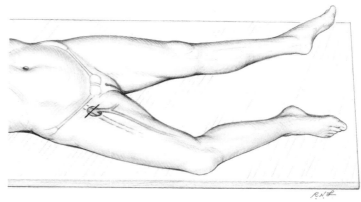

7

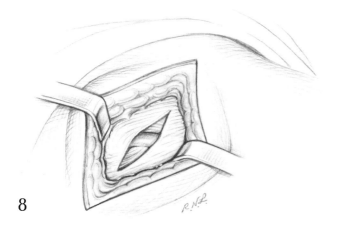

8

8

Division of membranous layer (Scarpa's) of superficial fascia

The superficial tissues are divided in the line of the skin incision, using the scalpel or scissors, until the deep layer of the superficial fascia is exposed. The bluish long saphenous vein can often be seen deep to this fascia. The membranous fascia is then divided in the line of the skin and no other tissues are cut so that there is no risk of damaging lymphatic vessels or nerves. Small skin retractors are manipulated by an assistant to expose the fascia and then the saphenous vein.

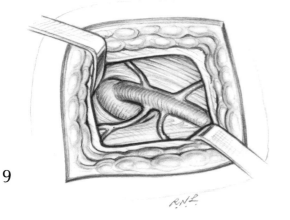

9

9

Exposure of saphenofemoral junction

After exposure, the saphenous vein is then cleaned both distally and proximally using a swab held in non-toothed (McIndoe) dissecting forceps. The tributaries are exposed and the termination of the saphenous vein at the femoral vein is exposed.

10

Division of long saphenous vein

When the saphenofemoral junction has been identified, the long saphenous vein is divided between straight artery forceps, so that the proximal stump can be elevated to aid isolation of the tributaries. If a small artery (superficial external pudendal) passes in front of the saphenous vein, the proximal saphenous vein stump can be passed under the artery, or else the artery is divided. Usually the artery passes through the angle of the saphenofemoral junction along the lower edge of the fossa ovalis.

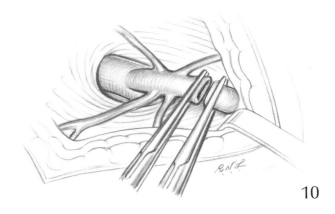

10

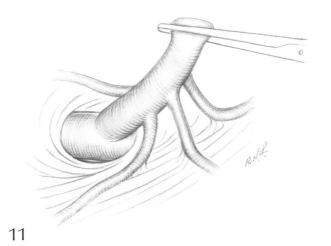

11

Division of tributaries

11

The proximal long saphenous vein stump is then lifted and the tributaries isolated by sweeping off the adjacent tissue using a swab. Although the position and number of tributaries are variable, four groups corresponding to the arterial branches must be identified and divided. On the lateral side the anterolateral tributary and superficial circumflex iliac vein must be found. These are sometimes flattened against the saphenofemoral junction and so overlooked and this is the commonest cause of recurrence.

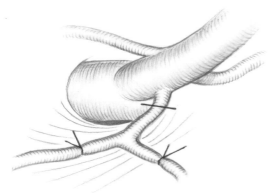

12

12

If there is a single lateral vessel, it must be followed until it divides, as overlooking this is another possible cause of persistent veins on the front of the thigh.

Proximally, the superficial inferior epigastric vein is easily found and divided. Medially, the superficial external vein is divided. Finally, the posteromedial tributary is found and divided between ligatures to avoid haematoma formation above the bandage. This large medial tributary usually passes down the back of the thigh to join the short saphenous vein and if it is not seen in the surgical field because of a lower termination it must be sought under the distal edge of the wound.

13

Exposure of saphenofemoral junction

After dividing all juxtafemoral tributaries, elevation of the long saphenous vein stump reveals the junction with the common femoral vein as a line of demarcation, the colour change being due to the different wall composition. Both the lateral and medial surfaces of the femoral vein must be seen to be clear of tributaries, to ensure a flush ligation. It is not necessary to divide the deep fascia and the deep external pudendal vein needs to be divided only if unusually large.

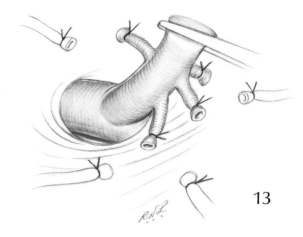

13

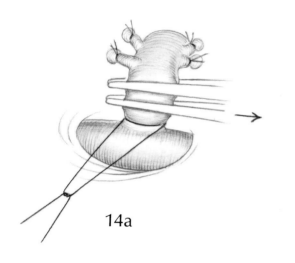

14a

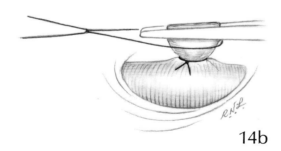

14b

14a & b

Ligation of saphenofemoral junction

Two adjacent forceps are placed on the termination of the long saphenous vein so that the proximal ligature is placed flush on the side of the femoral vein, taking care not to stenose this vein by excessive elevation of the junction. The vessel should not be transfixed because sometimes it is fragile and easily torn. There is no need to use non-absorbable sutures. For the proximal ligature chromic 0 catgut is used; for the second suture on the saphenous vein and for all other vessels and tributaries finer catgut is used (2/0 plain or 3/0 chromic). Once the saphenous vein is isolated the table can be tilted so that the legs are raised to an angle of 10°–20°.

15

Introduction of stripper

The stripper is then introduced into the upper end of the saphenous vein and passed towards the knee. It must be directed down the marked vein by manual manipulation. This is made easier by straightening the leg, and the stripper then passes to the upper calf. Here it often enters an anterior tibial tributary just below the knee and it must therefore be withdrawn and guided into the posterior arch vein tributary or long saphenous vein just below the knee. It is usually possible to pass the stripper down an incompetent saphenous vein and if the vein is duplicated or, rarely, triplicated each vein must be removed after passing strippers distally.

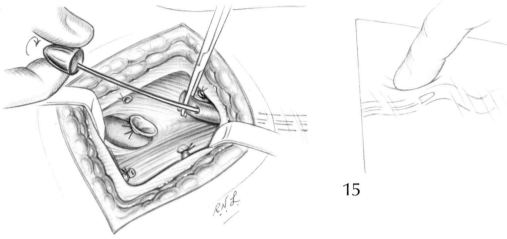

15

16 & 17

Exit of stripper

By twisting and manipulating the stripper with one hand and the vein with the other the tip of the stripper is advanced through the tortuous varicose vein to just below the knee. The perforating vein at the upper tibia must be reached but the long saphenous vein in the lower leg is seldom involved and is protected in a fascial tunnel passing along the tibial border. At this level the saphenous nerve has not joined the saphenous vein and damage to the lymphatic vessels in the lower leg is also avoided by not stripping below the upper calf. A small (1 cm) vertical incision is made over the tip of the stripper using a No. 15 scalpel blade. The vein is then exposed and divided; the distal end is ligated using 3/0 chromic catgut and the stripper brought out.

When the stripper has been pulled down until the head is flush at the upper end of the saphenous vein a ligature is placed around it, to secure the vein to the stripper. Normally a 9 mm head is used, but if the vein is very large a 12 mm head will prevent inversion, as will a double ligature.

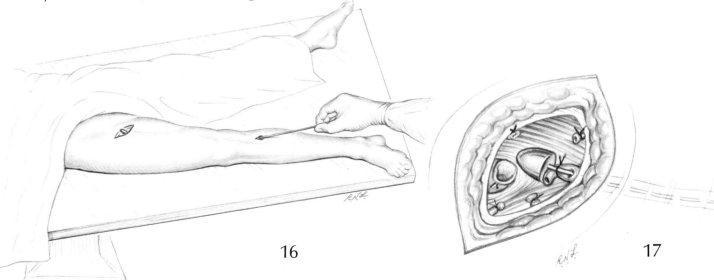

16   17

18

Closure of groin wound

After the head of the stripper has been tied into the vein and buried, the wound is closed in two layers. The membranous layer of superficial fascia is closed with two (occasionally three) interrupted 2/0 chromic catgut sutures which are placed so that the knot is deep.

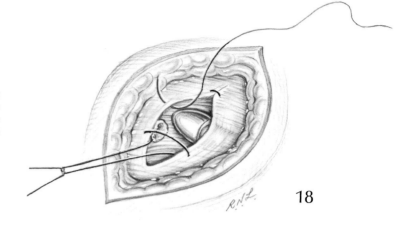

18

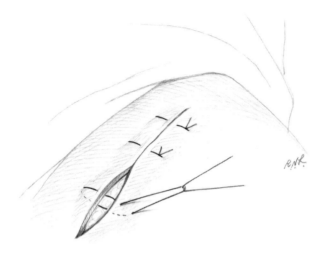

19

19

The skin is closed with three or four interrupted vertical mattress sutures using monofilament nylon, preferably 5/0 or 3/0 mounted on a fine straight needle.

20

Removal of vein and stripper

After the groin wound has been closed, the vein is removed by pulling the stripper from the wound in the upper calf. The stripper is pulled steadily and slowly and if the vein is bulky its removal through a small incision is made easier by pulling the corrugated vein down the stripper and out of the lower wound. Bleeding is usually minimal when the legs are elevated whilst stripping. Bleeding may occur if there is a large incompetent perforating vein in the lower thigh or upper calf, but this is immediately controlled by firm local pressure and further elevation of the leg.

Pulling the stripper downwards facilitates early closure of the groin wound and accurately selects the vein or veins to be removed. By not stripping the long saphenous vein from the lower leg, damage to the saphenous nerve is unlikely and this is further prevented by stripping in a downward direction so that the stripper head will not impact in the divisions of the saphenous nerve.

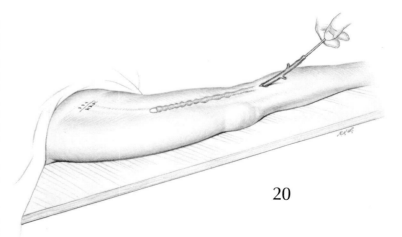

20

Passing the stripper upwards

Rarely is it impossible to pass the stripper in a downward direction and it may be convenient to pass the stripper up from an incision over the vein on the lower leg. Instead of stripping upwards, the head and tip can be removed and reversed, so that the vein is stripped in the usual downward direction. By stripping in a downwards direction much larger lengths of tributaries are removed.

21

Elevation of limb

Immediately after stripping the long saphenous vein and removing any other dilated veins, the table is lowered and the leg elevated. This, plus expression of any blood from the vein tract, controls bleeding and prevents haemotoma formation.

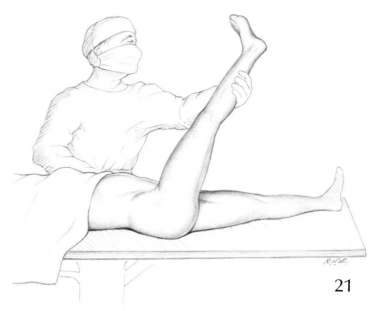

21

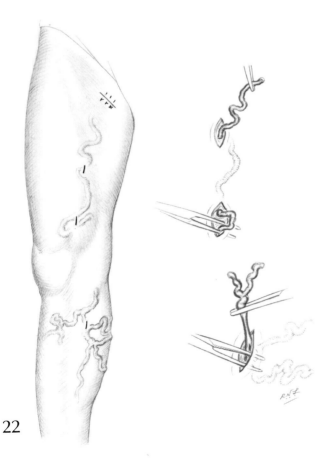

22

22

After the long saphenous vein has been withdrawn on the stripper, the various subsidiary varicose tributaries, which have previously been accurately marked, are withdrawn through a series of small stab wounds. These incisions are vertical, 0.75 cm in length, and made with a No. 15 scalpel blade. The veins are removed using straight artery forceps and care is taken that only veins are removed. Fine artery forceps are opened in each small incision to separate the subcutaneous tissue and isolate the vein. The vein is then grasped firmly and gently eased out; with care long segments of the tortuous veins are removed. The venous tributaries removed in this fashion include the anterolateral tributary on the thigh, the posterior arch vein on the calf and sometimes the anterior tibial tributary. Care is taken to make the small incisions vertical and not in the vicinity of joints.

Ligation of incompetent perforating veins

Incompetent perforating veins may be present as a primary and isolated problem but often they are secondary, either as the re-entry of a large saphenous vein reflux or secondary to deep vein pathology in the post-thrombotic syndrome. When associated with incompetence of the saphenous system, incompetent perforating veins can easily be dealt with during surgical treatment of the saphenous veins. There is no need for extensive subfascial dissections because significant incompetent perforating veins only occur in small numbers and can be ligated through small extrafascial approaches. In the post-thrombotic syndrome the secondary incompetent perforating veins are often associated with pathological changes in the skin and subcutaneous tissue (eczema, ulceration and lipodermatosclerosis) and surgery is best avoided in such tissue, particularly since the underlying problem cannot be cured.

23

When operating on primary varicose veins any grossly incompetent perforating veins are marked by a circle and these fascial defects are also points which control filling of the superficial veins. The typical sites are shown in Illustration 2.

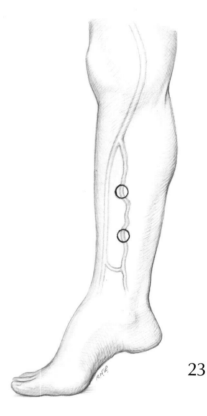

23

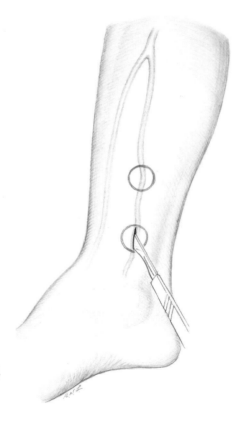

24

24

A 2 cm long vertical incision is made over the marked points and the vein isolated.

25

The superficial vein is dissected out proximally and distally until the T-junction with the perforating vein is found and isolated. The vein is divided and ligated on each side and the perforating vein freed down to the deep fascia; often there is an associated artery and when pulling on the vein it is possible to pull the deep vein and posterior tibial artery through the wide fascial defect.

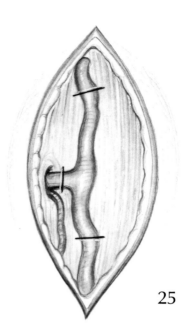

25

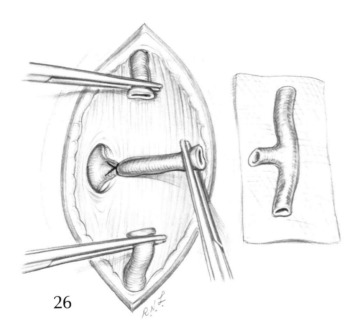

26

26

The perforating vein is ligated at the deep fascia close to its junction with the deep vein. Finally the fascial defect is closed with one or two chromic gut sutures.

27

Closure of wound

After expressing any blood and clots from the wounds the small incisions are closed with one or two interrupted vertical mattress sutures using fine monofilament nylon on a straight needle (3/0 or 5/0). No subcutaneous sutures are used, except for the deep fascia at the groin, popliteal fossa and perforating vein sites.

28

Bandaging

After all free blood has been expressed from the wounds on the elevated leg, the whole limb is covered with a pressure bandage using cotton crêpe bandages of limited stretch (STD Export or S&N Elastocrêpe). Dry dressings are placed over each wound and a 7.5 cm bandage is applied from the metatarsal heads to the upper calf. A 10 cm bandage then overlaps this and continues to the upper thigh.

A small Airstrip dressing is applied to the groin. No pins are used to fix the bandages on an anaesthetized patient. The foot of the bed is elevated 20° until the patient is fully conscious. When conscious the patient is instructed to walk every hour.

29a & b

POSTOPERATIVE CARE

The following morning all bandages and dressings are removed and the wounds covered by short lengths of 2.5 cm Micropore. An elastic stocking is then applied over these and the patient discharged home. The stocking can be removed at night and a bath or shower taken; the Micropore dressings are blotted dry and the patient can sleep without the stocking which is then replaced each morning. The leg should be treated as no more than a bruised leg and normal activities resumed as comfort allows.

On the seventh or eighth day the sutures are removed and the stockings discarded. Excessive bruising can be controlled by the use of bandages or a stronger elastic stocking (Scholl Duoten, Sigvaris).

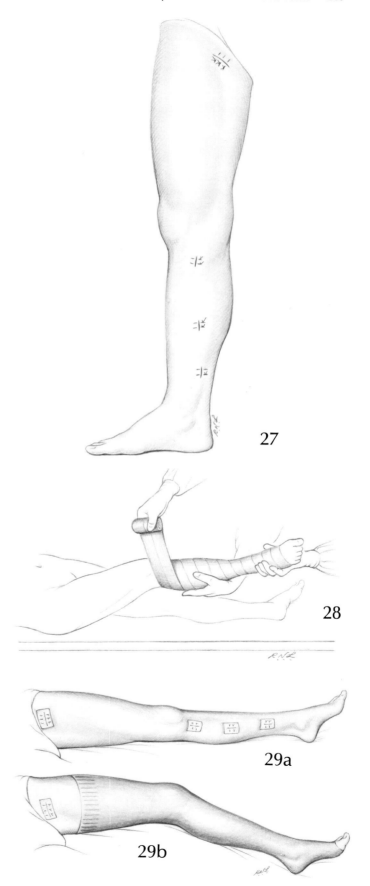

27

28

29a

29b

Operation for short saphenous vein incompetence

30

The patient is placed in the lateral position with the lower leg flexed and the upper leg extended; if the incompetence is unilateral the leg for operation is uppermost. A cassette containing a 30 cm × 40 cm X-ray film is placed under the upper leg and the X-ray tube positioned over the leg and centred on the knee joint. Sterile hypodermic needles are used as markers, being inserted intradermally, a 25 gauge needle at the highest point where the short saphenous vein was palpable and a 21 gauge needle at the knee crease (indicated by arrows in *Illustration 31a*).

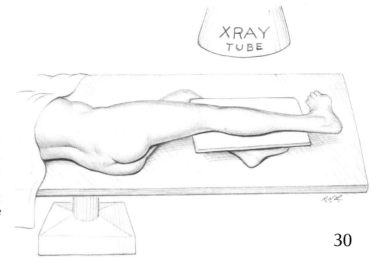

30

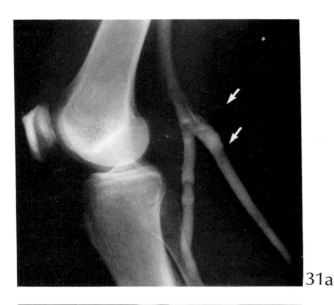

31a

31a, b & c

The film is exposed after injecting 10–15 ml of contrast media (Hexabrix is used because of its low osmolality which avoids irritant side-effects); during the second half of the injection of contrast media, central venous pressure is raised by obstructing respiration, so that the valves in the popliteal vein are demonstrated.

The injection of contrast is made directly with a 15 gauge needle if the vein is large or via a butterfly cannula (21 or 23 gauge) if the vein is tortuous. The X-ray film is then processed while the surgeon scrubs and prepares the patient.

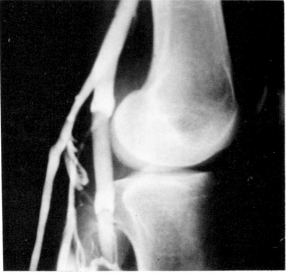

31b

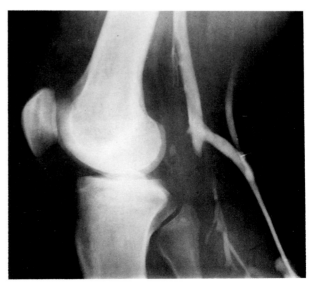

31c

32

The incision

Using the X-ray and skin marking needles as a guide, the surgeon makes a 2.5 cm transverse incision over the saphenopopliteal junction, which is usually on the back of the lower thigh, above the popliteal crease. The X-ray makes possible a small and accurately placed incision which is preferable to larger explorations. The popliteal fascia is exposed and often the underlying vein is visible; the fascia is divided transversely in the line of the skin incision to expose the fat and contents of the popliteal fossa.

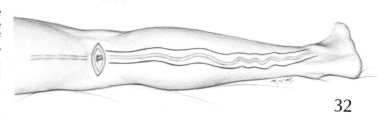

32

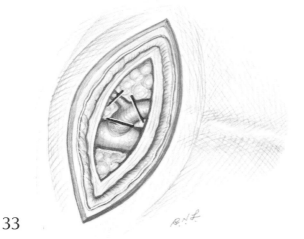

33

Flush ligation and stripping of short saphenous vein

33

The vein is isolated by blunt dissection and carefully separated from the closely applied sural nerve. The vein is lifted up and divided. There is usually a larger superior tributary which passes up the back of the lower thigh to communicate with the posteromedial tributary of the long saphenous vein, the profunda vein or sometimes the tributaries of the internal iliac veins. This vein must be divided to prevent recurrence.

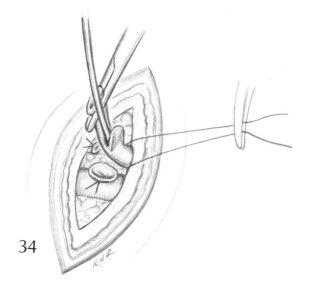

34

34

The termination of the short saphenous vein is located and a flush ligation on the popliteal vein is made using 2/0 chromic gut. A second 3/0 plain ligature is used as a safety measure. A stripper is then passed down the short saphenous vein to just above the lateral malleolus.

35

A small 1 cm vertical incision is made to expose the stripper. After the stripper has been pulled down, the head is tied in the upper end of the vein and the incision at the popliteal fossa closed in two layers: continuous 3/0 chromic gut to the popliteal fascia and three interrupted nylon sutures to skin. Stripping in a downward direction ensures removal of clearly marked veins. The wounds are closed as before.

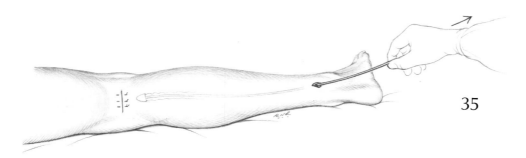

35

36

If the vein does not join the popliteal vein

When the short saphenous vein does not communicate with the popliteal vein, or else this connection is very small, there is no need to expose this area. Instead, the short saphenous vein is exposed above the lateral malleolus and a stripper inserted and passed up into the thigh. The termination may be in the back of the thigh or join the long saphenous vein via the posteromedial tributary. At the highest point a small incision is made over the tip of the stripper which is then brought out of the wound. The ends of the stripper are removed and exchanged. After placing the top end of the stripper (with the vein tied to it) below the deep fascia the wound is closed in two layers, using CGS for the fascia and 5/0 Ethilon for the skin. The stripper is then removed downwards with a gentle pull which avoids damage to the adjacent sural nerve.

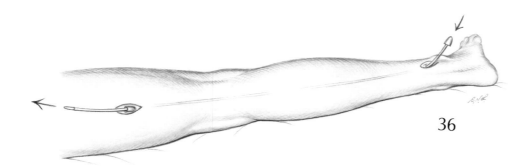

36

Recurrence at the groin

This occurs when a vein is left communicating with the femoral vein. Gross recurrence is immediate when the ligation is not flush and a long stump of saphenous vein with tributaries is present. Sometimes the second part of a double long saphenous vein is missed. Recurrence is most commonly caused by overlooking of the lateral tributaries which may be hidden by fascia during the initial ligation. This results in a tortuous mass of varicosities at the groin surrounded by scar tissue leading to recurrence of irregular varicose veins down the leg.

Because of the friable thin-walled veins, surrounded by dense scar tissue with distorted anatomy, a direct approach is very difficult. Therefore, it may be better to expose the femoral vein, and several approaches have been described. Many surgeons favour a high approach, exposing the femoral artery before the vein[1-4]. A lateral exposing the femoral artery before the vein[1-4]. A lateral vertical incision has been used[5] to expose the artery first and so avoid lymphatic damage. The previous scar was widely excised by Li[6] who also first exposed the femoral artery but recognized the increased risk of lymphatic damage. Foote[7] also reopened the original scar and extended it down medially to expose the femoral vein from below, but when great difficulty was encountered he exposed the femoral vein from above. Dodd and Cockett[8,9] have used a 10 cm long high transverse incision extended down medially for 5 cm as a 'hockey stick' to open the femoral sheath and expose the femoral vein from below. The disadvantage of the medial approach is damage to the important ventromedial bundle of lymphatic vessels[10].

The present author's method is as follows.

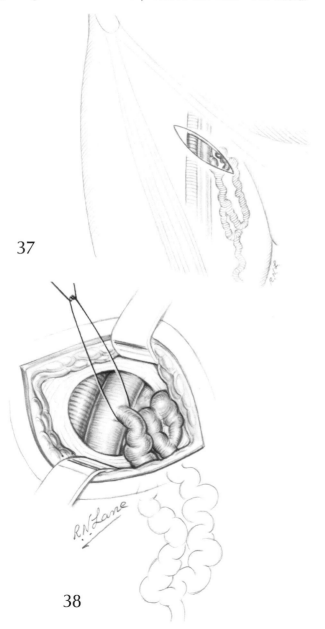

37

37

Incision for re-exploration at groin

The previous scar is excised, using a longer, 7.5 cm transverse incision placed over the saphenofemoral junction.

The femoral artery is identified by its pulsation lateral to the varicosities. An incision is made in the femoral sheath just medial to the artery, and the femoral vein is exposed below the saphenofemoral junction.

38

Dissection of saphenofemoral junction

The femoral vein is then carefully dissected upwards until the persistent tributaries and saphenofemoral junction are isolated. After ligating and dividing all persistent communications with the femoral vein, the incision is closed in two layers as before and the recurrent veins are removed from the leg through small incisions.

38

COMPLICATIONS

The most common difficulty, particularly for an inexperienced surgeon, is massive venous bleeding while dissecting out the saphenofemoral junction.

When this occurs, mild finger or swab pressure on the spot will control the haemorrhage while the table is tilted to raise the feet. When the pressure is released after a few minutes the bleeding is usually reduced to a trickle and can be accurately controlled either with an artery forceps or fine suture. Blind clamping should never be done as there is a real risk of further damage to the femoral vein or even the femoral artery.

Occasionally the stripper may pass into the deep vein via a wide short perforating vein. This occurs only when stripping up and it is therefore safer to pass the stripper downwards and always be able to feel the stripper beneath the skin.

Excessive sharp dissection in the groin, especially in large wounds, may disrupt some lymphatics and can occasionally result in the formation of a lymphocele. This should be aspirated.

Slight damage to cutaneous nerves is difficult to avoid completely. Therapy involves explaining to the patient the unavoidability and harmlessness of this small impairment. It will then be forgotten.

Arterial injuries, though serious, are extremely rare. They must be promptly identified and treated. An inexperienced operator must be able to identify them and transfer the patient to a vascular surgeon for urgent repair.

References

1. Luke, J. C. Management of recurrent varicose veins. Surgery 1954; 35: 40–44

2. Lofgren, E. P., Lofgren, K. A. Recurrence of varicose veins after the stripping operation. Archives of Surgery 1971; 102: 111–114

3. Nabatoff, R. A. Technique for operation upon recurrent varicose veins. Surgery, Gynecology and Obstetrics 1976; 143: 463–467

4. May, R. Surgery of the veins of the leg and pelvis. Philadelphia: Saunders, 1979

5. Junod, J. M., Varices et leurs complications: traitement chirurgical des cas difficiles. Helvetica Chirurgica Acta 1971; 38: 167–170

6. Li, A. K. C. A technique for re-exploration of the saphenofemoral junction for recurrent varicose veins. British Journal of Surgery 1975; 62: 745–746

7. Foote, R. R. Varicose veins. 3rd ed. Bristol: Wright, 1960

8. Dodd, H., Cockett, F. B. The pathology and surgery of the veins of the lower limb. Edinburgh: Livingstone, 1956

9. Dodd, H., Cockett, F. B., The pathology and surgery of the veins of the lower limb. 2nd ed. Edinburgh: Churchill Livingstone, 1976

10. Brunner, Phlebologie U. Prokt. 1975; 4: 266

Illustrations by Robert N. Lane

Injection treatment of varicose veins

W. G. Fegan MCh, FRCSI
Formerly Research Professor of Surgery, University College of Dublin,
Trinity College at Sir Patrick Dun's Hospital, Dublin, Irish Republic

General principles

Venous drainage

There is no such thing as venous drainage in the standing, walking or sitting patient. Blood in veins drains only when the bottom of the patient's bed is considerably elevated. Blood will move only from one segment of vein to the next when there is a favourable pressure differential. The haemodynamics of the venous segment of the perfusion arch of the tissues of the lower limb is as active and more complex than is the haemodynamics within an artery. The venous pumping system has to generate with each step a high systolic pressure to overcome gravity and a low diastolic pressure to allow for refilling and the development of a favourable gradient for tissue nutrient exchange.

Flow and pressure changes

Flow in a segment of vein can vary in eight different ways. It can flow in either direction at high pressure or low pressure, quickly or slowly, in a laminar or turbulent manner. Retrograde turbulent flow directed against one side of a vein will give rise to a blow out while failure to develop low pressure in the venules after the commencement of walking will interfere with tissue nutrient exchange.

If varicose veins were due to an alteration in the pressure pattern within the vein, the vein would react as a vein transplanted into the arterial tree. The changes in pressure would equally affect all surfaces of the vein resulting in uniform hypertrophy and later, symmetrical dilatation. This is not the ultimate derangement in the pathological vein.

Varicosity occurs usually on alternate sides of the vein, but it may also dilate in a 'barber's pole' fashion.

Valvular incompetence

The classic saphenovarix occurs at the apex of a reflux turbulent jet of blood due to valvular incompetence (primary or secondary) at the saphenofemoral junction. Where veins are not supported by Sherman's fascia, varicosity develops sooner. Turbulence is easily detected over these veins.

Turbulence would appear to be extremely damaging or injurious to the functioning of the muscle fibres and the elastic lamina of the vein wall. The muscle fibres decrease in number and the elastic lamina fragments at the apex of the turbulent jet. The difference in the overall thickness of the veins need not be impressive as the intima at this point thickens considerably. This would appear to be due to organization of layering thrombus as a result of turbulence. Such evidence leads us to the conclusion that asymmetrical dilatation (varicosity) in varices is a result of high velocity turbulent flow in poorly supported veins[1].

Flow in superficial varices is found to be turbulent when the velocity reaches certain critical points. These are: (1) shortly after assuming the erect position and (2) at the high velocity peaks developed after the commencement of walking[2].

Principles of treatment

Treatment is dependent on the type of pathology present.

Pronounced superficial varices are quite common in the symptomless leg (varicose veins). A patient with a leg seriously embarrassed with advanced signs and symptoms of chronic venous insufficiency occasionally has no varices (postphlebitic limb).

The two conditions can coexist in the same leg. This gives rise to the erroneous idea that they are sequential. In our opinion this confused thinking is responsible for much of the misunderstanding in the diagnosis and treatment of these conditions.

Incompetent perforating veins

A meticulous surgical dissection of the first group of varices to appear will usually demonstrate one incompetent perforating vein. This is not sufficient to interfere with pump reserve or efficiency, but it causes insidious upward uniform dilatation in the related superficial veins. With normal functioning valves in the superficial veins, alterations in pressure patterns due to incompetent perforating valves can only ascend. The superficial dilatation due to the inadequate drop in pressure after the commencement of walking gives rise to secondary valvular incompetence in the superficial veins[3] and when it involves a higher perforating vein valve a reverse high velocity circuit is established.

In some cases, if the incompetent perforating veins are tied off, the superficial varices disappear and the superficial veins return to normal, demonstrating the reversibility of secondary valvular incompetence[4]. Injection compression therapy takes advantage of the ability of superficial veins with secondary valvular incompetence to recover as one can give treatment and observe the effects before giving the next treatment.

Postphlebitic sydrome

When treating a patient who has primarily the postphlebitic syndrome[2] and in whom the varicose veins are either absent or of little importance, all efforts should be directed towards the restoration of the pump. The signs and symptoms of the postphlebitic syndrome are primarily due to the inability of the pumps to reduce the pressure after the commencement of walking to a point at which nutrient exchange will take place. One or two incompetent perforating veins do not necessarily render the pumps incapacitated because of the very considerable reserve pumping capacity, but the more valves that are damaged, especially in the deep perforating veins, the more the pumping capacity is reduced.

Management

The easiest method for the busy surgeon to distinguish these patterns from each other, is on the basis of symptoms. Patients with symptomless varices rarely have pump damage. Patients with signs and symptoms of the postphlebitic limb arising from venous derangement always have damage to the valves in the deep and perforating veins despite the presence or absence of varicose veins. The ideal management for both types of patient is, in our opinion, injection, compression and ambulation. The first treatment may be nothing more than compression and ambulation, but with meticulous palpation sites of incompetent perforators come to light which are subsequently injected.

Patients with symptomless varices can, with confidence, be promised a complete cure. Those with the postphlebitic syndrome can be rendered symptomless and thus clinically cured but the degree of normal pumping efficiency present before the first episode of deep-vein thrombosis can never be fully restored. These patients must be observed periodically and advised to maintain their pump muscles by walking and to remove unnecessary strain on the vein wall and valves by the avoidance of standing. The judicious periodic use of elastic stockings is advisable.

Pregnant patients who have varicose veins are treated routinely as frequently their veins do not return to normal in the puerperium and may continue to deteriorate past the point of recovery. Initially immediate supportive therapy is provided and any localized incompetent perforations are treated.

Specialist clinic

A clinic devoted entirely to the diagnosis and injection treatment of varicose veins is essential to ensure that the technique is carried out to perfection. It should be adequately staffed by the right proportion of experienced nurses, doctors and secretaries for maximum efficiency.

History

A history is taken with particular note of any past injury to the leg, thrombophlebitis or any previous episodes of deep-vein thrombosis. The patient is weighed and if overweight is strongly advised to diet. A blood sample is taken for the following tests: blood film, haemoglobin, W.R., Kahn white cell count and ESR and the patient is given written instructions to carry out throughout treatment.

Contraindications

1. Gross obesity – this makes it difficult to maintain adequate compression.
2. Inability or unwillingness to undertake the required amount of walking.
3. An allergic response to the sclerosant (sodium tetradecyl).
4. Oral contraceptives – whilst there is no evidence to suggest that patients taking oral contraceptive run a higher risk of developing deep-vein thrombosis and pulmonary embolism, treatment is not undertaken until the patient has stopped taking an oral contraceptive for 6 weeks.

Treatment

1

Materials

A stool and couch with swivel trays underneath containing bandages, Sorbo rubber pads and lint are required. A tray, containing four to six all-glass or disposable syringes with transparent shanks fitted with fine disposable needles and loaded with the sclerosant (0.5 ml of sodium tetradecyl) is at hand, as after commencing treatment the surgeon cannot move away from the patient.

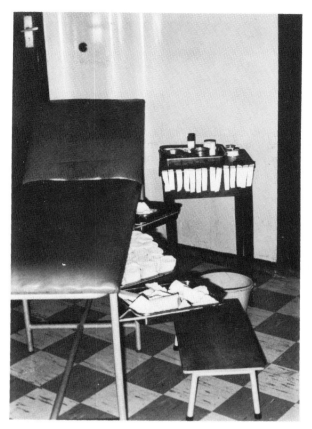

1

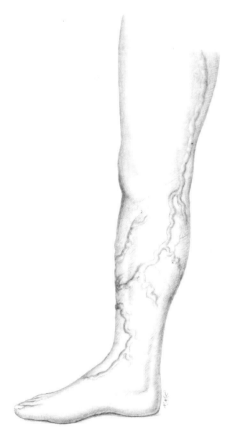

2

2

Varicose veins

Standing on the stool the patient shows typical varicose veins involving the long saphenous system with some perforator valvular incompetence.

3

Inspection and palpation

Veins are marked by inspection. Percussion of a dilated vein, while the other hand palpates the surface of the limb, will bring still more veins to light and when this mapping process is completed it is sometimes possible to suspect the site of the perforating veins with incompetent valves.

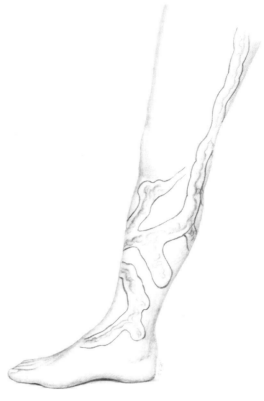

3

4

Areas of fascial deficiency

The patient lies down with the heel comfortably supported on the surgeon's shoulder. The limb is palpated with the flat of the hand until the muscles become flaccid. Now the surgeon's fingers are flexed and the tips should comb the leg in an effort to detect areas of fascial deficiency. These are marked with a grease pencil of a different colour.

4

5

Likely sites of retrograde filling

The tips of the fingers are pressed into as many as possible of these areas or orifices of fascial weakness.

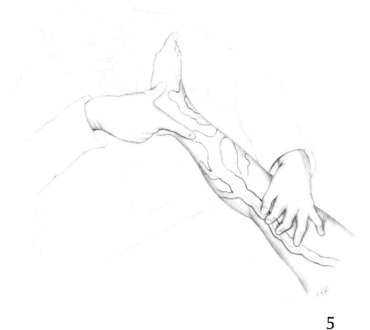

5

6

Filling of veins

The patient is now requested to stand and the lowermost fingers are removed first. If filling of the veins in the lower leg does not take place then it is reasonable to assume that there is no incompetent perforator at the site of this apparent fascial weakness but instead the fat in this area has been displaced by a bunch of dilated veins, creating the impression of fascial weakness.

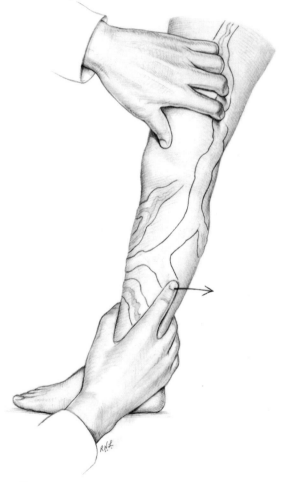

6

7

Selection of sites for injection

If, on the other hand, the veins fill immediately then it is reasonable to suspect that there is an incompetent perforator in this area. It is perhaps wise to consider these the sites at which pressure will control the filling of the superficial system. These we choose as the ideal sites for injection.

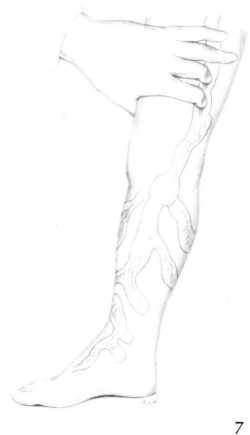

7

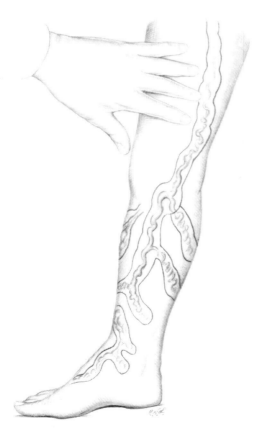

8

8

Removal of pressure

The illustration shows a further distension of the superficial system after removing the pressure from an incompetent Hunterian perforator.

9

Insertion of needle

With the patient lying horizontal it is quite easy to enter the vein and withdraw blood (the plunger of the syringe having been tested for freedom of movement). It should be noted here that the blood should not enter the syringe but only the transparent shank of the needle.

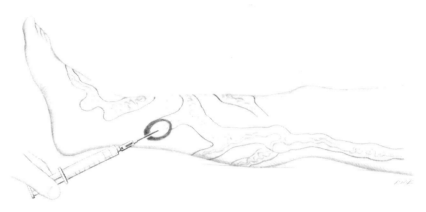

9

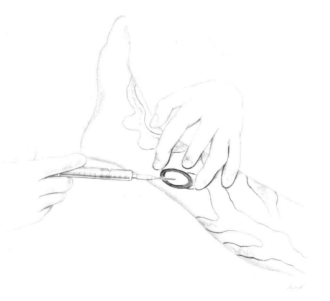

10

Injection of the sclerosant

The leg is elevated and placed against the shoulder or upper chest of the surgeon. The injection is given into a segment of vein isolated by the ring and index fingers compressing on either side in an attempt to restrict the sclerosant fluid (sodium tetradecyl) to the selected site. This would appear a pious hope but when the area is examined some weeks or months later the segment of superficial vein involved in the fibrosis matches exactly the gap between the ring and index fingers.

10

Bandaging

11

The syringe is withdrawn and bandaging above, below and over the site of injection is commenced. It is usually possible to apply one or two turns of the bandage above and below the compressing fingers before removing them.

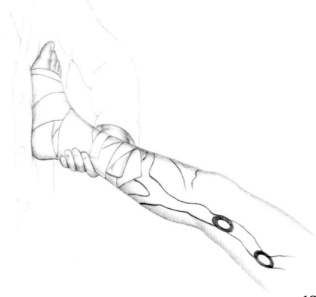

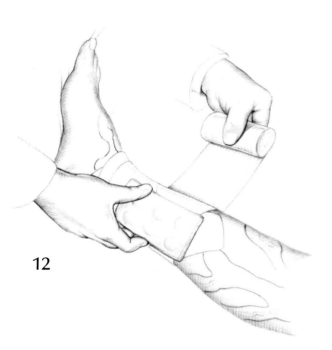

12

12

Sorbo rubber pad

A bevelled Sorbo rubber pad is bandaged immediately into position over the site of injection.

13

The importance of bandaging

The remainder of the bandage is applied to the foot excluding the toes. The bandager should not have a preconceived pattern into which he visually forces the bandage. The contour of the patient's leg should determine the pattern of the bandage and the pressure of both borders of the bandages should be exactly the same. Bandaging is more a sensory art using proprioceptive sensation rather than a visual art. It is the secret of the success of this technique and if the bandages have fallen off or have to be adjusted before the return visit then the surgeon has not mastered the technique and instead of a short segment of hard painless fibrotic veins patients will develop random areas of painful superficial thrombophlebitis which is certainly not the desirable end result.

13

14

Prevention of abrasion of the skin

To prevent the bandage in the region of the knee cutting the skin over the hamstring tendons it is necessary to place a Sorbo rubber pad in the popliteal fossa. This becomes an absolute necessity if pressure over the termination of the short saphenous controls the filling in the superficial veins; this is a frequently overlooked common incompetent perforator which responds very well to injection and compression.

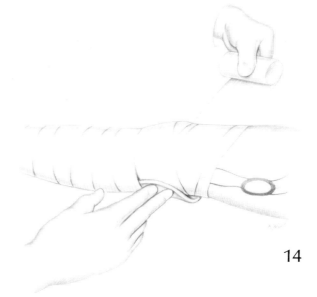

14

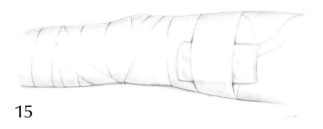

15

15

Traumatization of the long saphenous vein and thrombophlebitis

A pad is shown placed over an injected superficial vein in the region of the lower Hunterian incompetent perforators. It is important that the rubber pad protrude above the upper edge of the bandage; otherwise the bandage will roll down and form a sharp ropelike border which traumatizes the long saphenous vein and gives rise to the complication of ascending thrombophlebitis. Sometimes it is wise to use adhesive strapping to make sure that the bandage does not roll, nor the rubber pad slip out.

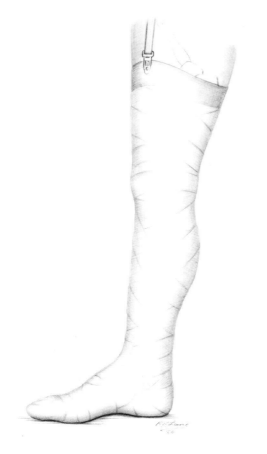

16

16

Elastic stocking

An elastic stocking is applied immediately after the last bandage is firmly anchored in position. It is most important that the patient should be able, fit and prepared to walk within seconds after the completion of treatment. Appointments for a return visit in 1–2 weeks should be made prior to commencement of treatment. We are convinced that the lack of complications in our clinic is due to the commencement of walking for 1 hour immediately following injection.

Post-treatment

Special care

The patient is instructed to walk for 1 hour immediately following injection and to continue to walk as much as possible on the day of injection and thereafter for 5 km (3 miles) a day. This does not include walking around the house. The most difficult point to get across to the patient is the avoidance of standing. Our patients are warned against the danger of standing and advised, if not walking, to sit preferably with legs elevated.

Pain

Pain may occur in the leg and the patient is advised to take analgesics and to increase the amount of walking. If this does not relieve the pain the bandage should be removed and the leg examined.

Superficial thrombophlebitis

Localized superficial thrombophlebitis may occur. This is usually caused by failure to use the empty vein technique, by inadequate compression or excessive use of the sclerosant.

Intra-arterial injection of the sclerosant

The accidental intra-arterial injection of the sclerosant in the hands of the experienced surgeon is a rare but serious complication. If this does occur injection of procaine around the artery, local cooling, systemic heparinization and infusion with low molecular weight dextran has been shown to be effective in preventing or minimizing permanent damage to the foot.

Advantages of injection compression sclerotherapy

The advantages to the patient of this method of treatment are that hospitalization and interruption of employment are avoided, treatment is immediate upon referral to the clinic and there are no resulting scars. Patients appear to prefer this method of treatment. The surgeon avoids an in-patient waiting list and therefore saves hospital bed occupation.

Provided it is practised by an expert, injection compression sclerotherapy can produce results which compare favourably with surgery[5,6] in terms of relief of symptoms and disappearance of obvious varicosities.

References

1. Sommervill, J. J. F., Byrne, P. J., Fegan, W. G. Analysis of flow patterns in venous insufficiency. British Journal of Surgery 1974; 61: 40–44

2. Fegan, W. G., Kline, A. L. The cause of varicosity in superficial veins of the lower limb. British Journal of Surgery 1972; 59: 798–801

3. Fegan, W. G., Fitzgerald, D. E., Beesley, W. H. Valvular defect in primary varicose veins. Lancet 1964; 1: 491–492

4. Quill, R. D., Fegan, W. G. Reversibility of femorosaphenous reflux. British Journal of Surgery 1971; 58: 389–393

5. Chant, A. D. B., Jones, H. O., Weddell, J. M. Varicose veins: a comparison of surgery and injection compression sclerotherapy. Lancet 1972; 2: 1188–1191

6. Heslop, J. H. The modern treatment of varicose vein disease. New Zealand Medical Journal 1977; 38: 389–394

Further reading

Fegan, W. G. Varicose veins, compression sclerotherapy. London: Heinemann, 1967

Venous ulcers

John T. Hobbs MD, FRCS
Senior Lecturer in Surgery, University of London;
Consultant Surgeon, St Mary's Hospital, London, UK

Introduction

Chronic leg ulcers are amongst the most mistreated of all chronic disorders and treatment is often inadequate, sometimes aggravating the situation.

The treatment of venous ulcers may be considered in three stages: (1) diagnosis; (2) management to effect healing; (3) prevention of recurrence by eliminating the cause.

Diagnosis of leg ulcers

Venous

Many causes have been listed for chronic leg ulcers, but in practice most are venous in origin. A careful assessment by history and physical examination should reveal the cause and special investigations are seldom necessary, other than for research purposes. In longstanding ulcers there are often multiple aetiological factors. Venous ulcers typically occur in the gaiter area above the ankle joint or below and behind the medial or lateral malleolus in the territory of the long and short saphenous veins. They vary greatly in size but are usually oval or serpiginous in shape and often multiple. They occur most commonly on the medial aspect below the site of the ankle-perforating veins. The edge of a venous ulcer is usually sloping and the base flat but covered with infected slough. During healing the slough is shed, healthy clean granulations develop and a pink rim of new epithelium begins to grow in from the edge or sometimes develops from islands in the ulcer. Venous ulcers are usually associated with other signs of venous hypertension such as induration, pigmentation, lipodermatosclerosis, eczema and oedema. Dilated varicose veins may be present but are often not apparent.

The precise mechanism has not been established but oedema and increased capillary permeability leading to fibrin cuffs are important and venous hypertension is the underlying cause; similar changes and ulcers are seen in association with arteriovenous fistulae where they have been reported at other sites than the lower leg.

Ulcers are sometimes due to a simple primary varicose vein occurring at the lower end of the incompetent long saphenous vein which has few dilated tributaries but a grossly dilated vein from the groin to the ulcer site. A similar ulcer may occur on the lateral aspect of the foot or below the lateral malleolus in an area of eczema and atrophie blanche associated with a grossly incompetent short saphenous vein. These ulcers are usually caused by trauma and fail to heal because of the venous hypertension due to gross saphenous incompetence.

The majority of venous ulcers are not associated with obvious varicose veins, although skin changes are always present. These are the end-stage of the post-thrombotic syndrome and in some cases there may be no previous history of deep venous thrombosis. After a deep vein (iliac, femoral or popliteal) thrombosis there is usually residual damage, in the form of a permanent occlusion or valvular incompetence, and usually a combination of both. These changes in the deep veins cause incompetence of the ankle-perforating veins which are the underlying cause of the ulcer because there is now ambulatory venous hypertension in the skin and subcutaneous tissues. Sometimes the deep vein thrombosis is limited to the calf but results in incompetence of the perforating veins.

Ulcers are often precipitated by minor trauma due either to a direct blow or scratching an eczematous area. A local dressing is applied by the patient but secondary infection soon occurs and the painful ulcer restricts mobility. Oedema increases and the ulcer becomes more purulent and more painful. The pain restricts movement of the ankle joint and the calf muscle may waste, so that a simple venous ulcer has become a stasis ulcer owing to the failure of the calf muscle pump mechanism.

Many longstanding ulcers, although of simple venous origin, cannot easily be cured because of gross wasting of the calf muscle associated with ankylosis of the ankle joint. The problem is aggravated by associated arthritis and anaemia in the elderly.

Ulcers complicating primary varicose veins are easily identified when there is a typical and gross primary varicosis.

Ulcers complicating the post-thrombotic syndrome may be identified from a careful history and physical examination. If there is doubt, laboratory investigations may be used. Venous pressure studies and venography are the most reliable methods of studying physiological and anatomical changes, but both are invasive.

Arterial

The history and physical examination may suggest an ischaemic element, particularly if the surrounding skin is healthy and the ulcer unusually painful. The foot pulses must be palpated and if there is any doubt they should be further investigated by examination with Doppler ultrasound and measurement of ankle systolic pressure. Sometimes there is an arterial element in a chronic venous ulcer, when care should be taken to avoid excessive compression.

Hypertension

Ulcers on the lateral aspect of the middle or upper calf may be seen in elderly patients, usually female, with a blood pressure greater than 200/100. These are often bilateral, though not always simultaneous.

Stasis

Patients with extensive arthritis affecting the feet, ankles or knee-joints may have poor mobility and gross muscle wasting, and the loss of an effective calf muscle pump is the cause of the chronic leg ulcer. The changes are most marked with rheumatoid arthritis where there are also skin changes and haematological factors.

Miscellaneous

Ulcers atypical in site and the appearance of the leg should alert the clinician to other causes, including thalassaemia and other haematological disorders, trophic causes, allergic vasculitis, diabetes and syphilis. An area of cellulitis, especially streptococcal, will break down and ulcerate spontaneously. Malignant change in chronic leg ulcers is usually obvious but extremely rare and is confirmed by biopsy.

Gross oedema may cause an ulcer to develop from a minor wound; this type of ulcer is more common in hot climates and heals quickly when the oedema is eliminated. Ulcers from different causes may occur simultaneously.

Treatment

PRINCIPLES

Many expensive preparations and techniques have been described but these are seldom, if ever, necessary. Simple methods, correctly applied, will normally be sufficient to heal most ulcers.

The direct cause is venous hypertension which must be controlled by elevation or compression bandaging to effect an initial healing; permanent cure requires elimination of the underlying venous problem.

Treatments aimed at the secondary effects (diuretics, antibiotics, local medicaments, fibrinolytics and drugs claimed to change capillary permeability) will not cure and may not help.

Many patients develop ulcers because they have sensitive skins and the allergic tendencies may be aggravated by topical preparations.

The basic principles of ulcer treatment are: cleansing of the ulcer, simple local dressing and adequate support. Normal activities can be continued, walking is encouraged and the interval between dressing changes is as long as possible, up to as much as 3 weeks. Except for ischaemic ulcers the pain is eliminated within hours of adequate cleansing and the application of sufficient support.

The bandages must be firm and one-way stretch weave will avoid constricting edges. They need not be excessively elastic or heavy. The medicaments added to impregnated bandages probably do little more than provide firmer longer-lasting support and prevent meddling.

Infection is secondary and rarely important despite the results of bacteriological studies. Routine swabbing and culture is not necessary unless specifically indicated by the appearance. Heavily infected ulcers with surrounding inflammation do require frequent cleansing and dressing changes for a few days. Most ulcers with profuse offensive discharges improve dramatically when the oedema is eliminated. The infection which must be recognized immediately and treated actively is that due to β-haemolytic streptococcus; here there is a serous discharge with an unhealthy purply red base; if this is not promptly treated a spreading subcutaneous infection will rapidly develop and this florid erysipelas will lead to large areas of tissue and skin loss.

Several methods are effective and if the rate of healing suddenly slows the treatment should be changed. A simple plan, which has been used successfully for many years, will be described.

MANAGEMENT

A venous ulcer can be induced to heal by supportive bandaging or by elevation. Elevation requires in-patient care and is rarely, if ever, required in the management of venous ulcers.

1

Cleaning of the ulcer

The ulcer is cleaned with cotton wool balls or pledgets soaked in a sterilizing solution of hydrogen peroxide 3 per cent (10 vol.) or Eusol.

If there is extensive eczema or infection, soaking the leg in weak potassium permanganate solution is an effective and painless method of cleansing.

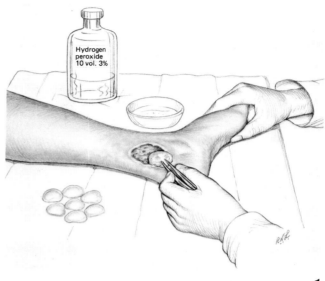

1

2

Mechanical debridement of ulcer

The slough and necrotic material is picked from the base using fine (McIndoe) dissecting forceps. When very firmly adherent it is separated by cutting where fixed. The dry scab is removed from the wound edge to aid epithelization. The ulcer is picked clean to a red base whenever possible. This mechanical debridement is far more effective than chemical debridement and is without the risk of allergic responses. Anaesthetics are not required and patients quickly tolerate it when they gain immediate relief from pain and can see the improved healing.

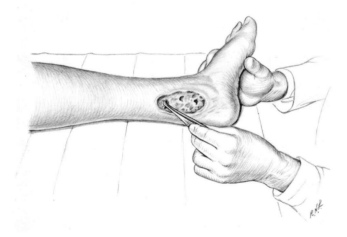

2

3

Application of gentian violet

The ulcer is then painted with a saturated solution (5 per cent) of gentian violet in spirit, covering all the raw areas.

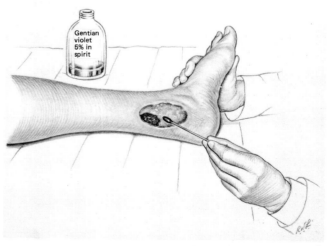

3

4

Ulcer covered with dry dressing

A dry dressing (such as Regal Swab 7.5 × 7.5 cm or 10 × 10 cm) is placed over the ulcerated area. Several pads are used if there is some oedema or much discharge. Although effective for burns and clean wounds, paraffin tulle and expensive preparations such as Melolin can do harm, if left *in situ* for extended periods, because any discharge is kept in contact with the normal skin around the ulcer and this may break down.

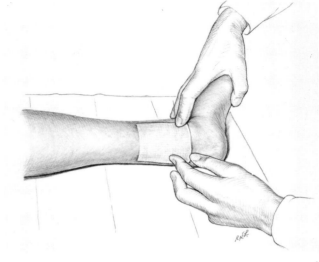

4

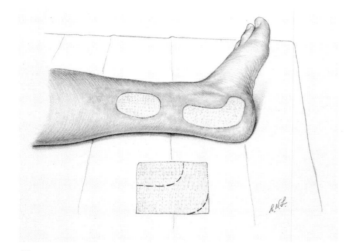

5

5

Pad cut to shape

If the ulcer is in a hollow or behind or below the malleolus, more pressure will be achieved if a pad of foam rubber or thick felt is cut to shape. This also helps in thin legs with fragile skin.

6

Protected length of padded tubular bandage

If the leg is thin and there is a risk of excessive pressure over tendons, e.g. tibialis anterior or the achilles tendon, or over the anterior border of the tibia, a length of Tubipad (size P4X) or thick pad is placed over the dressing before the bandages are applied. This should be reversed to avoid the polyurethane foam pad coming into contact with the skin.

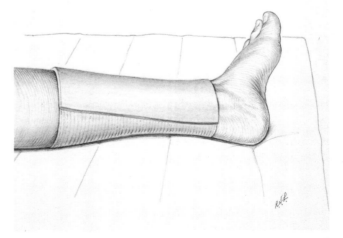

6

7

Cotton tubular bandage for delicate skin

If the skin is inflamed and delicate it may be protected by a sleeve of cotton gauze before the bandages are applied (e.g. Tubiton, Tubigauze).

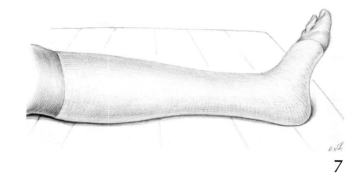

7

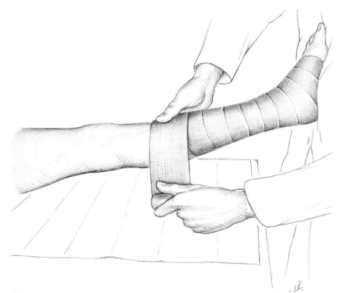

8

Application of bandages

The leg is then firmly bandaged from the head of the metatarsals to the upper calf, care being taken to avoid tight constricting turns and to ensure a reduced pressure up the leg. A 7.5 cm Elastocrêpe bandage is used first and over this is placed the whole or part of a 10 cm bandage.

8

9

Bandages covered by elasticated tubular bandage

Finally the bandages are covered with a length of flesh-coloured Tubigrip to hide the bandages, hold them in place and prevent rucking.

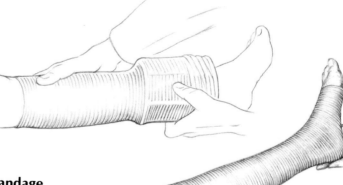

9

ALTERNATIVES

10

Application of povidone-iodine

Sometimes gentian violet does not seem effective, even when it has previously helped; it is then worth using a dry and safe alternative application. Povidone-iodine is often helpful in this situation.

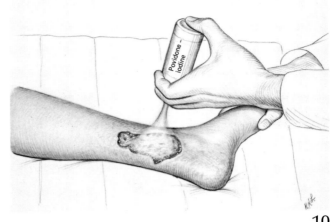

10

11

Use of sulphadiazine cream

If the discharge is greenish and the odour suggests a Gram-negative infection (Proteus, B. coli or Pseudomonas) sulphadiazine (Flamazine, Silvertone) cream is effective. It is applied with a wooden spatula to fill the ulcer crater. A dry dressing and the bandages are then applied in the usual way. After one or two applications the infection is cleared and gentian violet can be used again.

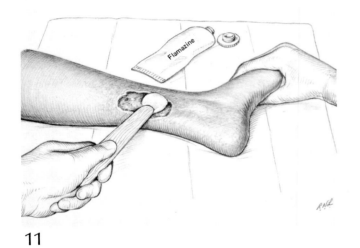

11

12

Dressing for a very dirty ulcer

Rarely a very infected ulcer can be quickly cleaned by the use of Debrisan or Iodosorb powder applied twice a day.

The ulcer is usually clean within 2 days and should then be dressed with gentian violet and bandaged at periods of 2–4 weeks, in the usual manner.

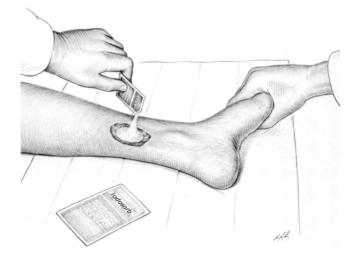

12

13

Application of glycerin and ichthyol

Extensive inflamed induration will often benefit from the application of glycerin and ichthammol on a pad over the ulcer previously covered with gentian violet, 5% in spirit.

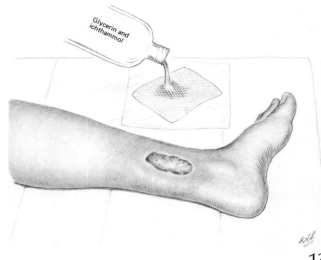

13

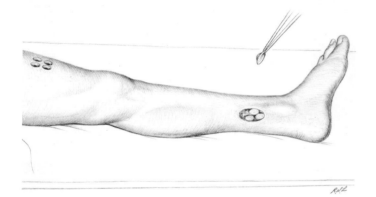

14

14

Application of pinch grafts

If an ulcer that has been healing well suddenly ceases to make progress and is reduced to a small fibrotic base, healing may be stimulated by the application of a few pinch grafts (1–5) taken from the thigh using local anaesthesia. Often these 'take' but even when they fail, they appear to stimulate rapid healing.

15

Use of elastic stockings

In frail legs of older patients, once the ulcer is healing well, bandages can be replaced by an elastic stocking placed over a cotton tube (Tubinette) holding the dressing in place.

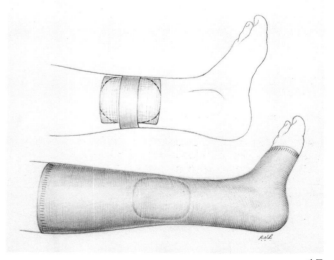

15

16

Soft bandage for frail legs

If support is necessary in fragile legs, the soft conforming Kendall Conform bandage is very effective, but care must be taken in view of its elasticity.

Application of medicated bandages

If the skin of the whole lower leg is not in good condition or if the bandages do not easily stay in place because of the shape of the leg or because of disturbance by the patient, medicated bandages may be preferable.

If bandages are applied in a continuous circular manner, a tight constricting band may easily occur. Because it is necessary to use scissors to remove the hard dry bandage the skin is easily damaged, resulting in additional wounds. Therefore, bandages should not be applied in this manner. They can be applied in short lengths which have been cut from the roll but this is time-consuming.

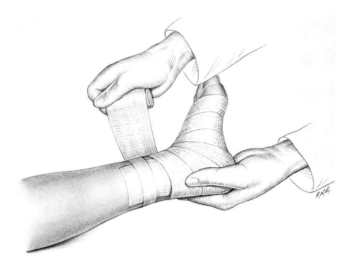

16

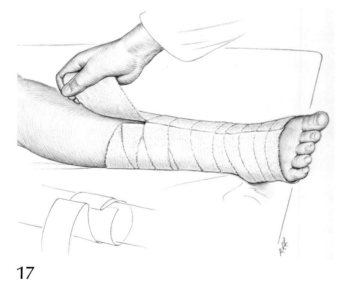

17

17

An effective method is to fold back the bandage with only a short overlap. This avoids any constricting rings and the bandage is easily removed by alternately folding back each side. After application, the medicated bandage is covered with a 7.5 cm or 10 cm bandage and Tubigrip as before.

Although there are many types of medicated bandages there is doubt about the specific benefits of the particular ingredients and some may easily cause a severe local reaction. As a guide the following medications may be used:

> Zinc paste with urethrane and calamine (Calaband), if much irritation.
> Zinc paste and ichthammol (Ichthaband, Icthopaste) if much induration.
> Zinc paste, calamine and iodochlorohydroxyquinolone (Quinaband) if florid infection is present.

All forms of gelatin boots shrink slightly as the paste gels (either by cooling or drying) and this explains their superiority over all other forms of compression dressings.

Probably the most effective medicated bandage is simple zinc oxide but it must be used in a composition which does not harden excessively (Viscopaste PB7) and therefore requires a firm overbandage. If there is much eczema, a very effective application is the Cortacream bandage (1 per cent hydrocortisone and silicone).

The bandage should be left in place as long as possible. It is normally changed initially after 1 or 2 weeks, and then when the ulcers are clean it can be left for 3, 4 or even 5 weeks.

18

Concomitant injection to speed healing of ulcer

If ulcers are clean but slow to heal despite the elimination of any oedema a dramatic improvement occurs if the vein adjacent to an ulcer is injected. This vein associated with an incompetent perforating vein is usually to be found just above the ulcer but sometimes it may be necessary to inject a vein in the base of the ulcer. The standard technique[1] is used, injecting 0.5 ml of 3 per cent sodium tetradecyl sulphate (STD, Trombovar or Sotradecol) into the vein with the leg elevated. A small cotton wool ball is held over the injection site with a strip of Dermicel, adjacent to the ulcer dressing. The leg is then bandaged in the usual way and it is not disturbed for 3 weeks.

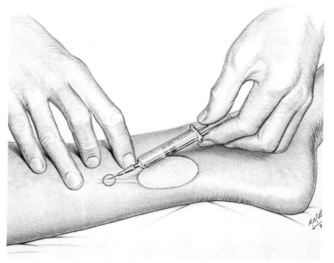

18

Prevention of recurrence

To prevent the ulcer recurring the underlying venous hypertension must be eliminated.

Varicose veins

If the hypertension is due to primary varicose veins the problem can be cured by surgery; this entails flush saphenofemoral ligation with stripping of the long saphenous vein down to the lower leg and sometimes directly to the ulcer, or flush saphenopopliteal ligation with stripping of the short saphenous vein down to a lateral ulcer. If a grossly incompetent perforating vein is present this can be ligated extrafascially through a small vertical incision placed directly over the junction at the time of surgery to the long saphenous vein. Any residual veins can later be dealt with by injection and, once the leg is clear of vein problems with a healthy skin, no further treatment is required.

Post-thrombotic syndrome

Ulcers associated with the post-thrombotic syndrome will require long-term care because the underlying problems in the deep veins cannot be cured. The skin can be protected from the deep vein pathology by interruption of the incompetent communicating veins between the deep and superficial system. Because treatment of these perforating veins cannot be achieved permanently at the first operation and, because it entails operating through damaged skin and tissue, surgery is best avoided. These incompetent perforating veins secondary to deep vein pathology are easily eliminated by effective sclerotherapy which allows normal life to continue. Therefore, in the post-thrombotic syndrome treatment should include the following.

1. Reduction of any excess weight especially on the trunk to enable the diaphragm to function most effectively in aiding venous return.
2. Exercise to encourage the muscle pumps and aid venous return.
3. Care of the skin to avoid and promptly treat infection or trauma.
4. Adequate support to prevent oedema. Strong elastic stockings must always be worn. These must be graduated and the pressure at the ankle should be sufficient to control the problem. This is likely to be 20–30 mmHg or more depending on the state of the veins and the size of the patient. Light-weight stockings can be used for brief social occasions, when there is no oedema and the skin is healthy.

If there are signs of deterioration or eczema, bandages should be used and Betnovate will control any eczema. As soon as significant veins redevelop or eczema appears the veins should be eliminated by further injection-compression.

Conclusion

Excision and skin grafting are not necessary for venous ulcers. Thus elimination of venous hypertension by removing the vein problem temporarily or permanently and the use of adequate support, as indicated, will prevent the recurrence of venous ulcers.

Reference

1. Hobbs, J. T. The treatment of varicose veins by sclerosing therapy. In: Rutherford, E. B., ed. Vascular surgery, 2nd ed., Ch. 135. Philadelphia: W. B. Saunders, 1984

Illustrations by Angela Christie

Ligation of the ankle-perforating veins

F. B. Cockett MS (Lond.), FRCS
Teacher and Examiner in Surgery, the University of London;
Consulting Surgeon, St Thomas's Hospital, London;
Consultant Surgeon to King Edward VII Hospital for Officers, London, UK

David Negus DM, MCh, FRCS
Teacher in Surgery, the University of London,
United Medical Schools of Guy's and St Thomas's;
Consultant Surgeon, Lewisham and Hither Green Hospitals, London, UK

Introduction

The direct ankle-perforating veins in the lower half of the leg are the main channels of venous drainage of the ankle skin into the deep veins of the calf. In the erect, exercising limb nearly all the venous blood from the superficial tissues drains this way. Incompetence or destruction of the valves in one or more of these veins allows a high-pressure reflux from the calf into the ankle skin and subcutaneous tissues, resulting in widespread venular dilatation and ankle swelling. As time goes on, such lesions as eczema, subcutaneous fat necrosis and fibrosis and ulceration may make their appearance (the so-called 'postphlebitic syndrome').

Indications

There are three main groups of cases in which incompetent ankle perforators occur, and in which exploration and ligation may prevent or cure ulcers. The best results of operation are obtained early, either when the pre-ulcer signs only are present, or when an ulcer has just appeared and has been present for a relatively short time (6 months to 2 years). After ulceration has been present unchecked for many years, irreversible local changes in the skin occur, and even radical perforating vein surgery may fail to heal the ulcer permanently.

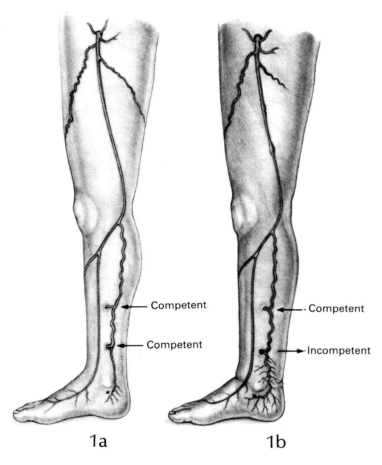

1a   1b

1a & b

Incompetent long saphenous and ankle-perforating veins

Patients with varicose veins may demonstrate primary long saphenous incompetence with normal competent ankle perforators, which siphon off the high venous pressure coming down the long saphenous branches and thus protect the ankle skin. Only excision of the long saphenous vein is necessary.

Other patients may demonstrate primary long saphenous incompetence with abnormal incompetent ankle perforators. The high venous pressure coming down the long saphenous branches is added to and increased by the ankle perforator incompetence, leading to venular dilatation at the ankle (the 'ankle flare'), together with oedema, eczema, pigmentation and eventually ulceration. In this type of case, ligation of the incompetent perforator, in conjunction with high ligation and stripping of the incompetent long saphenous vein (or short saphenous vein) gives the best results. In these cases the deep veins are normal, and so in many cases a permanent complete cure can be achieved.

2a & b

Incompetent deep calf veins and ankle perforators

During the acute stage of the peripheral type of deep-vein thrombosis involving the calf veins the thrombus may extend into the perforating veins. Following the acute stage the veins recanalize but the venous valves are rendered incompetent, including those in the ankle perforators. In these patients, who are left with minimal obstruction of deep veins, ankle-perforator ligation achieves good long-term cure of ankle ulcers.

3a & b

Iliac vein obstruction and incompetent deep veins

During the acute phase of extensive iliofemoral deep venous thrombosis, the perforating veins may also be involved. In the post-thrombotic phase there may be one or more incompetent ankle perforators. But the important factor is the permanent obstruction of the iliac vein.

Ligation of the ankle perforators must be approached with caution in these patients, as it is not the complete answer to the problem. Most of the high venous pressure at the ankle is due to the permanent obstruction to the iliac vein (usually at the iliac compression point, where the left common iliac vein is crossed and compressed by the right common iliac artery).

If the peripheral ankle perforators are large and obvious, a limited ligation of these may be undertaken to help control local skin deterioration in their immediate vicinity. However, in no sense is the operation a cure in these cases, and the patient always needs long-term management with compression bandages and postural treatment. In some cases a saphenous crossover graft (Palma operation) should be considered, to help relieve the iliac obstruction.

Preoperative

This operation must never be done when the leg is oedematous, in the presence of active eczema, or in the presence of open infected ulcer. The essential preoperative treatment is a period of pressure bandaging to control the oedema and to bring the ulcer into a healing phase. This must usually be supplemented by a few days' rest in bed, with the foot of the bed raised, before operation.

Sepsis is controlled by oral antibiotics. For local treatment a simple dry gauze dressing or one wrung out in normal saline is used. Strong local antiseptics and preparations containing antibiotics should not be used as local dressings as they tend to promote a local eczematous reaction.

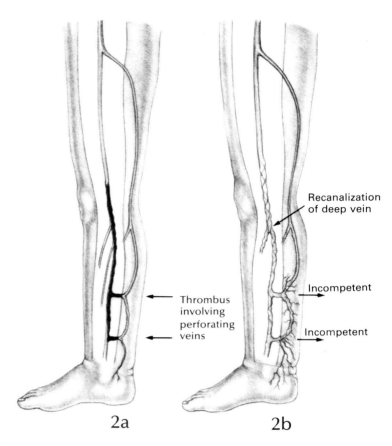

Recanalization of deep vein

Thrombus involving perforating veins

Incompetent

Incompetent

2a   2b

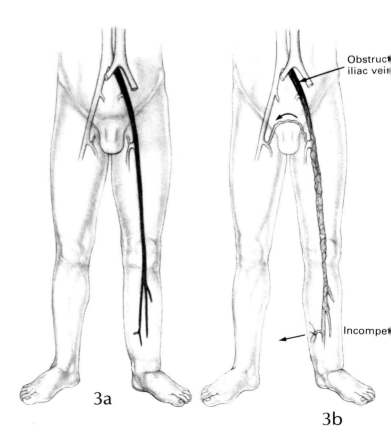

Obstruct iliac vei

Incompe

3a   3b

The operations

Position of patient

Operations on the perforating veins should be done with the patient lying flat on the back, with the legs widely apart on a foot board, and the table tilted head down about 20° to reduce the bleeding during the operation. The operator sits at the foot of the table.

4

Anatomy of the ankle-perforating veins

On the inner side of the limb there are two main direct perforating veins (2) emerging from holes in the deep fascia. They are situated behind the long saphenous vein (1). The upper one is approximately halfway up the leg. The lower one is four fingerbreadths above the internal malleolus. Note that the perforating veins communicate by fine venous arches, and also with the long saphenous vein, by a large constant posterior arch vein (3) rising at knee level.

On the outer side of the limb there is only one constant large perforator (5) which communicates directly with the short saphenous vein (4). Much less constant is the so-called mid-calf perforating vein (6), emerging close to the insertion of the gastrocnemius into the soleus tendon. When present, however, it is often large and important.

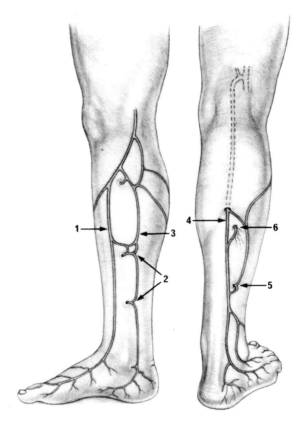

4

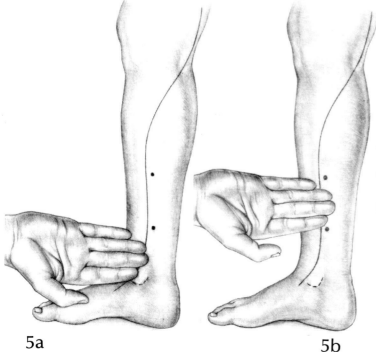

5a   5b

5a & b

Locating the ankle perforators

The 'hand's breadth' rule is very useful in indicating the location of the two main internal ankle perforating veins. The lowest main perforator is four fingers or a hand's breadth above the internal malleolus and the next perforator is a hand's breadth higher.

6a & b

The incision

The incision starts just above halfway up the leg, one fingerbreadth behind the medial subcutaneous border of the tibia. It is carried straight down to a point halfway between the medial malleolus and the tendo Achillis. The vertical incision must never be dropped beyond the internal malleolus, otherwise the lower part may exhibit delayed healing and a troublesome scar, sometimes with a keloid reaction.

If there is an unhealed ulcer in the ankle region, well localized and of long duration, then this may be completely excised to the full depth of the skin as part of the incision. This defect is then grafted 2–3 days later.

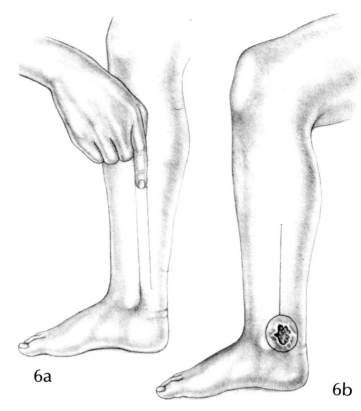

6a   6b

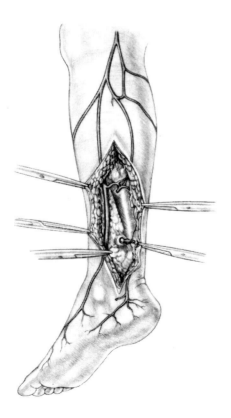

7

7

The extrafascial operation

When the subcutaneous tissues are in good condition, freely mobile and contain large palpable masses of veins, the extrafascial approach is used. The line of emergence of the perforators is cut down on, carrying the knife straight down the deep fascia. Any large vein in the subcutaneous tissues is then identified and followed up and down: it will lead to one or other of the enlarged perforating veins. Any lateral dissection is carried out mainly by gauze dissection right down on the deep fascia, sweeping the flaps medially and laterally. This is quite safe, but excessive local dissection in the subcutaneous plane may impair the arterial supply of the skin, leading to areas of skin necrosis in the incision and delayed healing. However, under the anterior flap the long saphenous vein can be identified and used to insert a stripper. Stripping of an incompetent long saphenous vein can thus be combined with ankle-perforator exploration.

The subfascial operation

8

This operation is performed through the same incision. It is more suitable for the case with the indurated leg in which the skin has been bound down to the underlying fascia. The knife is carried straight down through the deep fascia, exposing the muscle.

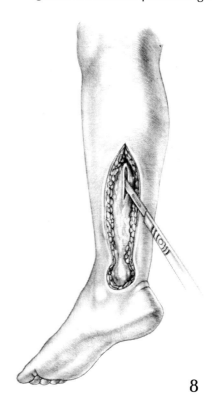

8

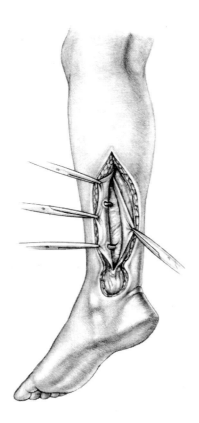

9

9

A number of artery forceps are then attached to the deep fascia of the anterior aspect and this flap is lifted up and the perforating veins sought as they pass from muscle to deep surface of fascia. In this plane wide lateral and medial dissection can be done without jeopardizing the blood supply of the skin. All ligating should be done with fine catgut; non-absorbable ligatures should never be used.

10

Closure

A few fine catgut sutures may be placed in the fascial layer to draw it together, but these are not strictly necessary. The skin is best closed by a few mattress sutures of nylon or silk. It is important to avoid excess tension on individual stitches as this may lead to localized skin necrosis. If the skin of the ankle cannot be closed without tension, it is best left open and the elliptical defect grafted at a later date.

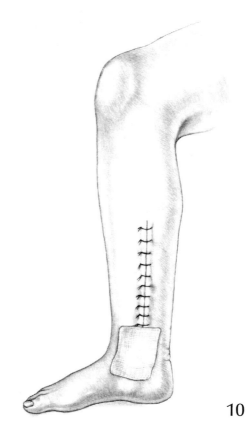

10

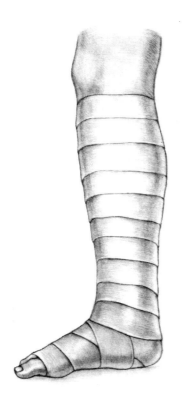

11

11

The limb is enclosed in a firm crêpe bandage. (Heavy duty webbing elastic bandages should never be applied to an unconscious patient as they may cause skin necrosis if too tight.)

The lateral and mid-calf perforating veins may be ligated through short vertical incisions over them.

Postoperative care

The limb is elevated while the patient is at rest in bed, and active ankle movements are encouraged.

Ambulation for short walking periods begins on the 2nd or 3rd postoperative day, with a firm webbing bandage for extra support when the patient is up.

Stitches are removed on the 10th postoperative day. By this time the patient is fully mobile, but he must wear the elastic webbing bandage over foot, ankle and leg constantly during the day for at least a month. After that it can be either discarded altogether (in most cases) or replaced by a light, openwork elastic stocking for a further period.

Further reading

Dodd, H., Cockett, F. B. The pathology and surgery of the veins of the lower limb. 2nd ed. Edinburgh: Churchill Livingstone, 1976

Haeger, K. Management of chronic venous insufficiency by ligation of incompetent perforating veins. In: Rutherford, R. B., ed. Vascular surgery. Philadelphia: Saunders, 1977: 1243–1246

May, R., Partsch, J., Staubesand, J., eds. Perforating veins. Munich: Urban & Schwarzenberg, 1981

Negus, D. The peripheral venous system. In: Keen, G., ed. Operative surgery and management. Bristol: Wright, P. S. G., 1981: 533–560

Venous thrombectomy

James A. DeWeese MD, FACS
Professor and Chairman, Division of Cardiothoracic Surgery,
University of Rochester Medical Center, Rochester, New York, USA

Preoperative

ILIOFEMORAL VENOUS THROMBOSIS

Iliofemoral venous thrombosis is characterized by massive painful oedema of the entire leg which may be accompanied by vasospasm and, in some instances, gangrene. The thrombosis is usually localized initially to the iliac and proximal femoral veins, but may also ascend from the calf veins. There is significant early morbidity and death may occur. There is usually late morbidity due to the postphlebitic syndrome[1-4].

Indications for thrombectomy[2]

Thrombectomy is indicated when the disease process is less than 7 days old and is still localized to the iliac and femoral veins as demonstrated by phlebography. Patent channels may be re-established immediately and the valves of the femoral and saphenous veins can be maintained. Early and late morbidity can be decreased.

Thrombectomy is also indicated when vasospasm or the cyanosis of extreme venous stasis does not respond to conservative treatment. Increased venous drainage from the leg can prevent loss of a limb.

Contraindications to thrombectomy[2]

1. Pelvic inflammatory disease or tumour.
2. Inability to mobilize patient due to age, debilitating illness, casts or traction.
3. Conditions which prevent use of anticoagulants.

Preoperative management

A phlebogram is obtained to determine the extent of the thrombosis. Patients with only proximal iliofemoral venous thrombosis are taken immediately to the operating theatre. If there is more extensive thrombosis, the patient is anticoagulated with heparin, placed in bed with the legs elevated at least a foot above the level of the heart and observed. If cyanosis or arterial pulsation do not improve within 6 hours, the operation is performed.

SUBCLAVIAN VEIN THROMBOSIS

Venous thrombosis of the upper limb classically occurs following unusual exercise of the arm. It is characterized by painful massive oedema of the arm and tenderness along the course of the axillary and subclavian veins. It is usual for the thrombus to be localized initially to the subclavian vein between the clavicle and first rib, but it frequently extends distally to the axillary vein. Pulmonary embolization occasionally occurs. There may be significant early and late morbidity due to persistent or intermittent pain and oedema[5,6].

Indications for thrombectomy

The presence of a thrombosis less than 7 days of age, particularly if the patient is young. The risk of the operation is minimal and early and late morbidity can be significantly decreased.

Preoperative management

A phlebogram is obtained to determine the extent of the thrombosis. Heparin anticoagulation is begun.

The operations

ILIOFEMORAL VENOUS THROMBECTOMY

Local anaesthesia is preferred. The groin and upper thigh are prepared. The entire leg is enclosed in sterile stockingette so that it can be manipulated during the procedure.

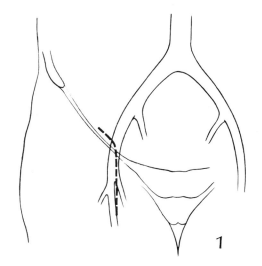

1

The incision

The incision is made along the inguinal crease from the midpoint of the inguinal ligament to within 1 cm of the pubic tubercle. If necessary it can be extended distally, medial to the course of the femoral vessels.

2

Mobilization of vessels

The femoral vein and its branches are carefully mobilized. Particular care is taken to identify and control the posterior branches which would otherwise cause unnecessary bleeding later in the procedure. A tape with its ends slipped through a short segment of rubber tubing is used for proximal and distal control. This allows occlusion of the vessel around intraluminal catheters.

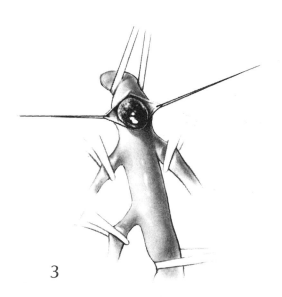

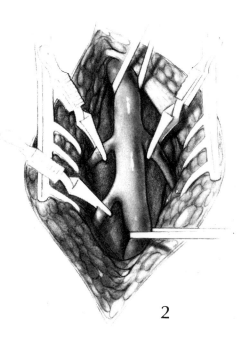

3

Venotomy

A longitudinal venotomy is made in the common femoral vein. Stay sutures are placed in the edges of the incised vein to minimize handling of the vein with instruments. The thrombus bulges forth and as much as possible is gently extracted with forceps. It is rarely possible to extract the clot completely by this method.

ILIAC THROMBECTOMY

4

Insertion of Fogarty catheter[7]

A Fogarty venous thrombectomy catheter is carefully passed alongside the thrombus to the level of the inferior vena cava.

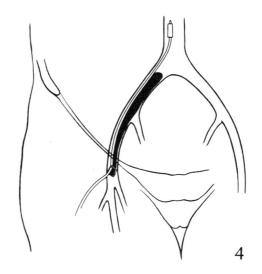

4

5

Inflation of balloon

The balloon on the tip of the Fogarty venous thrombectomy catheter is then inflated and the catheter removed. The thrombus is extruded from the venotomy incision ahead of the balloon.

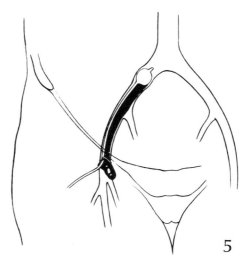

5

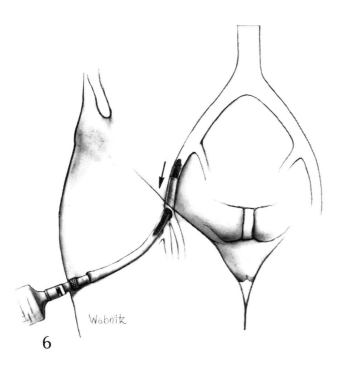

6

6

Use of alternative catheter

Older thrombi may be too adherent to the vein wall to be removed with the Fogarty catheter. In this case, a semi-rigid plastic catheter, which is slightly smaller than the vein and attached to a 50 ml syringe, is cautiously introduced until resistance is met. Suction is then applied to remove the remainder of the thrombus. Unnecessarily rigorous suction such as that provided by a high-power vacuum line should be avoided or the blood loss will be excessive. After the operator believes all of the thrombus is extracted, a phlebogram of the iliac vein should be obtained to demonstrate patency to the level of the vena cava. Further passages of the catheter may prove necessary.

FEMORAL THROMBECTOMY

7

The proximal femoral vein is occluded and the distal clamps removed. The leg is elevated and a tight rubber elastic bandage is wrapped tightly around the leg, beginning at the foot and ending just distal to the groin incision. It may be possible to remove all thrombi in this manner and obtain a brisk flow of blood.

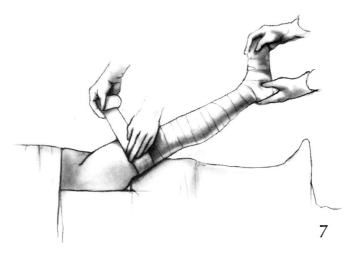

7

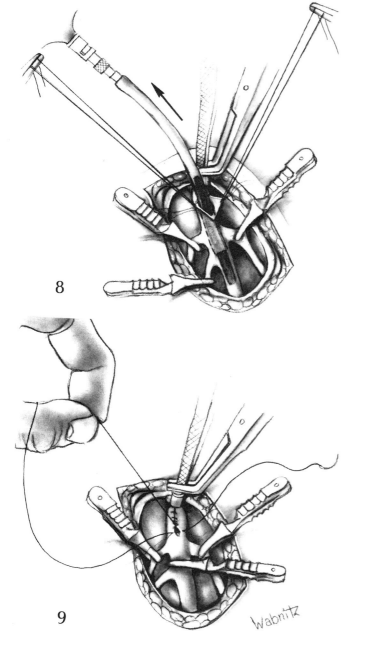

8

9

8

Passing of catheter

It may be necessary to pass catheters distally to remove all thrombi completely. Fogarty catheters can usually be passed to the level of the knee by gently manipulating the catheter tip through the valves. Plastic catheters can be introduced, if necessary, by intermittently distending the vein with a saline solution as the catheter is inserted.

9

Closure

The venotomy is closed with fine monofilament suture on atraumatic needles, using stay sutures at each end of the incision and a continuous running stitch. If a satisfactory flow of blood cannot be established from one of the branches, it is ligated flush with the femoral vein. The wound is closed with interrupted sutures without drainage.

SUBCLAVIAN VENOUS THROMBECTOMY[6]

A general anaesthetic is preferred. The neck and upper chest are prepared and draped.

10

The incision

The incision is begun at the medial head of the clavicle and carried along the clavicle to its midpoint.

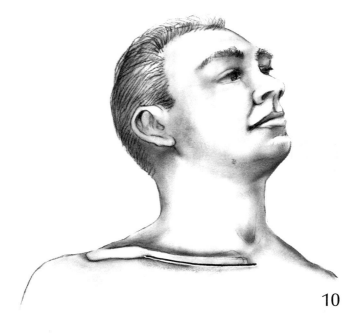

10

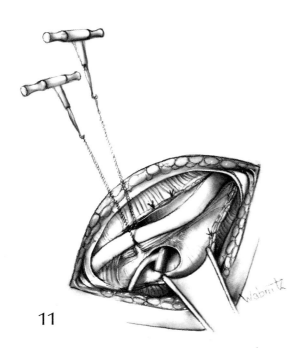

11

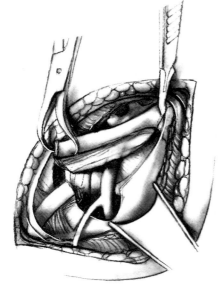

12

11

Excision of medial half of clavicle

Although the operation can be performed without the removal of the clavicle, the exposure is superior when it is resected. There is surprisingly little deformity or morbidity associated with the absence of the medial half of the clavicle.

The insertion of the sternocleidomastoid muscle into the superior border of the clavicle is incised. The insertion of the pectoral muscle into the inferior border of the clavicle is incised and the muscle retracted inferiorly to expose the clavipectoral fascia and costocoracoid ligament. The clavicle is divided with a Gigli saw just lateral to the junction of the cephalic vein with the axillary vein.

12

Division of subclavius and clavipectoral muscles

The subclavius muscle and clavipectoral fascia are divided at the level of the insertion of the cephalic vein. The clavipectoral fascia is incised medially along the inferior border of the costocoracoid ligament to the point where it inserts into the first rib and this insertion is divided. The costoclavicular ligaments and sternoclavicular ligaments are similarly divided. The medial half of the clavicle, subclavius muscle and clavipectoral fascia are then retracted anteriorly as posterior attachments are divided, including the insertion of the sternohyoid muscle.

13

Exposure of subclavian vein

The entire course of the subclavian vein is now exposed. The internal jugular, innominate, axillary and other significant branches such as the external jugular vein are occluded and a longitudinal incision made in the subclavian vein. The thrombosis is usually surprisingly localized to the subclavian vein beneath the clavicle. Thrombus which has propagated distally can usually be manually expressed through the venotomy. The use of plastic catheters or the Fogarty catheter is rarely necessary.

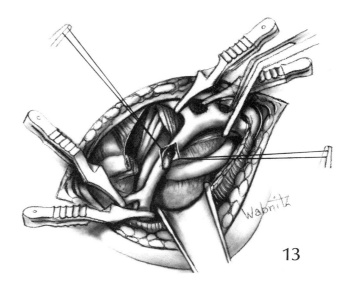

13

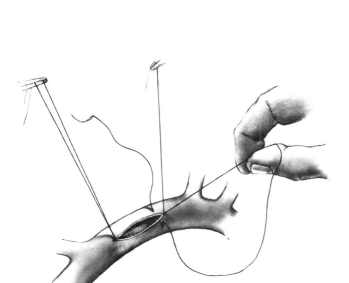

14

14

Closure of arteriotomy

The venotomy is closed with fine sutures on atraumatic needles, using a continuous stitch between two stay sutures.

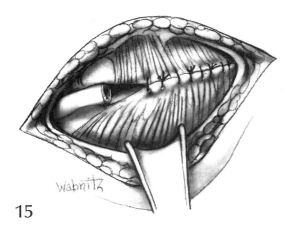

15

15

Closure of wound

The fascia of the sternocleidomastoid muscle and the pectoralis major muscle is approximated. The subcutaneous tissue and skin are closed in layers.

Postoperative care

If the patient has undergone iliofemoral venous thrombectomy, he remains in bed with the feet elevated 30 cm (12 in) until the oedema subsides. He is then allowed to get up and walk with elastic support from the toes to the upper thigh. He is not allowed to sit for 2 weeks. Elastic support is not necessary after that time if the thrombectomy has been completely successful.

Following thrombectomy for iliofemoral or subclavian venous thrombosis, the patient is placed on continuous intravenous heparin anticoagulation which maintains partial thromboplastin times 1½ to 2 times normal for 7 days. Warfarin is begun on the 4th postoperative day and prothrombin times 1½ to 2 times normal are maintained for at least 6 weeks.

References

1. DeWeese, J. A. Thrombectomy for acute iliofemoral venous thrombosis. Journal of Cardiovascular Surgery 1964; 5: 703–712

2. DeWeese, J. A. Iliofemoral venous thrombectomy. In: Bergan, J. J., Yao, J. S. T., eds. Venous Problems. Chicago Year Book Medical Publishers, 1978: 421–440

3. Mavor, G. E., Galloway, J. M. D. Iliofemoral venous thrombosis: pathological considerations and surgical management. British Journal of Surgery 1969; 56: 45–59

4. Edwards, W. H., Sawyers, J. L., Foster, J. H. Iliofemoral venous thrombosis: reappraisal of thrombectomy. Annals of Surgery 1970; 171: 961–970

5. Adams, J. T., McEvoy, R. K., DeWeese, J. A. Primary deep venous thrombosis of upper extremity. Archives of Surgery 1965; 91: 29–42

6. DeWeese, J. A., Adams, J. T., Gaiser, D. L. Subclavian venous thrombectomy. Circulation 1970; 41 & 42: Suppl., II 158–II 164

7. Fogarty, T. J., Dennis, D., Krippaehne, W. W. Surgical management of iliofemoral venous thrombosis. American Journal of Surgery 1966; 112: 211–217

Illustrations by Anita Matthews and Robert Wabnitz

Interruptions of the inferior vena cava and femoral veins

James T. Adams MD
Professor of Surgery, University of Rochester Medical Center, Rochester, New York, USA

Historical background

Since the turn of the century it had been recognized that pulmonary embolism was a cause of death following operations, injuries, severe illnesses and prolonged bed rest. Because autopsy studies demonstrated thrombi in the veins of the lower extremities, Homans[1], in 1934, suggested ligation of the femoral veins for the prevention of pulmonary embolism. In some patients, however, thrombosis extended proximally beyond the femoral vessels or was located in the pelvic venous beds so that ligation at the femoral level was inadequate. This prompted Homans[2], in 1944, to recommend ligation of the inferior vena cava. Subsequently, vein ligation became a frequently performed operation. Yet, although the procedure prevented pulmonary embolism, the ensuing venous obstruction and propagation of the thrombosis distal to the site of ligation resulted in a significant incidence of lower extremity morbidity. This morbidity, referred to as the postphlebitic syndrome and characterized early by leg swelling and pain, and late by pigmentary changes and ulcerations of the skin was appreciable enough after vein ligations to constitute a real disadvantage. In order to prevent or minimize the adverse effects of vein ligation, techniques of partial interruption were devised[3-7]. These techniques consisted of the extraluminal application of sutures or plastic clips which narrowed or compartmentalized the vein sufficiently to prevent passage of potentially fatal pulmonary emboli without interfering significantly with blood flow. More recently, methods of intraluminal partial interruption of the inferior vena cava have been described[8-10]. A major advantage of the intraluminal techniques is that they can be done under local anaesthesia so that a major surgical procedure can be avoided in poor risk patients who require caval interruption.

Indications

Anticoagulation combined with a short period of bed rest and followed by ambulation with elastic support of the legs is the treatment of choice for patients with acute venous thrombosis with pulmonary embolism. Unfortunately, anticoagulation does not always prevent recurrent pulmonary emboli and by far the most frequent indication for vein interruption is recurrent embolism in patients receiving adequate anticoagulation therapy. A second major indication for vein interruption is when anticoagulation therapy is contraindicated in a patient who has suffered a pulmonary embolus. Such patients include those with an ulcerative lesion of the gastrointestinal tract or who have recently had urological or neurosurgical operative procedures. Less frequent indications for vein interruption are: (1) in high risk patients during the course of certain surgical procedures such as pelvic or groin lymph node dissection for cancer, resection of abdominal aortic aneurysm, or operations for trauma to the major abdominal veins; (2) in cases of suppurative pelvic thrombophlebitis with septic pulmonary emboli; (3) in cases of chronic or recurrent multiple small pulmonary emboli causing progressive cor pulmonale; and (4) following pulmonary embolectomy.

Site of interruption

The majority (90–95 per cent) of pulmonary emboli come from sites of thrombosis in veins drained by the inferior vena cava with about 65 per cent coming from veins below the inguinal ligaments. Therefore, interruption of the inferior vena cava clearly offers the greatest protection against recurrent pulmonary embolism. However, interruption of the femoral vein in the groin is reasonable when positive identification of thrombi in the deep veins of the lower extremity has been made by phlebography. The advantages of femoral vein over caval interruption include: (1) femoral vein procedures can be done safely in poor risk patients under local anaesthesia whereas vena caval procedures require general anaesthesia; (2) anticoagulation must be discontinued for a vena caval interruption but can be continued if the femoral vein is interrupted; (3) patients with pre-existing cardiac disease do not tolerate sudden interruption of the total venous return from both lower extremities if the cava is ligated or a site of partial interruption becomes occluded by a detached thrombus; (4) femoral vein interruption preserves the total venous return from the opposite extremity when unilateral limb thrombosis has been demonstrated on phlebograms. Interruption of the inferior vena cava is indicated when there is clinical or phlebographic evidence of pelvic vein thrombosis, if thrombosis extends above the level of the inguinal ligaments, or if bilateral phlebograms fail to demonstrate any source of venous thrombosis in the lower extremities.

Types of interruptions

Most surgeons now prefer partial interruption of the femoral vein or inferior vena cava rather than ligation because of the reduced incidence of late lower extremity morbidity. The methods of partial interruption include: (1) application of an external clip with two serrated edges which divide the vein into channels each measuring 3 mm in diameter[5]; (2) application of an external plastic clip with two smooth edges which narrows the lumen of the vessel to a width of 2.5 mm[6]; (3) plication of the vein with two or three mattress sutures which divide the lumen into compartments each measuring about 3 mm in diameter[7]; (4) creation of a grid-filter by inserting mattress sutures across the lumen of the vein so that strands are 2 or 3 mm apart and tied loosely so that the vein lumen is not constricted[4]; and (5) application of a plastic clip with one flat and one serrated edge which divides the vein into

compartments measuring 3 mm in diameter[3]. All of the techniques of partial interruption appear equally capable of trapping potential lethal emboli without interfering with venous flow. In general, the methods of partial interruption of the inferior vena cava using external plastic clips are superior to suture techniques because they do not injure the luminal surface, are more reliable in compressing or dividing the vein into channels of appropriate size, and are technically easier to perform.

The Adams–DeWeese clip[3] is preferred for interruption of the vena cava because of its ease of application. The grid-filter suture technique is preferred for partial interruptions of the femoral vein because clips do not seat properly in the narrow femoral space and thus cause angulation and occlusion of the vein. Of the several methods of intraluminal interruption of the inferior vena cava described, the most popular is insertion of a device which has an umbrella design consisting of sharp metallic spokes radiating from a central hub. This is covered by a thin circular sheet of Silastin that has perforations to allow the passage of blood. These three methods of venous interruption will be described although the other methods of partial interruption or ligation can be used if preferred.

Preoperative preparation

Patients with underlying cardiac disease who are in congestive failure as a result of the embolic episode should be fully digitalized and an adequate diureses. If the vena cava is to be interrupted, the bleeding and prothrombin time of patients on anticoagulants achieved should be corrected by the administration of Vitamin K or protamine sulphate intravenously. Anticoagulation can be maintained if interruption is to be carried out at the femoral vein level. In the operating room, the lower extremities should be wrapped with elastic bandages from the toes to below the groin and the legs elevated at least 15° to allow maximal venous return.

Local anaesthesia can be used for femoral vein interruption and for intraluminal interruption of the inferior vena cava. General endotracheal anaesthesia is used for extraluminal interruption of the vena cava.

The operations

EXTRALUMINAL INTERRUPTION OF INFERIOR VENA CAVA

1

The incision

The inferior vena cava can be approached either transperitoneally or extraperitoneally. The transperitoneal approach is preferred because it facilitates exposure of the vena cava at the level of the renal veins, a level which cannot easily be achieved through the standard extraperitoneal approach. Ligation just below the entrance of the renal veins avoids the creation of a cul-de-sac wherein inflow is sluggish and thus conducive to thrombosis should the site of partial interruption be subsequently occluded by thrombosis or a detached clot. The transperitoneal approach also enables simultaneous ligation of the ovarian (or testicular) veins through which emboli may pass from sites of pelvic vein thrombosis.

With the patient in a supine position, either an upper midline or right subcostal incision can be used. With a subcostal incision, the right rectus muscle is transected; with a midline incision the peritoneal cavity is entered through the linea alba.

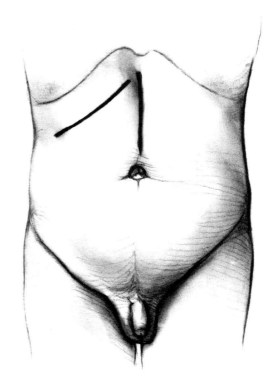

1

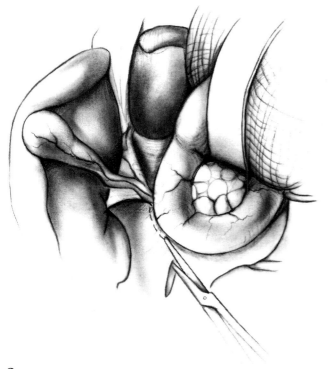

2

Exposure of inferior vena cava

The viscera are packed out of the right upper abdomen in a manner similar to that used for a cholecystectomy. The peritoneum lateral to the second portion of the duodenum is incised and the retroperitoneal space entered. By blunt dissection the duodenum and head of the pancreas are then mobilized toward the midline. This manoeuvre exposes the inferior vena cava and both renal veins as they enter the vena cava.

2

3

Mobilization of inferior vena cava

The fascia over the inferior vena cava is carefully incised, after which a long-limb, right-angle clamp is passed around the cava just below the entrance of the right renal vein. The clamp is passed from the right side of the vena cava and directed behind it by finger palpation to protect the aorta. Care must be taken to avoid injury to the nearby paired upper lumbar veins.

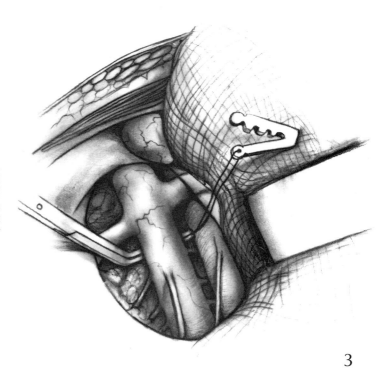

3

4

4

PASSAGE OF CLIP AROUND THE CAVA

A 4/0 nylon suture threaded through the small perforation in the open end of the smooth limb of the clip is grasped by the clamp and drawn through behind the cava. With traction on the suture, the smooth limb of the open clip is gently guided behind the vena cava.

5

5

Securing the clip

The suture is then passed through the perforation in the serrated limb of the clip and, after positioning of the clip just below the entrance of the renal veins, the clip ends are approximated by tying the suture. A second 4/0 nylon suture tie is applied around the end of the clip and seated in opposing grooves on the outer edge of each limb. The interruption procedure is completed by ligating the left ovarian (or testicular) vein as it enters the left renal vein. Since the right ovarian vein enters the vena cava below the level of the clip it does not require ligature. The abdominal incision is then closed in layers, without drainage, to complete the operation.

INTRALUMINAL INTERRUPTION OF INFERIOR VENA CAVA

6

The incision

The patient is placed in a slight Trendelenburg position to protect against accidental air embolism during insertion of the applicator catheter. With the head rotated to the left, an oblique or transverse incision is made on the right side of the neck over the clavicular head of the sternomastoid muscle. Separation of the muscle fibres exposes the internal jugular vein.

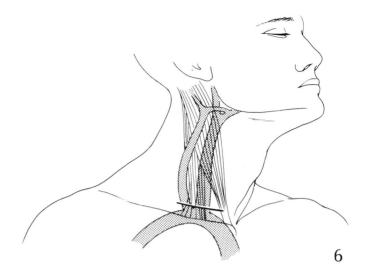

6

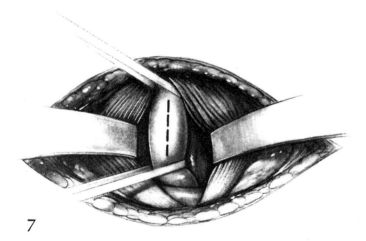

7

7

Isolation of vein

The fascia over the internal jugular vein is incised and about 3 cm of the vein mobilized. Two umbilical tapes are passed around the vein to be retained as keepers to control any subsequent bleeding. A longitudinal incision is then made in the internal jugular vein between the umbilical tapes. The catheter capsule, which contains the folded umbrella filter attached to a guide wire, is inserted into the vein.

8

Passage of catheter

Under fluoroscopic control, the catheter is advanced successively through the superior vena cava and right atrium and into the inferior vena cava. The distal end of the capsule is positioned below the level of the right kidney pelvis. This level is determined by obtaining a preliminary intravenous pyelogram.

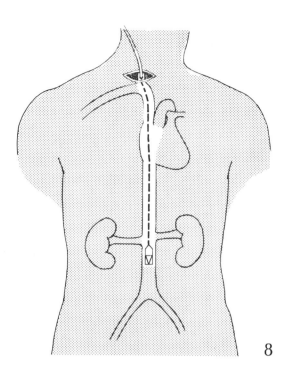

9

Insertion of umbrella

The guide wire is then thrust forward through the catheter allowing the umbrella to be ejected from the capsule. When the umbrella springs open its pointed spokes penetrate the wall of the vein.

10

Fixation of umbrella

The umbrella is fixed in place by slight upward traction on the guide wire. The guide wire is then unscrewed from the umbrella and it, along with the catheter, is removed. The incision in the internal jugular vein is closed with fine plastic vascular suture material and the wound closed in layers without drainage. At the conclusion of the operation, a plain roentgenogram of the abdomen is obtained to verify the position of the umbrella in the inferior vena cava.

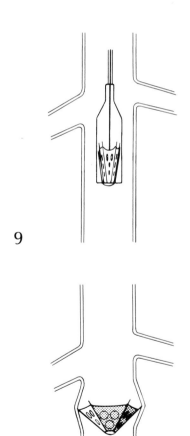

PARTIAL INTERRUPTION OF FEMORAL VEIN

11

The incision

An incision is made in the skin crease just below the inguinal ligament and extending medially nearly to the pubic tubercle.

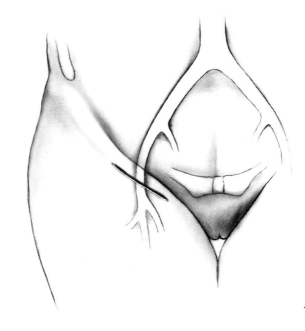

11

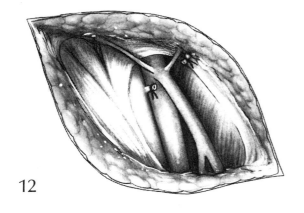

12

12

Exposure of femoral vein

The saphenous vein is identified and followed to the fossa ovalis where it joins the common femoral vein. The small superficial external pudendal artery, lying just beneath the saphenous vein, is ligated and divided. The fascia over the common femoral vein is then incised.

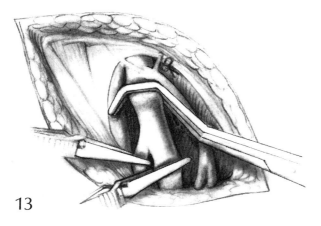

13

13

Isolation of femoral veins

The superficial femoral and deep femoral veins are mobilized and occluded with bulldog clamps. A vascular clamp is then applied across the common femoral vein immediately below the entrance of the greater saphenous vein.

14

Insertion of sutures

Mattress stitches of 4/0 or 5/0 nylon are passed through the common femoral vein just below the occluding vascular clamp. The strands are placed approximately 2 or 3 mm apart. Generally two, and no more than three, sutures are required.

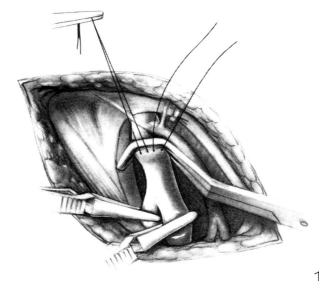

14

15

Tying of sutures

The clamps are removed from the vein and the sutures are individually tied to provide slight tension without significantly compressing the vein. Tying the sutures over a No. 34 hard rubber catheter avoids excessive narrowing of the vein. (The inset indicates the cross-sectional appearance of an ideal filter.) The wound is then closed in layers after meticulous haemostasis has been obtained. If the patient has been maintained on anticoagulants, a small plastic catheter can be brought out of the subcutaneous tissue through a stab incision inferior to the wound and connected to constant low pressure suction for 24–48 hours.

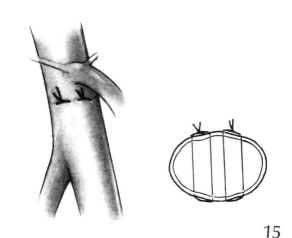

15

Postoperative care

Postoperative management is principally directed towards the prevention of oedema in the lower extremities and the prevention of further thrombosis or new thrombosis. Lower extremity oedema can be minimized by elevation of the lower extremities 15–20° above the heart level and restricting ambulation until all pre-existing leg oedema has disappeared. When the patient becomes ambulatory, support elastic stockings should be worn at all times. The patient should be instructed against prolonged standing or sitting with the legs dependent for 1–4 weeks.

When not contraindicated, anticoagulation therapy should be instituted in the postoperative period. This is initiated using concentrated aqueous heparin given intravenously to achieve a clotting time two or three times above control. The patient is maintained on heparin for 7–10 days and then switched to warfarin sodium for an additional 8–12 weeks. The purpose of postoperative anticoagulation is to prevent progressive thrombosis below the interruption site which will contribute to the postphlebitic syndrome.

Results

Operative mortality

The operative mortality following any type of vein interruption procedure is related primarily to the severity of the underlying cardiac disease and the degree of incapacitation resulting from the episode of pulmonary embolism which led to vein interruption[11, 12]. Significant pre-existing cardiac disease has been associated with a 30 per cent mortality rate following inferior vena caval interruption compared to 3–7 per cent mortality rate in patients without cardiac disease. Early mortality as a direct result of or failure of the operative procedure itself is usually from two sources: recurrent pulmonary embolism and fatal shock. Fatal embolism following either ligation or partial interruption of the inferior vena cava is extremely rare and indicates that thrombosis was present or had formed in a vein proximal to the site of interruption or that the interruption site had become disrupted. Fatal shock is almost exclusively a complication of vena caval ligation. This is the result of sudden pooling of blood in the lower extremities causing a critical decrease in venous return to the heart. This complication is rare following partial interruption procedures.

In-hospital mortality following interruption of the femoral vein varies between 5 and 15 per cent and is also related primarily to the severity of underlying myocardial disease[13]. The incidence of recurrent fatal embolism subsequent to interruption at the femoral level is somewhat higher than that following interruption of the inferior vena cava.

Late complications

Recurrent non-fatal pulmonary embolism following either ligation or partial interruption of the inferior vena cava has been reported in between 5 and 15 per cent of patients[11, 12]. Recurrent non-fatal embolism after femoral vein interruption occurs in 10–25 per cent of patients[13].

Lower extremity swelling immediately following surgery occurs frequently following vein ligation or when a site of partial interruption becomes suddenly occluded by embolus or thrombosis. Elevation of the lower extremities and early reinstitution of anticoagulation postoperatively will prevent or minimize the development of this early oedema. Significant late extremity morbidity has been reported in up to 30 per cent of patients following femoral or vena caval interruption with a lower incidence in patients undergoing partial interruption procedures[11, 12]. Most late morbidity is secondary to pre-existing thrombosis or to progression of this thrombosis. In most large series, 60 to 70 per cent of partial interruption procedures have remained patent by phlebography and in these patients there has been a reduced incidence and severity of the postphlebitic syndrome[12].

References

1. Homans, J. Thrombosis of the deep veins of the lower leg causing pulmonary embolism. New England Journal of Medicine 1934; 211: 993–997

2. Beall, A. C., Fred, H. L., Cooley, D. A. Pulmonary embolism. Current problems in surgery. Chicago: Yearbook Medical Publishers, 1964; February

3. Adams, J. T., DeWeese, J. A. Partial interruption of the inferior vena cava with a new plastic clip. Surgery, Gynecology and Obstetrics 1966; 123: 1087–1088

4. DeWeese, M. S., Hunter, D. C., Jr. A vena cava filter for the prevention of pulmonary embolism: a five-year clinical experience. Archives of Surgery 1963; 86: 852–868

5. Miles, R. M., Chappell, F., Renner, O. A partially occluding vena caval clip for prevention of pulmonary embolism. American Surgeon 1964; 30: 40–47

6. Moretz, W. H., Rhode, C. M., Shepherd, M. H. Prevention of pulmonary emboli by partial occlusion of the inferior vena cava. American Surgeon 1959; 25: 617–626

7. Spencer, F. C., Quattlebaum, J. K., Quattlebaum, J. K., Jr, Sharp, E. H., Jude, J. R. Plication of the inferior vena cava for pulmonary embolism: a report of 20 cases. Annals of Surgery 1962; 155: 827–837

8. Greenfield, L. J., McCurdy, J. R., Brown, P. P., Elkins, R. C. A new intracaval filter permitting continued flow and resolution of emboli. Surgery 1973; 73: 599–606

9. Hunter, J. A., Dye, W. S., Javid, H., Najafi, H., Goldin, M. D., Serry, C. Permanent transvenous balloon occlusion of the inferior vena cava: experience with 60 patients. Annals of Surgery 1977; 186: 491–499

10. Mobin–Uddin, K., McLean, R., Bolooki, H., Jude, J. R. Caval interruption for prevention of pulmonary embolism. Archives of Surgery 1969; 99: 711–715

11. Adams, J. T., Feingold, B. E., DeWeese, J. A. Comparative evaluation of ligation and partial interruption of the inferior vena cava. Archives of Surgery 1971; 103: 272–276

12. Donaldson, M. C., Wirthlin, L. S. Donaldson, G. A. Thirty-year experience with surgical interruption of the inferior vena cava for prevention of pulmonary embolism. Annals of Surgery 1980; 191: 367–372

13. Adams, J. T., DeWeese, J. A. Comparative evaluation of ligation and partial interruption of the femoral vein in the treatment of thromboembolic disease. Annals of Surgery 1970; 172: 795–803

Venous reconstructive procedures

E. A. Husni MD
Associate Director, Department of Surgery, Huron Road Hospital, Cleveland, Ohio, USA

Introduction

Three decades of experimental and clinical trials of venous reconstruction have greatly enriched our knowledge of the anatomy and physiology of veins in health and disease. These endeavours have also helped dispel the fear of thromboembolism long, though unjustifiably, regarded as the nemesis of vein surgery[1,2]. Pitfalls in patient selection and technical shortcomings of venous reconstruction have also been fairly well identified, so that the vascular surgeon is now better able to choose the candidates, and select and execute the correct operative procedure.

Preoperative

Patient selection

The principal guidelines for patient selection are: (1) the nature and extent of venous disease; (2) the degree of venous hypertension; and (3) the duration of the disease.

In the lower limb, the nature and degree of disease is determined by a contrast phlebogram obtained with and without a Valsalva manoeuvre. The examiner's attention is drawn to pressure defects, abnormality of valves, presence of thrombus, recanalization and the size of collateral channels.

Determinations of the venous pressure[3] are then made through the same cannula in the supine resting position (RVP), in the standing position (SVP) and after active ambulation (AVP). The examiner must keep in mind that the RVP is elevated only in acute or subacute occlusion of the deep veins, as seen in phlebitis, traumatic interruptions and massive extraluminal compression. The SVP varies with the person's height and is ordinarily unaffected by any disease process. The AVP, which should normally be <50 per cent of the SVP, varies directly with the extent of the occlusive process and the paucity of collateral channels[2]. The ideal candidate for venous reconstruction has segmental rather than generalized disease, coupled with a marked degree of venous hypertension (AVP >80 per cent of SVP). The high AVP provides the pressure gradient, the driving force behind the venous blood flow, to maintain patency of the reconstructed veins. It was primarily this basic principle that inspired the concept of creating an arteriovenous fistula distal to the reconstruction in an effort to enhance vein graft patency[4,5] by to establishing both a high pressure gradient and an increase in the rate of venous return.

In cases of trauma, venous reconstruction should be undertaken soon after the injury and prior to the onset of venous thrombosis. Repair of the damaged vein can avert acute venous insufficiency that may jeopardize survival of the limb, especially when the concomitant artery is also injured[6,7] and will help prevent future post-thrombotic changes in the limb.

In postphlebitic disease of the lower limb, surgical intervention may be contemplated 8–12 months after onset of the acute process. This is the time required for the recanalization process and the optimum enlargement of collateral channels.

Basic principles of venous reconstruction

1. During the operative procedure anticoagulation with heparin sodium (100 u/kg) is recommended about 10 minutes before the anastomosis is begun. Protamine sulphate (0.5–1.0 mg/kg) is administered to neutralize the heparin 15–20 minutes after anastomosis is completed.

2. The vein and surrounding tissues should be handled gently and meticulously. Excessive injury to the intima by crushing instruments, and excessive pulling and stretching by forceful irrigation is a sure invitation to thrombosis. The vein should be handled by its adventitia, using fine-tipped forceps, atraumatic rubber-shod clamps and Silastic loops for control of bleeding. Overdistension should be avoided when irrigating the veins. Rough and meandering dissection will invite excessive tissue reaction, turgor and tension, providing an inhospitable environment for the low pressure vessel, compressing it and jeopardizing its patency.

3. There should be no tension on the reconstructed vein. Since it is the intraluminal pressure that keeps the vessel open, when that pressure is exceeded by the stretching pressure or the surrounding tissue pressure, the vessel will collapse. Unlike grafts placed in an arterial bed, where the intraluminal pressure is considerably higher, the margin of error in venous reconstruction is very narow. To avoid a graft under tension (a short graft) the surgeon should consider two technical points: first, the vein graft should always be longer than the segment it is intended to replace; and second, the length of the bypass should be estimated without pulling or overdistension with irrigation fluid. The latter manoeuvres will add misleading dimensions to the bypass and selecting the desirable length under these conditions will result in a short graft under tension.

1a, b & c

4. The anastomosis should be ample and performed with precision. To avoid stenosis at the site of anastomosis, two technical points are helpful: start with an anastomotic circumference slightly larger than that of the involved vessel as a certain amount of scarring and shrinkage will accompany the healing process at suture lines; maintain a loose, running suture with two or more anchor points to avoid the pursestringing effect of a tight continuous suture.

   Several manoeuvres have been successfully utilized to enlarge the anastomotic area: the diagonal (a), the fishmouth (b) and the trumpet cut (c). The suturing is performed with precision using a 6/0 vascular suture, with no more than 1 mm between successive bites. Close bites provide better intima-to-intima approximation, result in less crimping at the suture line and a smoother luminal surface.

   In the young patient, repair of vessels should be undertaken with interrupted suture, rather than continuous suture, to allow for future growth without stenosis as was clearly demonstrated by Ducharme[8] in his work on puppies.

5. Experience has shown that, in postphlebitic disease, the results of venous reconstruction can be greatly enhanced by the methodical removal of secondary varicose veins and ligation of the incompetent perforating veins. Meticulous haemostasis must be established before wounds are closed.

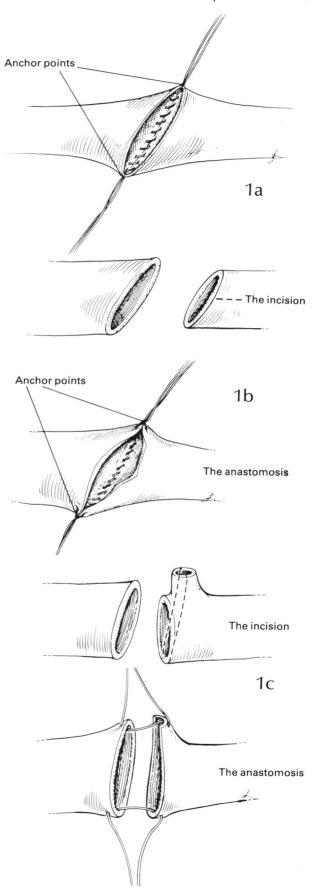

Anchor points

1a

– – – The incision

Anchor points

1b

The anastomosis

The incision

1c

The anastomosis

The operations

THE FREE GRAFT

The free sleeve graft is utilized to replace devitalized venous segments or to bypass venous disease[9]. Vascular prostheses have been successfully substituted for large veins in the body cavities but have not fared as well in the limbs[2], and autogenous veins remain the preferred substitute.

In harvesting the vein, it is essential to use meticulous technique and to follow the correct sequence of steps in the operative procedure: (1) the vein is removed together with ample perivenous adventitia, just prior to its insertion into the venous circuit, in order to maintain maximum viability and minimum ischaemic damage to its structure. (2) Harvesting is accomplished through a single incision or multiple shorter incisions in close proximity. The object is to free the vein without pulling to guard against intimal tears. (3) Tributaries are ligated with 4/0 vascular suture a comfortable 1–1.5 mm away from their junction point in order to avoid 'banding' at the site of ligature when the vein is fully dilated. (4) The vein is irrigated with blood or Ringer's solution containing 0.01 per cent papaverine hydrochloride and 0.01 per cent heparin sodium. It is kept moist with that solution until the procedure is completed.

2a–d

In cases of great disparity between the diameter of the graft and that of the host vein, two or more panels are sewn together to construct a sleeve of the desired dimensions. The two vein segments are opened longitudinally to prepare two panels (a), which are then approximated with suture (b, c). The completed panelled graft restores continuity to the popliteal vein (d). Two panels of saphenous vein will provide a lumen adequate for most purposes.

Construction of a spiral venous conduit[10] is another technique to achieve a free graft of variable dimensions. The surgeon is reminded that when a devitalized venous segment is resected, the edges of the transected vessel will pull apart significantly, and therefore the replacement should be adequate to fill the gap in order to avoid a short graft under tension.

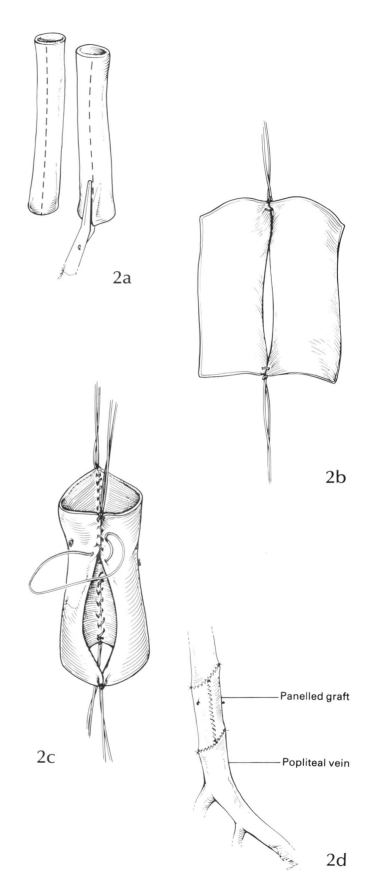

2a

2b

2c

Panelled graft

Popliteal vein

2d

THE CROSS-PUBIS (CROSS-OVER) BYPASS GRAFT

This modality, an ingenious imitation of natural collaterals, was devised by Palma and Esperon[11] to reroute venous drainage from the diseased limb to the contralateral limb utilizing the contralateral saphenous vein. This is currently the choice of procedure to bypass lesions of the iliac and femoral veins. The author has used this method in 90 cases with a patency rate of 75 per cent and a follow-up ranging from 6 months to 16 years. The standard tehnique is as follows.

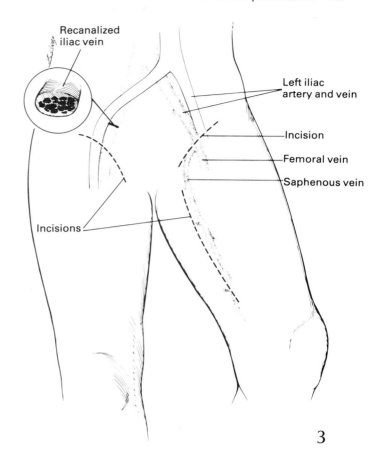

3

3

On the side of venous disease an incision is made along the inguinal crease overlying the femoral pulsation and carried medially and vertically. This provides adequate exposure to the common, superficial and deep femoral veins. Care must be taken to preserve large collateral channels and establish meticulous haemostasis. A similar incision is made on the contralateral side to expose the saphenous vein and the saphenofemoral junction. One or two additional incisions are made along the course of the long saphenous vein to secure the desirable length for a relaxed bypass.

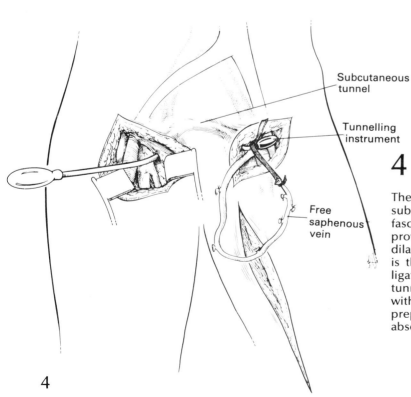

4

4

The two groin incisions are then connected with a subcutaneous tunnel running on the surface of the deep fascia. The tunnel is made with a blunt instrument providing ample dimensions to accommodate the fully dilated bypass. The distal end of the free saphenous vein is then transected between ligatures, its tributaries are ligated and divided and the free vein is passed through the tunnel to the opposite side without disturbing its junction with the common femoral vein. It is then irrigated with the prepared solution with minimum distension to ensure the absence of kinks and twists.

5

The free end is then transected diagonally at a point chosen to provide a relaxed bypass with preservation of the natural saphenofemoral junctional angle. The femoral vein is opened between clamps or vessel loops at a site that is relatively free of disease and that will provide maximum drainage from the deep femoral tributaries. A wedge of femoral vein 1.5 × 0.2 cm is removed and an end-to-side anastomosis is accomplished with 6/0 vascular suture, utilizing two anchor points along the anastomosis. Just prior to completion, clamps are released to flush out clots and trapped air.

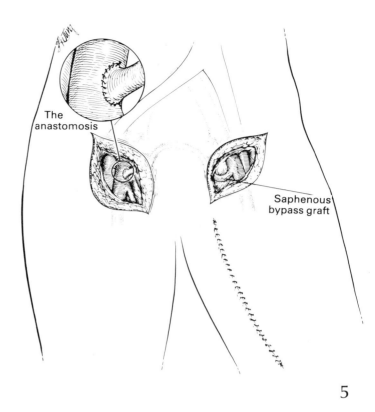

5

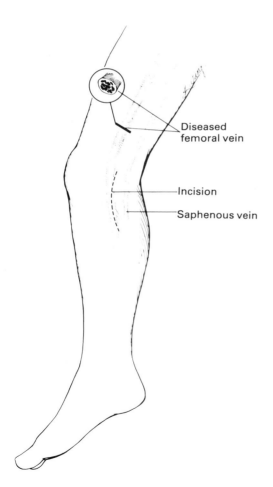

6

THE *IN SITU* SAPHENOPOPLITEAL BYPASS GRAFT

This procedure was designed to bypass the diseased superficial femoral and/or popliteal veins[12].

6

An incision is made on the medial aspect of the upper leg with the knee flexed at 120°.

7

It is carried through the fascia to expose the popliteal vein and its tributaries. Care must be taken to avoid injury to the saphenous vein, the saphenous nerve and its genicular branch that are intimate with the fascia at that level. The saphenous vein is then freed, its tributaries ligated and its main trunk transected at a level yielding the desired length.

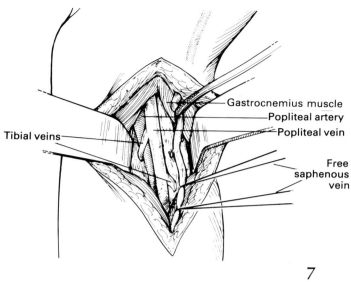

7

8

The anastomotic site is chosen in the popliteal vein or one of its large tributaries, depending on the disease process. The free end of the saphenous vein is approximated to that point and transected at a level allowing a gentle loop formation. An end-to-side anastomosis is then accomplished with 6/0 vascular suture. Clots and trapped air are flushed before completion. Over the last 15 years, 26 such procedures have been performed by our vascular service with a patency rate of 63 per cent.

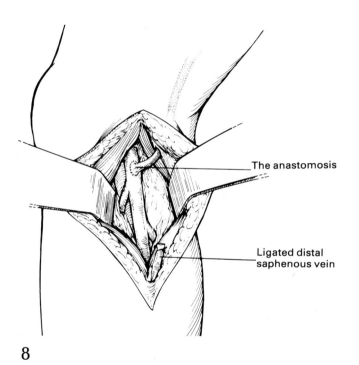

8

RECONSTRUCTION AND TRANSPOSITION OF VALVES

It has long been recognized that the integrity of valves in the femoral and popliteal veins is essential for venous return from the lower limb against the pull of gravity. In an effort to restore competence to damaged veins, several innovative procedures have been introduced over the years with limited success. These include muscle slings around the popliteal vein[13], direct repair of incompetent valves[14] and transposition of venous segments bearing competent valves into the incompetent venous system at the groin level[15]. While in very highly selected cases repair of the incompetent femoral vein valve may have some merit, the results of reconstruction and transposition of valves have been generally disappointing[16]. This is readily understandable since venous competence and haemodynamics are not the function of a single valve, but rather the outcome of the harmonious interplay of all the valves of the limb, especially those in the popliteal and femoral segments.

THE ADJUVANT ARTERIOVENOUS FISTULA

By establishing a steep pressure gradient across a fistulous tract in proximity to a venous bypass, an arteriovenous communication can effect a 500–700 per cent increase in the rate of blood flow through that bypass[17, 18]. This remarkable flow rate, coupled with an increase in the local venous pressure, may help maintain patency of the vein graft during the critical postoperative phase of tissue reaction and oedema and may therefore improve the potential for long-term success.

Data yielded by analysing 18 cases of venous reconstructive procedures that included an adjuvant arteriovenous fistula were not conclusive[18]. That notwithstanding, it is the author's impression that this modality has merit in cases where (1) the bypass is of small calibre (<3 mm in diameter); (2) when thrombectomy or endophlebectomy is undertaken and when artificial prostheses are utilized as venous conduits. Furthermore, a subtle and welcome byproduct of arteriovenous communication is the enlargement of collateral channels that may enhance venous return from the limb[18].

9

The fistula is constructed a minimum of 5–10 cm distal to the venovenous anastomosis. This location will spare the area of venous repair the additional tissue reaction incident to the fistula. It will also eliminate the possibility of inadvertent injury and further trauma to the reconstructed vein when repair of the fistula is undertaken. An interposition graft of autogenous vein, 4–5 mm in diameter, will serve the purpose very well in cases of femoral, iliac or inferior vena caval reconstructions.

Upon completion of the arterial connection, the graft is flushed to allow the escape of thrombus and trapped air, and then allowed to distend with arterial blood by placement of a vascular clamp on its free end. With this manoeuvre the desired loop of the prepared fistula is fashioned and the venous end is sutured to the chosen location in the femoral vein. An intraoperative femoral arteriogram is then undertaken to ascertain the satisfactory function of the fistula and the bypass. Repair of the arteriovenous communication is performed 2–4 months later, depending upon the degree of local and/or systemic reaction to the fistula.

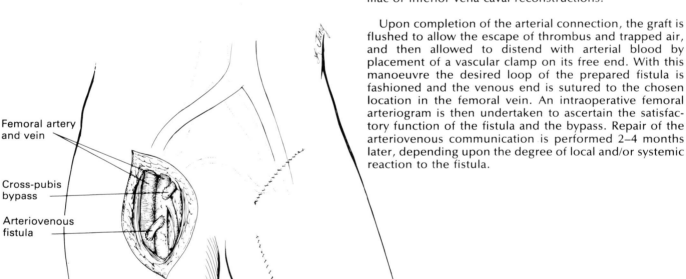

Femoral artery and vein

Cross-pubis bypass

Arteriovenous fistula

9

Postoperative care

Immediately after the incisions are closed, a pneumatic boot is applied to the limb and intermittent external pneumatic compression (IPC) is begun at 30 mmHg pressure with a cycle providing effective compression for 30–40 s/min. IPC, toes to upper calf and toes to upper thigh for popliteal and iliofemoral reconstructions respectively, is continuous for the first 24 hours. Beyond that period, the boot is removed periodically to allow the patient bathroom privileges, and it is discontinued when the patient is fully ambulatory after the third or fourth postoperative day. The limb is then provided with knee-high elastic support.

Conclusions

While venous reconstruction has earned a well deserved place in the annals of vascular surgery, it must not be regarded as a panacea for venous disease. In well selected cases, successful reconstruction can indeed prevent, reverse and even completely restore, pathological venous haemodynamics to normal, but offers little towards the amelioration of long-standing incompetence of the perforating veins, the vital link in postphlebitic disease[19, 20]. Time-honoured measures to deal with this problem must still be employed and elastic support will be needed by a large percentage of the patients. Finally, objectivity must be maintained in these endeavours as a responsible legacy to future generations of vascular surgeons.

References

1. Rich, N. M., Hughes, C. W., Baugh, H. J. Management of venous injuries. Annals of Surgery 1970; 171: 724–730

2. Husni, E. A. Issues in venous reconstruction. Vascular Diagnosis and Therapy 1981; 3: 37–48

3. Husni, E. A., Ximenes, J. O. C., Goyette, E. M. Elastic support of the lower limbs in hospital patients. Journal of the American Medical Association 1970; 214: 1456–1462

4. Bryant, M. F., Lazenby, W. D., Howard, J. M. Experimental replacement of short segments of veins. Archives of Surgery 1958; 76: 289–293

5. Hobson, R. W., Wright, C. B. Peripheral side to side arteriovenous fistula: hemodynamics and application in venous reconstruction. American Journal of Surgery 1973; 126: 411–414

6. Hughes, C. W. Arterial repair during the Korean war. Annals of Surgery 1958; 147: 555–561

7. Rich, N. M., Jarstfer, B. S., Geer, T. M. Popliteal artery repair failure causes and possible prevention. Journal of Cardiovascular Surgery 1974; 15: 340–351

8. Ducharme, J. C. End to end venous anastomoses in small puppies. Techniques, results, growth and some factors influencing thrombus formation. Ohio Medical Journal 1961; 57: 777–783

9. DeWeese, J. A., Niguidula, F. The replacement of short segments of veins with functional autogenous vein grafts. Surgery, Gynecology and Obstetrics 1960; 110: 303–308

10. Wright, C. B., Doty, D. B. Spiral vein grafting: the technique. In: Bergan, J. J., Yao, J. S. T. eds. Operative Techniques in Vascular Surgery. New York: Grune and Stratton, 1980: 307–310

11. Palma, E. C., Esperon, R. Vein transplants and grafts in the surgical treatment of the postphlebitic syndrome. Journal of Cardiovascular Surgery 1960; 1: 94–107

12. Husni, E. A. In situ saphenopopliteal bypass graft for incompetence of the femoral and popliteal veins. Surgery, Gynecology and Obstetrics 1970; 130: 279–284

13. Psathakis, N. Has the 'substitute valve' at the popliteal vein solved the problem of venous insufficiency of the lower extremity? Journal of Cardiovascular Surgery 1968; 9: 64–70

14. Kistner, R. L. Surgical repair of the incompetent femoral vein valve. Archives of Surgery 1970; 110: 1336–1342

15. Queral, L. A., Whitehouse, W. H., Flinn, W. R., Neiman, H. L., Yao, J. S. T., Bergan, J. J. Surgical correction of chronic deep venous insufficiency by valvular transposition. Surgery 1980; 87: 688–695

16. Johnson, N. D., Queral, L. A., Flinn, W. R., Yao, J. S. T., Bergan, J. J. Late objective assessment of venous valve surgery. Archives of Surgery 1981; 116: 1461–1466

17. Pokrovsky, A. V., Klioner, L. I. Reconstructive surgery for occlusions of the major deep veins. In: Hobbs, J. T., ed. The Treatment of Venous Disorders. London: MTP Press, 1977: 308–319

18. Husni, E. A. Arteriovenous fistula in venous reconstruction. In: Loose, D. A., ed. Vorsorgemassnahmen zur Ertassung der Getässkrankheiten. Reinbek: Einhom-Presse Verlag, 1983

19. Husni, E. A. Surgical management. In: Ban, N. U., Glover, J. L., Holden, R. W., Triplett, D. A., eds. Thrombosis and Atherosclerosis. Chicago: Year Book Publishers, 1982: 283–300

20. Husni, E. A. Reconstruction of veins: the need for objectivity. Journal of Cardiovascular Surgery 1983; 24: 525–528

Portal hypertension

Seymour I. Schwartz MD
Professor of Surgery, University of Rochester School of Medicine and Dentistry,
Rochester, New York, USA

Introduction

Portal hypertension is an elevation of pressure, that is, greater than 250 ml of saline, in the portal venous system. It is associated with the clinical manifestations of oesophagogastric varices, ascites, hypersplenism, and portal systemic encephalopathy. The causes of portal hypertension may be categorized conveniently as suprahepatic, intrahepatic and infrahepatic in origin. Well over 90 per cent of cases are due to an intrahepatic block, postsinusoidal in nature, and related to cirrhosis. A presinusoidal block may occur intrahepatically in patients with schistosomiasis or hepatic fibrosis, but is most frequently due to thrombosis or cavernomatous transformation of the portal vein. The rarest of the aetiological factors occur suprahepatically and are associated with the Budd-Chiari syndrome of endophlebitis of the hepatic veins[1].

The modern era of clinical application of shunting procedures dates to the reports in 1945 of Whipple[2] and Blakemore and Lord[3] demonstrating the feasibility of an operation. Initially there was increasing enthusiasm and indications for surgical intervention were extended from the therapy for bleeding oesophageal varices to the treatment of ascites and prophylactic shunts for varices which had not bled. As data have been analyzed, it is now felt that bleeding oesophageal varices represent the sole indication for a decompressive procedure with the exception of a rare case of Budd-Chiari syndrome.

A wide variety of portal systemic shunts have been performed to reduce portal hypertension and decompress oesophageal varices. The use of either small vessels, or 'make-shift' shunts which employ larger collaterals, is generally regarded as inappropriate, since the reduction of portal pressure is relatively insignificant and rarely permanent. The shunting procedures which have significantly and persistently reduced portal pressure include: the end-to-side portacaval shunt, with or without arterialization of the distal portal vein; the side-to-side portacaval shunt, either as a direct anastomosis or employing a graft between the portal vein and the inferior vena cava; the splenorenal shunt using the central end of the splenic vein; the central side-to-side splenorenal shunt; the selective splenorenal shunt using the splenic end of the splenic vein combined with ligation of the coronary vein and devascularization of the stomach; and anastomoses between the inferior vena cava and superior mesenteric vein, either as a direct end-to-side anastomosis or with the interposition of an 'H' graft.

Selection of procedure

In most instances, preference for a given surgical procedure is based on personal experience and it is now felt that it is difficult, if not impossible, to select a procedure based on preoperative haemodynamic studies. With a readily accessible and 'shuntable' portal vein, the end-to-side portacaval shunt is the most commonly performed. It is the easiest shunt to carry out and is generally associated with the lowest incidence of thrombosis. The presence of a large caudate lobe is less compromising to this procedure than to the side-to-side shunt.

In patients with extensive adhesions from previous operations in the right upper quadrant, the splenorenal or mesocaval shunts are generally easier to perform. Thrombosis, with or without recanalization of the portal vein (cavernomatous transformation), generally precludes a portacaval anastomosis and requires either a splenorenal or a mesocaval shunt[4]. The Budd-Chiari syndrome with massive ascites dictates a side-to-side shunt to decompress the liver[5]. Most patients' thrombocytopenia will be corrected by any decompressive procedure, but in the rare circumstance of a platelet count approaching zero and diffuse bleeding a splenectomy and central splenorenal shunt may be most expeditious.

Ascites is no longer considered a significant factor in determining the type of shunt to be performed. Massive ascites is considered a contraindication for a selective splenorenal shunt. Similarly, whether previous encephalopathy is an important determinant in the decision to shunt has not been resolved. Since it is felt that reduction in total effective hepatic blood flow is an important factor in the development of encephalopathy, arterialization of the distal portal vein has been advised to prevent this complication, as has the selective splenorenal shunt. The selective splenorenal shunt is attractive on a theoretical basis and reduced rates of encephalopathy have been reported, particularly in non-alcoholic cirrhotics. In time, following a selective splenorenal shunt, adhepatic portal flow may disappear and negate the theoretical advantage. The procedure has not improved survival of alcoholic patients.

Selection of patients

It has long been appreciated that the status of a patient's liver function is a critical factor in his ability to tolerate a portal-systemic decompressive procedure. Ascites which fails to respond to medical therapy, markedly reduced serum albumin, a bilirubin greater than 5 mg/dl, and a prothrombin time which is two and a half times prolonged and does not respond to vitamin K, plus the presence of encephalopathy after a bleeding episode has been controlled, portend poorly for the patient as an operative risk[6].

Attempts have been made to evaluate the dynamics of hepatic flow so that this can be used as a method of determining which shunt should be performed. Unfortunately, it remains difficult to determine which patients will tolerate a shunt or which is the appropriate shunt.

Portcaval shunts

END-TO-SIDE PORTACAVAL SHUNT

1

The operation is generally performed through a generous right subcostal incision which transects the medial portion of the left rectus, the entire right rectus, and extends around to the right flank. With this incision, the patient is either supine, or the right side may be slightly elevated.

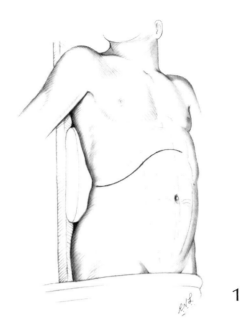

1

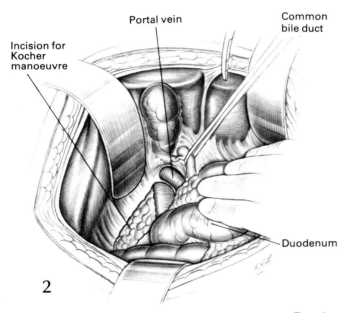

2

2

The liver is retracted craniad and a Kocher manoeuvre is performed to permit mobilization of the duodenum. Dissection is then begun in the hepatoduodenal ligament, and the portal vein is approached from the posterolateral aspect.

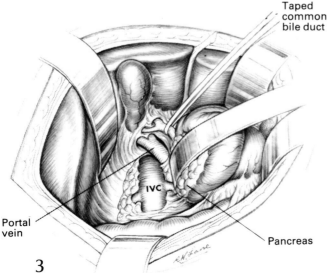

3

3

The portal vein is dissected free along its entire course from its retropancreatic origin to its bifurcation in the porta hepatis. Occasionally a cystic vein and small pyloric veins require ligation, but it is not usual for the entire portal vein to be freed without ligation of any branches. It is extremely important to transect or remove the fibrous and adipose tissue which constitutes the posterior portion of the hepatoduodenal ligament, posterior to the portal vein, in order to avoid angulation of the portal vein by this tissue.

4

After the entire length of the portal vein has been freed, attention is directed to dissection of the inferior vena cava. The incision in the retroperitoneum is extended, and the anterior, lateral and medial aspects of the inferior vena cava are exposed from the renal veins to the point where the vessel passes retrohepatically. A partially occlusive vascular clamp is applied to the anterior aspect of the vena cava and the tissue incorporated within the clamp is incised. The length of the incision in the inferior vena cava should be approximately one and a half times as long as the diameter of the portal vein. It is not necessary to remove an ellipse.

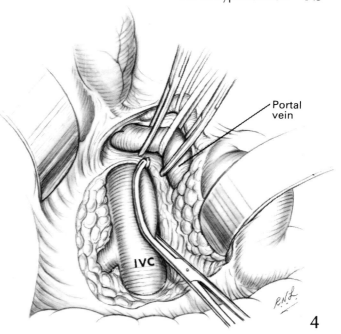

5

Vascular clamps or bulldog clamps are applied to the portal vein just above its origin and just below the bifurcation in the porta hepatis. The portal vein is then transected as far craniad as possible; the distal end is oversewn with vascular suture.

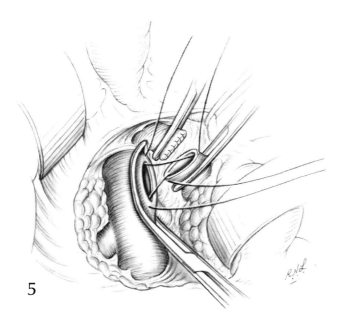

6

Two guide sutures are placed in the cut end of the portal vein, which is then turned down to the inferior vena cava. The upper end of the portal vein is then secured to the portion of the inferior vena caval incision.

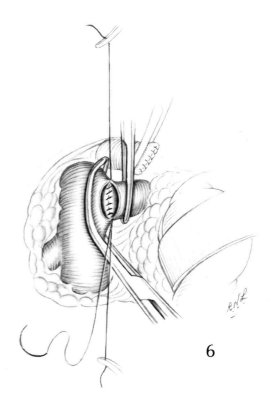

7

This craniad suture is then passed through the posterior wall of the portal vein into its lumen. The next suture passes from the inside out on the portal vein and outside in on the inferior vena cava, to facilitate the placement of a continuous suture along the posterior aspect of the anastomosis. After this suture has run the entire length of the lumen, it is then passed outside again on the portal vein and tied to the inferior stay suture.

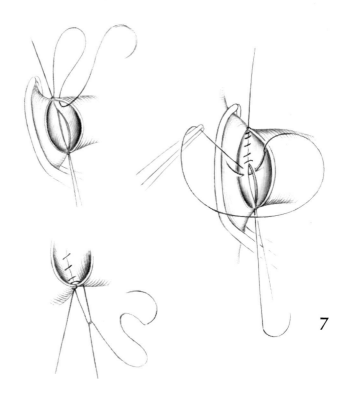

7

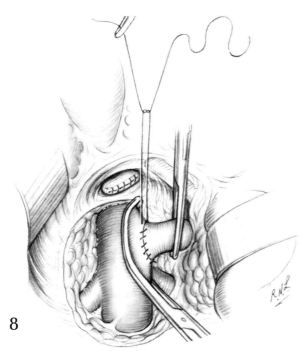

8

8

The anterior row of the anastomosis is then performed with a continuous or interrupted suture and tied eventually to the superior stay suture.

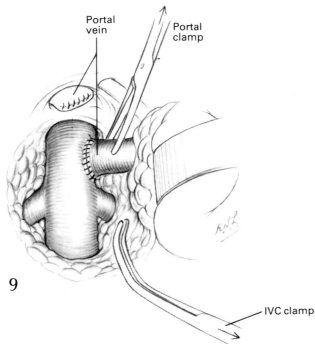

Portal vein

Portal clamp

9

IVC clamp

9

After completion of the anastomosis the clamp is removed from the inferior vena cava first, followed by removal of the clamp from the portal vein. The pressure is recorded directly from the portal vein to define the efficacy of the shunt. There should be less than a 5 cm gradient between the portal vein and inferior vena cava.

10

SIDE-TO-SIDE PORTACAVAL SHUNT

The initial stages of the operative procedure are identical to those described for the end-to-side portacaval shunt. A partially occlusive clamp is applied to the anterior medial aspect of the inferior vena cava, and bulldog clamps or occlusive umbilical tapes are applied to the upper and lower end of the portal vein to occlude this structure. A longitudinal incision of equivalent length to that made in the inferior vena cava, that is, approximately one and a half times the diameter of the portal vein, is then made in the lateral aspect of the portal vein. An elliptical segment may be excised, but this is not necessary. Non-absorbable 5/0 vascular sutures are placed at the upper and lower ends of the stoma. A continuous technique similar to that described in the end-to-side portacaval anastomosis is employed to the posterior row. After this suture is tied, an anterior continuous suture is placed.

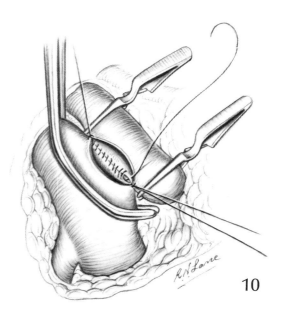

10

'H' GRAFT INTERPOSITION BETWEEN THE PORTAL VEIN AND THE INFERIOR VENA CAVA

After a partially occlusive clamp has been applied to the inferior vena cava as described above, and bulldog clamps are applied to the upper and lower portions of the portal vein, a No. 19 conduit Dacron tube is sutured first to the inferior vena cava as an end-to-side shunt, then to the portal vein as an end of prosthesis to side of portal vein shunt. The conduit should be constructed so that the shortest possible length is utilized. It is possible to use jugular vein rather than prosthesis for this shunt.

CENTRAL SPLENORENAL STUNT[7]

11 & 12

The operation is performed with patient supine or the left side slightly elevated. A left subcostal incision is used transecting the medial portion of the right rectus and extending well around to the left flank. A thoraco-abdominal approach may be employed if there is massive splenomegaly.

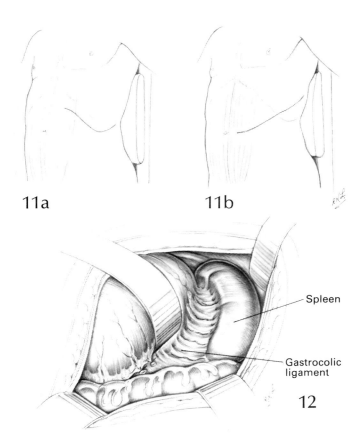

11a　　　　　11b

12

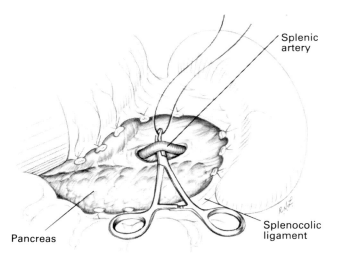

Splenic artery

Splenocolic ligament

Pancreas

13

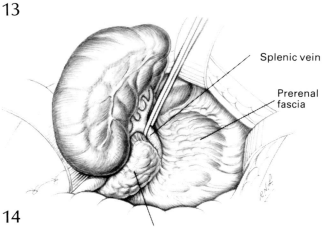

Splenic vein

Prerenal fascia

14

13

The transverse colon and splenic flexure are mobilized and retracted caudad. The short gastric vessels are doubly ligated and transected. Division of the splenophrenic ligament and splenic artery results in the establishment of an ultimate pedicle of splenic vein.

14

This is freed along the course of the pancreas by entering the avascular plane between the posterior surface of the pancreas and the posterior abdominal wall.

15

In order to perform a central splenorenal shunt, the splenic vein is dissected free to its junction with the superior mesenteric vein.

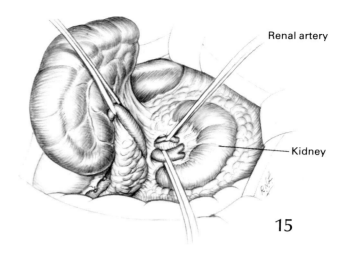

Renal artery

Kidney

15

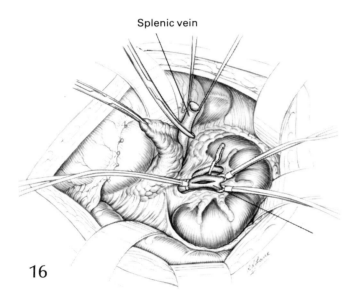

Splenic vein

16

16

A vascular clamp is applied centrally, the splenic vein is transected and the spleen removed. Stay sutures are placed in the stoma of the splenic vein. The peritoneum is incised just medial to the hilus of the kidney, and the left renal artery and vein are dissected free. Umbilical tapes are passed around the main renal vein and the major branches in the hilus of the kidney. It is preferable to occlude the renal vein with the umbilical tapes, but a partially occlusive clamp may be utilized. An incision is made on the anterior–superior aspect of the renal vein, measuring approximately one and a half times the diameter of the splenic vein. The renal artery is occluded temporarily with a bulldog clamp prior to this manoeuvre. The cut end of the splenic vein is brought down to the stoma on the anterior–superior aspect of the renal vein.

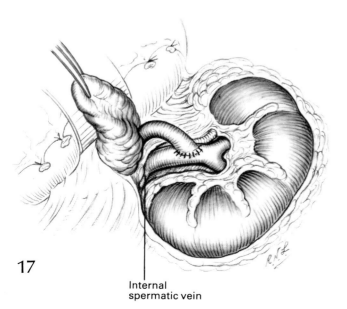

17

Internal
spermatic vein

17

An end-to-side anastomosis is performed by initially securing the two stay sutures and completing the posterior layer in the same fashion as described for the end-to-side portacaval shunt. Anastomosis of the anterior layer is then accomplished with a continuous 5/0 vascular suture. The occluding tapes around the renal vein are released first, and then the central clamp is removed from the splenic vein. Finally the bulldog clamp is removed from the renal artery.

Cavamesenteric shunts

END-TO-SIDE CAVAMESENTERIC SHUNT

18

The peritoneal cavity is entered via a midline or paramedian incision.

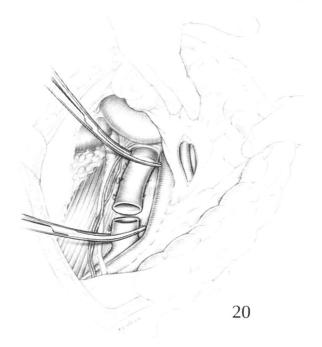

18

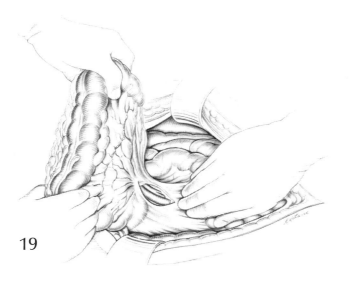

19

19

Upward traction is exerted on the transverse colon in order to expose the superior mesenteric vessels. The peritoneum is incised in the region of the superior mesenteric arterial pulse and the superior mesenteric vein is identified to the right of the artery. The colic vessels are preserved and the right side of the vein is carefully dissected. Tapes are passed around the mesenteric vein.

20

The lateral reflection of the ascending mesocolon is then incised along its entire length to permit medial displacement of the ascending colon, ascending mesocolon and transverse colon. This results in exposure of the inferior vena cava and the third portion of the duodenum. The inferior vena cava is mobilized from its origin at the convergence of the two common iliac veins up to the entrance of the right renal vein. In the course of this dissection, the paired lumbar veins are ligated in continuity and transected. After the infrarenal vena cava has been freed along its entire length, a vascular clamp is applied immediately below the renal veins.

20

21

Generally it is preferable to preserve a segment of the right common iliac vein to achieve added length. Therefore, the left common iliac vein is oversewn, and the right common iliac vein is transected as far distally as possible.

22

In turning the inferior vena cava up, there should be a gentle curve around the caudad portion of the third part of the duodenum. The inferior vena cava is then passed through a window which is created in the small intestinal mesentery between the ileocolic vessels and the origin of the main ileal trunk. This permits approximation of the end of the inferior vena cava to the right posterolateral aspect of the superior mesenteric vein. Anastomosis is usually performed proximal to the right colic vein. A partially occlusive clamp is positioned on the right side of the superior mesenteric vein, and an ellipse is removed from the right posterolateral aspect. This should result in a stoma one and half times longer than the diameter of the inferior vena cava. The anastomosis is performed with vascular silk, using a continuous suture posteriorly, interrupted at either end, and a continuous suture anteriorly. The opening of the peritoneum at the base of the transverse mesocolon is repaired, the ascending colon is repositioned in its natural location, and the lateral reflection of the ascending colon is sutured back in place.

'H' GRAFT MESOCAVAL SHUNT[8]

23

The superior mesenteric vein is isolated as described above for the classic cavamesenteric shunt. The tunnel is established directly through the right transverse meso-colon to permit visualization of the anterior surface of the inferior vena cava. At this point there is complete mobilization of the third and fourth portions of the duodenum, including the ligament of Treitz, in order to permit the duodenum to be moved craniad and prevent possible obstruction of the low-lying duodenum by the graft. The length utilized ranges between 5 and 8 cm and knitted Dacron with a diameter of 19–22 mm is employed. Autologous vein may be used and is associated with a lower thrombosis rate[9]. The caval anastomosis is effected first, utilizing a partially occluding atraumatic vascular clamp placed on the anterior surface of the vena cava. A single row of 4/0 vascular suture is used, interrupted at the craniad and caudad ends.

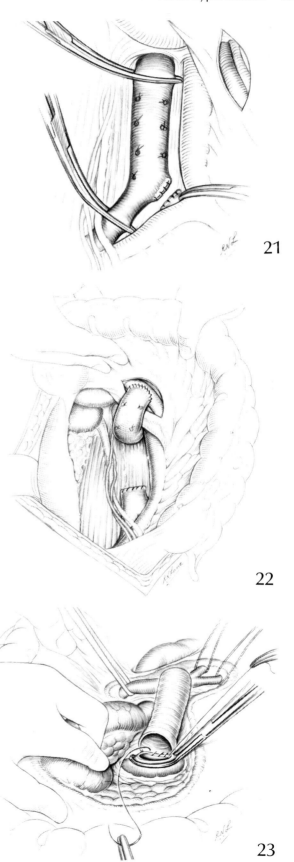

21

22

23

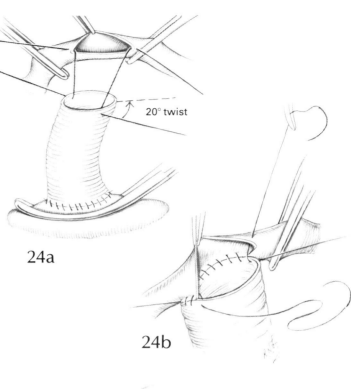

24a

24b

24 & 25

The graft is then trimmed to the adequate length to avoid both tension and excessive length. In view of the normal course of the superior mesenteric vein in relation to the inferior vena cava, it is considered advisable to rotate the graft clockwise approximately 20° prior to initiation of the anastomosis of the superior mesenteric vein. A venotomy approximately one and a half times the diameter of the superior mesenteric vein is made after proximal and distal occlusion. A single-layer anastomosis is then effected between the prosthetic conduit and the superior mesenteric vein.

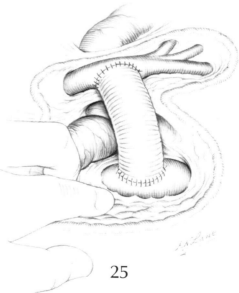

25

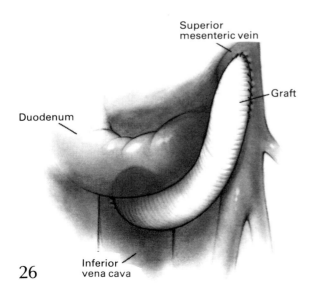

Superior mesenteric vein

Graft

Duodenum

Inferior vena cava

26

26

A longer C graft may be used to permit a gentle curve around the third portion of the duodenum and an anastomosis to the superior mesenteric vein where it crosses the duodenum[10].

Procedures directed at preserving portal flow

ARTERIALIZATION OF THE PORTAL VEIN[11]

Following the establishment of the end-to-side portacaval shunt, arterialization of the stump of the portal vein can be achieved by using the splenic artery or the gastro-duodenal artery turned up as a graft into the portal vein stump. Another approach to achieving arterial flow is direct interposition of a small conduit (8 mm) between the aorta and the portal vein stump.

SELECTIVE SPLENORENAL SHUNT[12]

27

The selective splenorenal shunt, when combined with partial gastric devascularization and ligation of the coronary vein, provides an important physiological advantage because oesophagogastric varices are decompressed, while splanchnic venous flow through the superior mesenteric vein is unaltered. In addition, there is a persistence of splenic venous hypertension. It is felt that the combination of maintenance of adhepatic flow through the portal vein and the splanchnic venous hypertension reduces the incidence of hepatic encephalopathy.

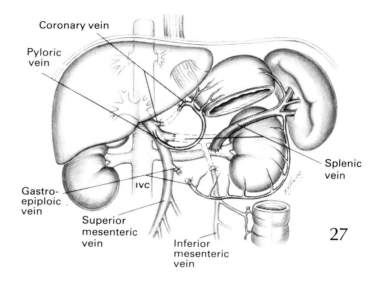

27

28

The operation is performed through a left subcostal incision which then curves under the right costal margin and transects the right rectus muscle. The lesser sac is entered by dividing the gastrocolic ligament from the lowest short gastric vein to the pylorus. The lower border of the pancreas is mobilized along its entire length. The splenic vein is dissected, removing the adventitial tissue, beginning dissection with the posterior surface.

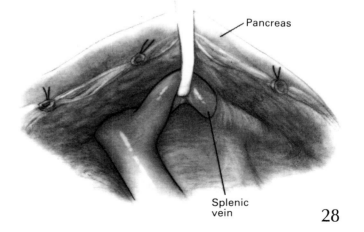

28

29

Dissection is carried out from the junction with the mesenteric vein in a lateral direction towards the hilum. The inferior mesenteric vein is doubly ligated and transected.

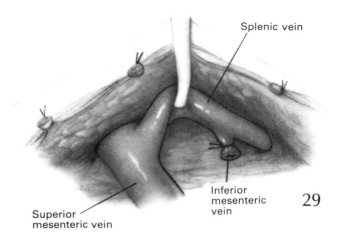

30

After clamps are applied the splenic vein is divided close to its junction with the superior mesenteric vein. Branches to the pancreas are ligated in continuity and divided.

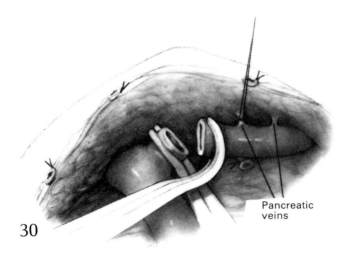

31

The left renal vein is then dissected free from surrounding tissue and a partially occlusive clamp applied to its anterior surface. An incision measuring approximately one and a half times the width of the splenic vein is made.

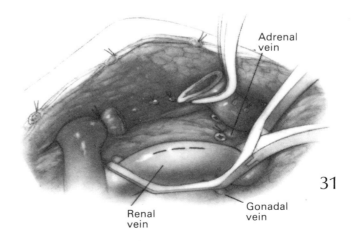

32

An anastomosis is carried out between the splenic vein and the renal vein, using fine sutures posteriorly in a continuous fashion, and interrupted anteriorly.

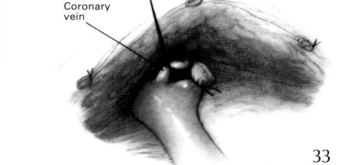

32

33

The pancreas is retracted craniad and the coronary vein is doubly ligated and transected where it enters the portal vein. As an alternative, the coronary vein can be exposed along the lesser curvature of the stomach and ligated along with small vessels near the gastro-oesophageal junction.

Coronary vein

33

References

1. Schwartz, S. I. Surgical diseases of the liver. New York: McGraw-Hill, 1964

2. Whipple, A. O. The problem of portal hypertension in relation to the hepatosplenopathies. Annals of Surgery 1945; 122: 449–475

3. Blakemore, A. H., Lord, J. W. The technique of using vitallium tubes in establishing portacaval shunts for portal hypertension. Annals of Surgery 1945; 122: 476–489

4. Grauer, S. E., Schwartz, S. I. Extrahepatic portal hypertension: a retrospective analysis. Annals of Surgery 1979; 189: 566–574

5. Orloff, M. J., Johansen, K. H. Treatment of Budd-Chiari syndrome by side-to-side portacaval shunt: experimental and clinical results. Annals of Surgery 1978; 188: 494–512

6. Malt, R. B., Malt, R. A. Tests and management affecting survival after portacaval and splenorenal shunts. Surgery, Gynecology and Obstetrics 1979; 149: 220–224

7. Linton, R. R., Ellis, D. S., Geary, J. E. Critical comparative analysis of early and late results of splenorenal and direct portacaval shunts performed on 169 patients with portal cirrhosis. Annals of Surgery 1961; 154: 446–459

8. Drapanas, T. Interposition mesocaval shunt for treatment of portal hypertension. Annals of Surgery 1972; 176: 435–448

9. Thompson, B. W., Casali, R. E., Read, R. C., Campbell, G. S. Results of Interposition 'H' grafts for portal hypertension. Annals of Surgery 1978; 187: 515–522

10. Cameron, J. L., Zuidema, G. D., Smith, G. W., Harrington, D. P., Maddrey, W. C. Mesocaval shunts for the control of bleeding esophageal varices. Surgery 1979; 85: 257–262

11. Adamsons, R. J., Kinkhabwala, M., Moskowitz, H., Himmelfarb, E., Minkowitz, S., Lerner, B. Portacaval shunt with arterialization of the hepatic portion of the portal vein. Surgery, Gynecology and Obstetrics 1972; 135: 529–535

12. Warren, W. D., Millikan, W. J. Selective transplenic decompression procedure: changes in technique after 300 cases. Contemporary Surgery 1981; 18 (3): 11–32

Lymphography

John H. N. Wolfe MS, FRCS
Consultant Surgeon, St Mary's Hospital, London, UK

Introduction

Clinical lymphography was introduced by Kinmonth in 1952. It may elucidate the cause of leg oedema but its major role in vascular surgery is in differentiating between the various types of primary lymphoedema. When clinical assessment is combined with lymphography an accurate prognosis may be obtained in many patients[2] and once the exact anatomical lymphatic abnormality is defined, appropriate operations may be carried out.

Other uses of lymphography include the identification of the specific leak causing a chylothorax of chylous ascites. Lymphadenograms, taken 24 hours after lymphography show the lymph nodes and can thus display anatomical or pathological abnormalities.

Preparation

Before investigation the girth of the limb should be reduced by bed rest with the foot of the bed elevated. Intermittent compression with a pneumatic boot is also of considerable assistance[3]. Cellulitis and areas of infection in the foot should be treated prior to lymphography.

Special equipment and materials

Lipiodol (Ultra Fluid Lipiodol; UFL) is now the contrast agent most widely used; it gives good anatomical detail of lymphatic vessels and nodes. However, being oil-based, it is not cleared rapidly and the quest continues for better contrast solutions. Direct injection into lymphatics can be difficult and it is to be hoped that good anatomical detail will eventually be achieved by subcutaneous injection. Encouraging results using this route have been achieved in animals, using various water-soluble media, but attempts to use them in patients have been disappointing. Radioactive isotopes have been used but their clearance lacks specificity and no detail can be expected with the present compounds and techniques.

Lipiodol lymphography therefore remains the method of choice for obtaining accurate data on the anatomy of the lymphatic system.

Short skin hooks are useful as skin edge retractors and microvascular scissors for the dissection; a dissecting microscope is imperative for difficult cannulations. A fine needle (30 s.w.g.) on polyvinyl tubing attached to a constant infusion pump with variable speed settings is used for the infusion. Castro Viejo needle-holders (with the ratchet removed) can be used to hold the needle, and fine Hoskins forceps to hold the perilymphatic tissues.

Technique

1

Anaesthesia and positioning

Cannulation of a normal lymphatic, as in the investigation of lymphoma, is relatively simple and can be performed using local anaesthesia. However, in the lymphoedematous limb, the search may be protracted and uncomfortable. For this reason and because any movement of the patient can dislodge the cannula, lymphography for lymphoedema should be performed under a light general anaesthetic.

It is essential to anchor the foot sufficiently to eliminate movement. A length of ribbon gauze ties the great toes together and is then fixed to the table. This also produces good plantar flexion which helps cannulation of the lymphatics.

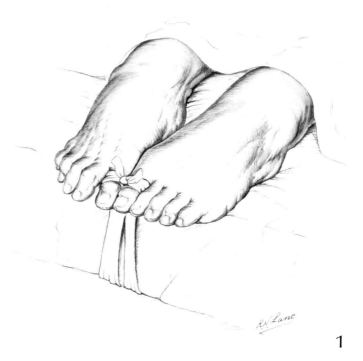

1

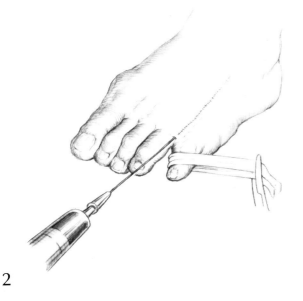

2

2

Demonstration of lymphatics

Approximately 0.2 ml of 11 per cent Patent Blue dye is injected just beneath the dermis in the web between each toe and also lateral to the fifth toe. Both legs are always investigated. Thus a total of 2 ml of Patent Blue Violet is used. When removing the needle, slight suction avoids spillage of the dye over the skin. A swab is used to massage the injection site and care should be taken not to wipe dye onto the dorsum of the foot.

This highly diffusible dye will, in normal circumstances, be carried rapidly to lymphatic collecting vessels. Normal lymphatics become visible as green-blue lines converging on the dorsum of the foot between the first and third metatarsal heads.

3

Dermal back flow

If the collecting vessels are inadequate or obliterated the dye may diffuse through the dermal plexus of lymphatics and produce a blue marbled appearance in the skin described as dermal back flow. It has been suggested that further lymphography is unnecessary if dermal back flow is present, but this is not a reliable test. Furthermore, identification of pelvic obstruction or hyperplastic lymphatics is of assistance in managing the patient.

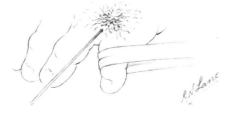

3

4

Dissection of lymphatics

A transverse incision is made over a stained lymphatic. In a lymphoedematous limb, when no lymph vessels can be seen, a transverse incision is made on the dorsum of the foot in order to dissect the lymphatics lying between the first and third metatarsal heads. These lymphatics eventually pass up the medial side of the leg alongside the great saphenous vein. Lymphatics travelling with the small saphenous vein are found immediately behind the lateral malleolus.

The incision is taken just through the dermis, and beneath this the lymphatic collecting vessels are sought. In the lymphoedematous foot bleeding may impair vision but diathermy should be used very sparingly and accurately; bleeding usually stops with pressure.

A small vein can easily be mistaken for a lymphatic. However, the vein appears thicker walled and a darker grey-blue.

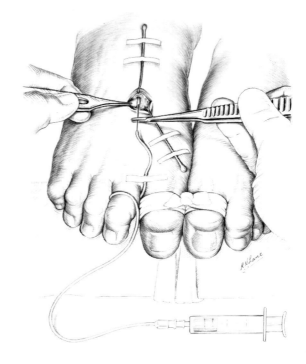

4

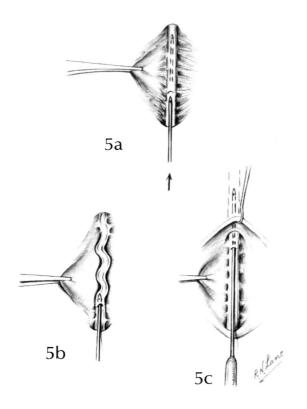

5a

5b

5c

5a, b & c

Cannulation of the lymphatic

(a) Once the lymphatic has been located it is teased out of the tissues and should be handled as little as possible. Only two-thirds of the circumference of the vessel wall should be dissected free since an isolated diseased lymphatic tears easily and the mobility hinders cannulation (b). The lymphatic may also go into spasm. This spasm may be relieved by a little 4 per cent procaine in the wound. If only a short length is isolated the cannulating needle disappears beyond the operator's vision and may transfix the vessel (c). The cannula should not be tied into the lymphatic. This is unnecessary and may damage the vessel. Occasionally there is considerable leakage of Lipiodol through the puncture site, a single throw using silk may reduce this.

Injection

When the needle is primed with contrast medium a small amount of air should be left in the attached polyvinyl tubing so that an air bubble can be seen passing up the lymphatic when the pump is switched on. Slight extravasation of air into the wall may allow manipulation and subsequent successful injection but extravasation of Lipiodol ends any further attempts to cannulate that particular lymphatic. An injection pump is necessary and should be set at a rate of 12 ml/hour; otherwise, the diseased, narrow lymphatic will rupture or there may be extravasation of dye as it passes up the lymphatic. As Lipiodol forms fat emboli in the lungs no more than 7 ml should be injected into each leg, that is 14 ml for a single investigation.

6a & b

Inguinal node lymphography

Obliterated lymphatics in the foot may be associated with normal pelvic lymphatics and a good prognosis; or with abnormal and obliterated pelvic lymphatics and a consequent poor prognosis. For this reason, direct injection of inguinal lymph nodes may be valuable where foot lymphography has failed.

A small (2 cm) incision is made over an inguinal lymph node which should be exposed with a minimum of dissection. Once its superficial surface is exposed it can be stabbed with the cannulating needle and lymphography performed. Prior injection of Patent Blue dye into the thigh may allow a lymphatic entering the node to be seen and cannulated, thus producing a better lymphogram.

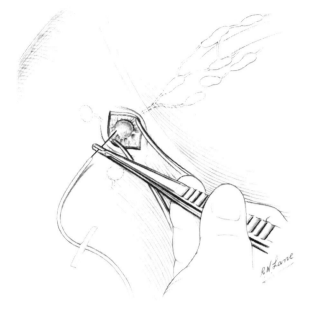

6a

Lymphography

Following injection either into the foot or into the inguinal lymph nodes, a radiograph should be taken within a few minutes to ensure that the lymphatics are filled with Lipiodol. If there is any evidence of globules of contrast media (*caviare sign*) the injection should be stopped immediately since this is diagnostic of an intravenous infusion. Further lymphangiograms (films of the lymphatic collecting vessels) should be taken as required. When the infusion is complete, massage and movement of the leg improves visualization of the thoracic duct which is best shown by a right oblique chest X-ray. Lymphadenograms should be taken 24 hours later.

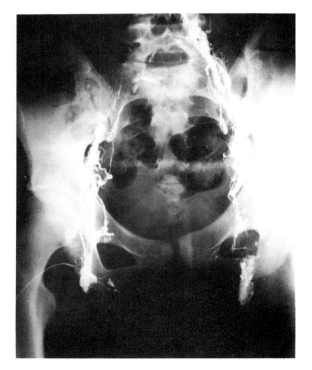

6b

Complications

Anaphylactic reactions to Patent Blue Violet and Lipiodol are rare. However, patients have developed pulmonary oil embolism leading to a pyrexia and diffuse pulmonary infiltration on the chest X-ray. Providing that no more than 14 ml of Lipiodol are used this does not occur. If Lipiodol is seen intravenously then the investigation should be terminated immediately. Lipiodol should not be infused following lung irradiation since cerebral oil embolism may occur in these circumstances.

LYMPHOGRAPHIC ABNORMALITIES

7

Primary lymphoedema – distal obliteration

Hypoplastic lymphatics confined to below the groin are illustrated in the right leg and are also demonstrated by the lymphogram (a). Normal lymphatic anatomy is outlined in the left leg (b). Distal hypoplasia is usually seen in females with bilateral distal oedema. This is the most common form of the disease and is usually mild and non-progressive, responding well to conservative treatment.

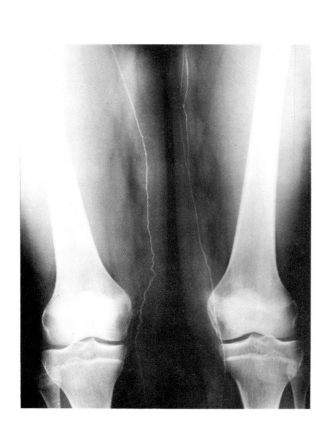

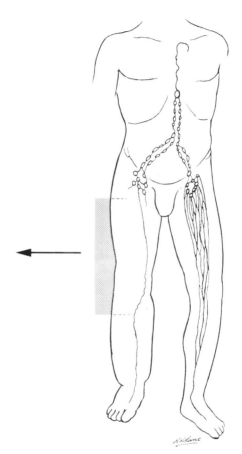

7

8

Pelvic obstruction

This is often found where there is whole leg unilateral oedema; males and females are equally affected. In these patients the lymphographic abnormality is in the pelvis and is associated with adequate distal lymphatics and a normal thoracic duct. If the patient is treated early in the process a small bowel mesenteric pedicle graft may be successful[4]. However there is now evidence that delay may make this impossible because of secondary obliteration of distal lymphatics[5]. Some patients have both *proximal and distal hypoplasia* and a normal thoracic duct.

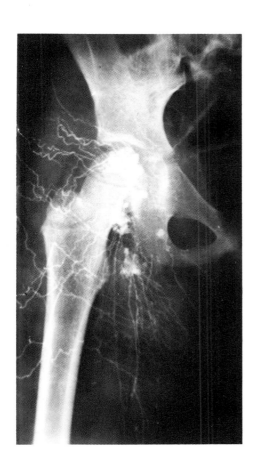

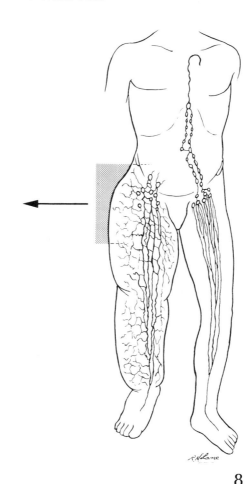

8

9

Megalymphatics

Occasionally varicose lymphatics may be seen. This abnormality allows reflux of chyle or lymph and may produce vesicles on the limbs or genitalia. It may also produce chylothorax, chylous ascites, or chyluria. This type of lymphoedema may be treated by ligation of the lymphatics which have been identified by lymphography[6].

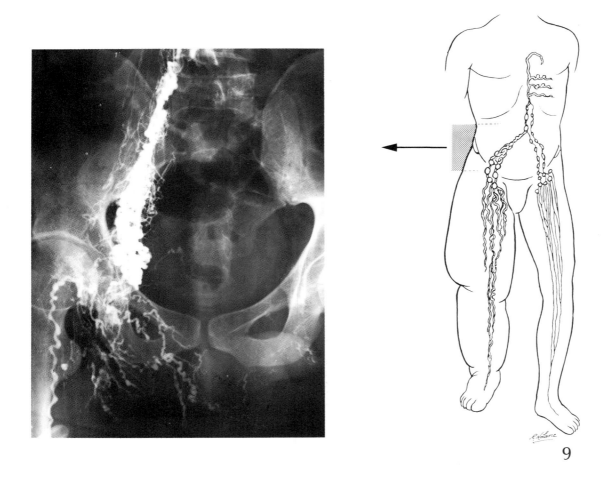

9

10

Bilateral hyperplasia of lymph vessels

Bilateral hyperplasia of lymph vessels is the other form of primary lymphographic abnormality that may be identified. In these patients the abnormality appears to be in the thoracic duct with secondary distension, tortuosity and collateral formation in the vessels distal to this. A lymphonodal venous or lymphaticovenous shunt may be helpful in these patients[7,8].

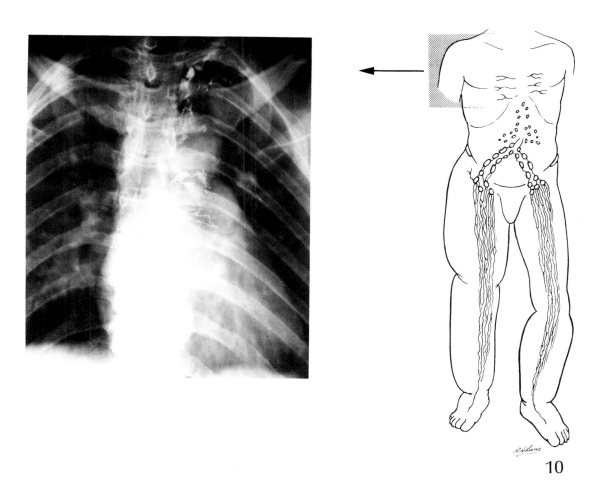

10

References

1. Kinmonth, J. B. Lymphangiography in man. A method of outlining lymphatic trunks at operation. Clinical Science 1952; 11: 13–20

2. Wolfe, J. H., Kinmonth, J. B. The prognosis of primary lymphedema of the lower limbs. Archives of Surgery 1981; 116: 1157–1160

3. Zelikovski, A., Manoach, M., Giler, S., Urca, I. Lympha-press, a new pneumatic device for the treatment of lymphedema of the limbs. Lymphology 1980; 13: 68–73

4. Kinmonth, J. B., Hurst, P. A., Edwards, J. M., Rutt, D. L. Relief of lymph obstruction by use of a bridge of mesentery and ileum. British Journal of Surgery 1978; 65: 829–833

5. Fyfe, N. C., Wolfe, J. H., Kinmonth, J. B. 'Die back' in primary lymphoedema – lymphographic and clinical correlations. Lymphology 1982; 15: 66–69

6. Kinmonth, J. B. The lymphatics: surgery, lymphography and diseases of the chyle and lymph system. 2nd ed. London: Edward Arnold 1982: 227

7. Nielubowicz, J., Olszewski, W., Muszynski, M., Sawicki, Z. Late results of lymphovenous anastomosis. Journal of Cardiovascular Surgery 1973; Special No. 113–120

8. O'Brien, B. McC., Shafiroff, B. B. Microlymphaticovenous and resectional surgery in obstructive lymphoedema. World Journal of Surgery 1979; 3: 3–15

Illustrations by Jorge Perez-Vela

Direct operations on the lymphatics

J. Leonel Villavicencio MD, FACS
Professor of Surgery, F. Edward Hébert School of Medicine,
Uniformed Services University of the Health Sciences, Bethesda, Maryland;
Director, Vein and Lymphatic Clinic, Walter Reed Army Medical Center, Washington, DC, USA

Introduction

The medical literature is rich in references to the multiple medical and surgical procedures which have been used with varied results in the management of the challenging diseases of the lymphatic system.

The lymphatic system is the 'poor relative' of the well-to-do family of the circulatory system. The last decades have witnessed unparalleled progress in the management of diseases of the arterial and venous systems, and there have been remarkable achievements in surgery of the heart. Despite all of these glittering successes in the field of cardiovascular surgery, patients suffering from diseases involving the lymphatic system still constitute a formidable challenge for the medical profession.

Progress in the understanding and management of lymphoedema of the upper and lower extremities has been slow. A great step forward in the knowledge of the pathology and aetiology of the lymphatic diseases was the introduction of lymphangiography into the clinical arena by Kinmonth[1,2] in the early fifties. From the visualization of the lymphatics in different clinical groups arose a classification of lymphoedemas that has furthered understanding of the pathophysiology of the disease and helped to establish guidelines for prognosis and treatment of the different types of lymphoedema encountered in clinical practice.

Classification of lymphoedema

Using clinical, lymphangiographic and histopathological studies, Kinmonth[3] classified lymphoedemas into primary and secondary. Cordeiro[4], in Brazil, who has worked extensively in the field of lymphatic disorders, based his classification on a large clinical experience with 453 cases of lymphoedema.

It is important to stress the value of the classification of lymphoedemas because of its surgical implications. In both classifications the following are considered to be *primary lymphoedemas*.

1. Milroy or familial lymphoedema.
2. Gonadal Dysgenesis-Turner Syndrome, which is associated with webbing of the neck, short stature, cubitus valgus and genital anomalies.
3. Lymphoedema praecox.
4. Lymphoedema tarda (Cordeiro uses the term to describe all those cases which appear after puberty. Kinmonth uses it to describe all cases appearing after 35 and uses lymphoedema praecox for those appearing before that age).

In all primary lymphoedemas one or more of the following lymphographic anomalies is present: megalymphatics or hyperplastic trunks with valveless, refluxing vessels; hypoplasia or aplasia, where there is an absence or a reduction in the number of lymphatic trunks and/or lymph nodes.

Secondary lymphoedemas include the following:

1. Those due to tuberculosis, filariasis, infections and neoplasia.
2. Post-traumatic: surgery with destruction of lymphatic channels and/or lymph nodes, fractures, burns, blunt trauma, animal bites, radiation, etc.
3. Post-chylous reflux, chyloedema.

The illustrations that follow show the most common clinical disorders of the lymphatic system based on lymphangiographic and histopathological studies.

ANATOMY AND PATHOLOGY OF THE LYMPHATIC SYSTEM

1

Normal lymphatic vascular system

Eight to eleven lymphatic channels are present in the lower extremity along the course of the saphena magna. The number of lymphatic trunks increases as they become more proximal. The number and size of the inguinal lymph nodes are important as in some cases they may be the site of chronic inflammation and obstruction of the lymph flow. Along the course of the short saphenous vein, there is an important lymphatic pathway which drains into the popliteal nodes of the deep system.

In the upper extremity, lymphatic channels course along the main veins and have a small number of epitrochlear nodes interposed.

Lymphatics have valves which are of great importance in the dynamics of the lymphatic circulation. The lymphatics of upper and lower extremities have a dermal valveless network which drains into the deeper valved channels.

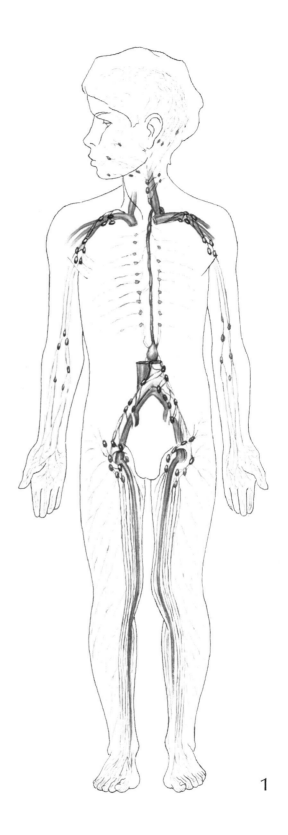

1

2

Hypoplasia of the lymphatic system

The number of lymphatic collectors is reduced to two or three. The lymph nodes may also be reduced in number and size. In the lower leg, usually on the external aspect, there is dermal back-flow when patent blue dye is injected to visualize the lymphatic system.

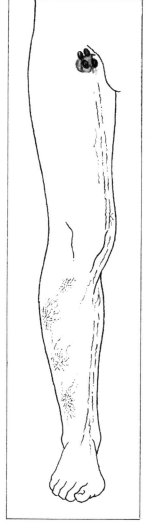

2

3

Aplasia of lymphatic channels and lymph nodes

Patent blue dye is seen in the dermal plexus of the lower leg as a sign of reflux into the skin caused by abnormal development of the lymphatic system. Reflux is also observed in cases of secondary lymphoedema with obstruction to the lymph flow at the groin or pelvis.

In a high percentage of cases of primary lymphoedema, lymphangiography and lymphochromy reveal a defect in the anatomy of lymph nodes and collectors.

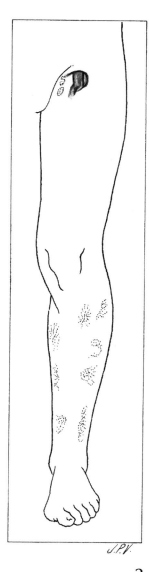

3

ANATOMY AND PATHOLOGY OF ABDOMINAL AND THORACIC LYMPHATICS

4

Normal lymphatic system of thoracic and abdominal cavities

A normal number of collecting ducts and a normal number and size of lymph nodes (no more than 20 mm in size) can be seen. A number of trunks originating from the femoral and iliac nodes drain lymph from the extremities and pelvis and course along the major abdominal vessels. The cisterna magna or cisterna of Pecquet collects lymph from abdominal and lumbar lymphatics and serves as a station for the transportation of intestinal lymph towards the thoracic cavity where the thoracic duct will drain the lymph flow (about 4–5 litres of lymph in 24 hours in a 70 kg man) coming from the lower half of the body and the lymph flow originating from the intrathoracic organs.

It is important to notice that there is also a right thoracic duct draining into the right subclavian vein. The main thoracic duct drains into the left subclavian vein.

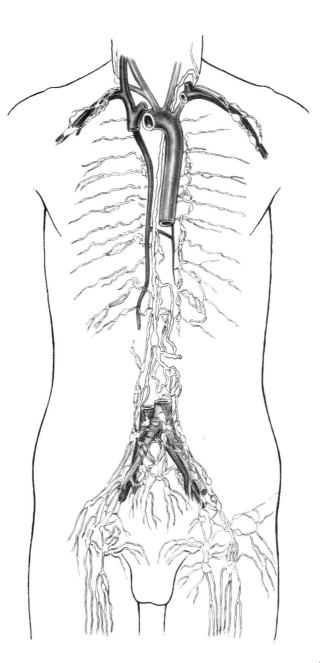

4

5

Normal intestinal lymphatics and mesenteric nodes

The blind-ended villous intestinal lymphatics will transport fatty acids, cholesterol and other fatty products which are responsible for the characteristic milky aspect of the intestinal chyle that was observed and described by Aselli of Pavia in 1627 in dogs who had recently eaten[5,6].

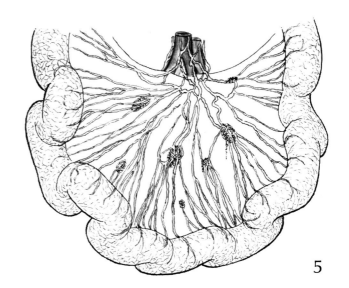

5

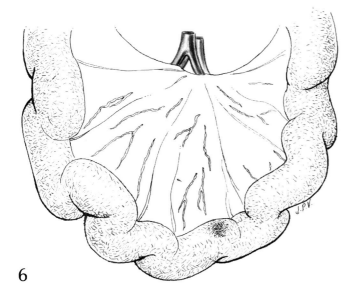

6

6

Hypoplasia of intestinal lymphatics and mesenteric nodes

Hypoplasia is found in some cases of chylous ascites. In these cases, chyle exudes from the intestinal wall and cannot be collected adequately. In other cases, a chylous fistula causes intraperitoneal collection of lymph. Refluxed lymph can leak through the inguinal spaces and produce chyloedema of thigh and lower leg as we have observed in one of our young patients.

SURGICAL PROCEDURES FOR LYMPHOEDEMA

The surgical procedures designed to treat the lymphatic disorders can be classified into two main categories: excisional procedures; and procedures designed to drain the lymphatic fluid towards non-affected areas.

This chapter describes a technique from the second group – the direct lymphovenous shunt. This reproduces most closely the normal physiological drainage of lymph into the venous system. In this operation, the lymphatic trunks distal to a site of obstruction are inserted into the neighbouring veins, thus bypassing the area of damaged lymphatic tissue. We have used this technique both in the upper and lower extremities during the last 6 years in Mexico City and more recently in the United States.

One of the largest experiences with direct lymphovenous anastomosis has been reported by Cordeiro[4] and Degni[8] from Brazil. In Mexico, Tijerina and Sanchez-Fabela (cited by Cordeiro[7]) have also accumulated considerable experience.

Cordeiro and Baccarat[7] reported their experience with 293 patients operated upon for lymphoedema since 1967. There were 191 procedures for lymphoedema of the lower extremities and 102 involving the upper extremities.

Preoperative

Selection of patients for direct operations on the lymphatics

Most of the patients suffering from lymphoedema of the extremities can be reasonably controlled with non-operative measures. Only 12 per cent of our patients have been considered to be candidates for direct lymphovenous shunts.

Indications

The following are considered most suitable for direct lymphatic surgery.

1. Patients with secondary lymphoedema.
2. Patients who have not responded to comprehensive and well controlled conservative treatment.
3. Patients without fibroedema. This means patients without chronically and irreversibly indurated tissues. Patients with fibroedema benefit by excisional surgery.
4. Non-obese patients.
5. Some patients with lymphoedema tarda in whom we suspect anomalies of the lymph nodes either alone or in combination with a possible diminution in the number or size of the lymph collectors. We have been able to operate successfully in some of these cases. It is important in these patients (usually females) to try to elicit a history of pelvic, urinary or genital infections which trigger the appearance of distal oedema (usually unilateral). It is possible that the lymphadenitis secondary to chronic or repeated infections in those areas, together with a congenitally insufficient lymphatic collector system, is the aetiological factor responsible for the appearance of lymphoedema after puberty.

Contraindications

1. The operation is not indicated in cases of chronic edema in which the lymphatic system is not primarily involved (cardiac, renal, etc.)
2. Patients with primary lymphoedema are not good candidates for this type of surgery.

Preoperative preparation

Lymphangiography and ascending phlebography are necessary studies in every patient considered for lymphovenous shunts. These studies should be performed 2–3 months before surgery to avoid operating on vessels which might have been recently irritated or inflamed by the contrast medium. As this operation is always performed electively, there should be sufficient time to study the case and carefully plan the procedure with the best possible knowledge of the lymphangiographic anatomy and phlebographic visualization of the venous trunks most suitable for the shunt. In some patients with secondary lymphoedema it is not possible to obtain visualization of the lymphatic system. We have operated on this type of patient and have always found satisfactory lymphatic trunks in cases of both lower and upper extremity lymphoedemas. Therefore, even though lymphangiography is extremely useful and should always be attempted, an operation can still be carried out with certain technical considerations (see below) when lymphangiography is unsuccessful.

If the patient is overweight, every effort should be made to have the weight reduced to a level as close as possible to the ideal weight for the patient's age and height. Obese patients tend to retain more fluid and to drain lymph with more difficulties than normal individuals.

Intensive preoperative efforts should be made to reduce induration and oedema as much as possible. To accomplish this the following care is recommended.

Patients should sleep with the foot of bed elevated 20–25 cm (Trendelenburg position).

Wash the extremity daily with soap and water and lubricate the skin thoroughly with lanolin or any other good skin softener.

Massage gently from foot to thigh or from hand to shoulder for 30 minutes twice a day, working specially over the areas which show more induration (usually the posterior aspect of the limbs).

Take immediate care of any skin lesions or fungus infections. Use prophylactic antibiotics (penicillin or cephalosporins) whenever an infectious process is discovered. We have seen acute episodes of lymphangitis occurring in the course of an ear, tooth or paranasal sinus infection.

Reduce salt intake and use diuretics judiciously. Diuretics are not used routinely and should only be employed when the accumulation of fluid in the extremity seems to be larger than usual.

Use external pneumatic compression and elastic external support. There are several good mechanical devices available commercially. They have sleeves for the upper extremity or boots of different sizes for the lower extremity. The magnitude of the pressure applied and the duration of the compression cycle can be varied and adjusted individually. They should be used daily, for periods of 1–2 hours, preferably before the patient goes to bed.

There are automatic pumps which deliver intermittent sequential pneumatic compression, literally milking the oedema fluid from foot to groin or from hand to shoulder. The daily use of these compression devices should be followed by the application of a firm elastic, rubberized bandage which must be worn from morning to evening. The elastic bandage should be wrapped from toes to groin or from wrist to shoulder (with special compression gloves for the hand). A period of rest of about one hour with the legs elevated without bandages is recommended 4–5 hours after its morning application.

We have been able to obtain better control of the oedema and greater reduction of the limb's size using a well applied, firm elastic bandage, carefully wrapped and held in place by a non-elastic regular nylon stocking or pantyhose, than with the use of the commercially available elastic stockings. Therefore, in the preparation of the lymphoedematous limb for an operation, we always substitute the elastic stocking for the rubberized bandage. The patient should be assured that the added trouble of applying the bandage and keeping it in place is well worth the effort!

Immediate preoperative measures

The patient should be admitted into the hospital 5–6 days before surgery. Careful daily measurements of the extremity should be recorded. It is important to mark the sites where the measurements are made. The circumference of the limb at midfoot, ankle, midcalf and lower and midthigh are recorded. For the upper extremity, the measurements are made at midhand, wrist, proximal third of forearm and midarm.

Bedrest is mandatory with the bed placed in the Trendelenburg position although bathroom privileges are granted. In cases of upper extremity lymphoedema, the arm should be elevated over pillows or suspended from a special frame placed over the bed. The straps holding the extremity should be carefully padded.

Daily massage, washing of the extremity and one hour of intermittent pneumatic compression twice a day should be continued until the day before the operation.

Prophylactic antibiotics are initiated the night before surgery.

With this regimen, the patient usually reaches a plateau where the maximum reduction of oedema and limb circumference is obtained. Any further reduction of oedema and limb measurements in the postoperative period can then be attributed to the surgical procedure.

One hour before surgery, 1–2 ml of 11 per cent patent blue dye is injected intradermally into the first interdigital space of hand or foot. Gentle massage and active movements of joints and muscles are recommended. The dye injection helps the surgeon to identify the lymphatic channels in the inguinal region or at midarm; these will be seen as bluish conduits.

Instruments

Visual magnification (×3.5–4.5) is essential. Good illumination with a headlight is very useful.

The instruments that we have found necessary for this operation are: self-retaining retractor (Whitlander), Miller-Semb three-prong tissue retractors, both sharp and blunt, Adson tissue forceps, fine DeBakey tissue forceps, fine blunt-tip dissecting scissors, curved mosquito forceps, Castroviejo needle holders and 7/0 or 8/0 double-armed monofilament sutures.

Special grooved needles or grooved Teflon catheters of different gauges are essential. They are described in the section on surgical technique (see *Illustration 10*).

Anaesthesia

Procedures involving the lower extremities can be performed under good epidural or spinal anaesthesia supplemented by the necessary sedation. If the patient is apprehensive, light general anaesthesia is preferable.

In operations for lymphoedema of the upper extremity, light general anaesthesia is always preferable.

The operation

The patient· is placed in a supine position with the operating table in the Trendelenburg position (15°). This position is not necessary in procedures involving the upper extremity.

7

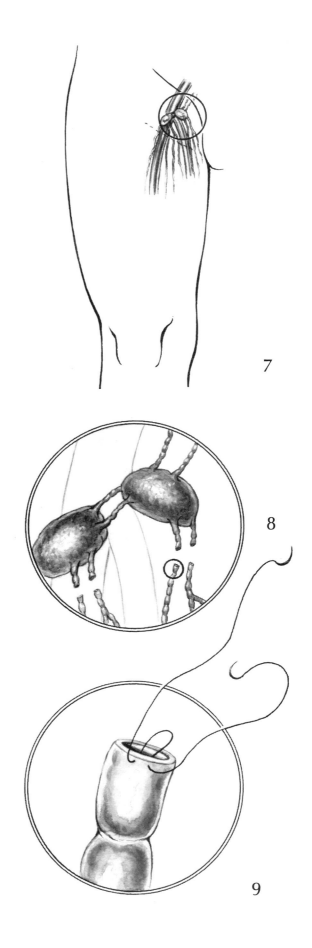

Skin incision and identification of lymphatics

A 5 m skin incision is performed about 3 cm below the saphenofemoral junction and parallel to the inguinal ligament. It is important that the incision be made only through skin. With visual magnification and good illumination, blunt careful dissection is carried out parallel to the saphenous vein. The subcutaneous tissue (where most of the lymphatics are located) is gradually separated and teased away using blunt fine scissors or, preferably, fine curved mosquito forceps. The incision is *gradually* and *carefully* deepened as the longitudinal dissection-separation of the subcutaneous tissue progresses. In cases where attempts to perform a lymphangiogram were unsuccessful, it is wise to locate the lymph nodes and try to identify the afferent lymphatic trunks arriving at them. Usually, lymphatics appear as pearly, bluish, thin structures. They should be carefully handled and dissected free for 4–5 cm. In secondary lymphoedema, 8–11 lymphatic trunks can be identified, some larger than others. The larger trunks are isolated and identified by passing a 5/0 silk around them.

8

Selection of lymphatics and vein dissection

The selected lymphatics (which should be as many as possible: 4–8) are now ready for their insertion into the vein. The saphenous vein should be dissected carefully for about 5–7 cm and vessel loops passed proximally and distally to achieve atraumatic control of the vein. If the saphenous vein is not available, the femoral vein should be dissected. A good branch of the femoral vein can also be utilized. The lymphatic trunk is divided and the proximal end is tied with 4/0 or 5/0 Dexon.

9

Preparing the distal end of the lymphatic trunk

The distal end of the lymphatic trunk is then held very gently with fine tissue forceps (Adson) and a 7/0 to 9/0 double-armed monofilament suture is passed from outside through the adventitia or through the upper lip of the lymphatic vessel. Sometimes, especially in very small lymphatics, we have found that it is easier to pass the two needles through the adventitia, *before* dividing the lymphatic. If we do this, the division of the trunk is made flush to the site where the sutures exit from the lymphatic wall.

10

Preparation and insertion of the special grooved needle

Once the lymphatic has been prepared with a double-armed suture, a place is selected on the vein for insertion of the special grooved needle which will facilitate the introduction of the lymphatic trunk into the vein.

The needle, which is illustrated here, has a groove 12 mm long and 2 mm wide placed 0.5 cm from the tip. Cordeiro and Degni have their own custom-made stainless steel needles of different lengths and diameters. We have made our own grooved catheters following Sanchez-Fabela's modification of Cordeiro's needles[4].

To prepare the grooved catheter we utilize intravenous Teflon catheters 16, 18 and 20 gauge, depending on the vein size. With the metal guide or stiletto inside the catheter, a 12 mm lateral segment of the catheter is excised with a No. 11 surgical blade, beginning 0.5 cm from the tip. The result is a grooved flexible catheter which is ready for insertion.

The catheter is inserted with the aid of the sharp stiletto into a site on the vein wall close to the selected lymphatic trunk to avoid tension in the anastomosis. The groove should be halfway into the vein and halfway outside the vein wall. Bleeding can be easily controlled with traction on the vessel loops.

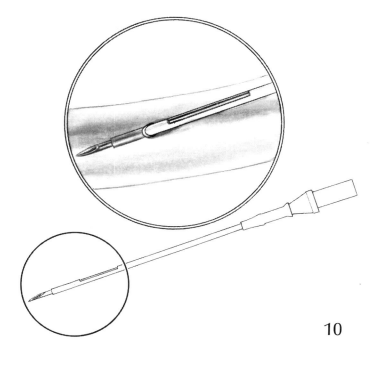

10

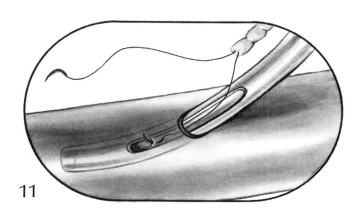

11

11

Passing the first needle through the lymphatic and vein

With the grooved catheter inside the vein, the lymphatic trunk that has been previously prepared with a double-armed suture is approximated to the vein wall. One of the two needles is passed from inside to outside the venous wall using the groove as a stent and guide to facilitate the introduction of the needle through the orifice made by the insertion of the Teflon catheter. The needle should exit from the venous wall about 4 mm from the entrance site as shown in the illustration.

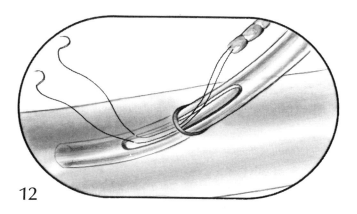

12

12

Passing the second needle into the vein and approximation of the lymphatic to the vein

With the assistant controlling the vein to avoid bleeding from the punctured venous wall, the second needle is passed from inside to outside in a manner similar to that shown in *Illustration 11*. The needle should exit about 1 mm lateral to the previous suture. The lymphatic trunk is then brought closer to the vein as the two ends of the suture are gently pulled.

13

Insertion of lymphatic trunk into the vein

In this illustration, the lymphatic trunk has been inserted into the vein by: (1) gently pulling the two ends of the suture; and (2) sliding the lymphatic trunk into the groove of the catheter through the orifice in the vein wall. Once the lymphatic is within the vein lumen, the two needles are cut and the suture tied loosely to avoid constriction of the lymphatic lumen.

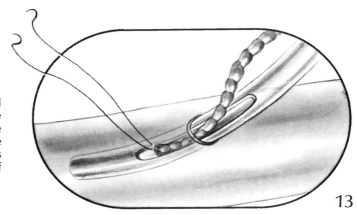

14

Removal of grooved catheter

The lymphatic trunk is seen within the venous lumen, being held against the vein wall by the loosely tied suture. Just before securing the knots, the Teflon catheter should be removed by twisting it 180° to avoid damage to the inserted lymphatic.

The lymphatic channel will fit nicely in the orifice of the vein, since the muscular venous wall tends to close the site of puncture. Any bleeding can be easily controlled with finger pressure. It is not advisable to apply pressure with sponges, since this may disrupt the lymphovenous shunt.

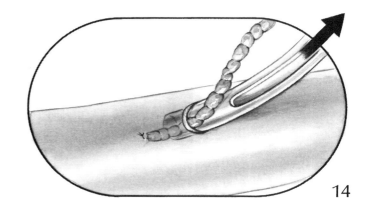

15

Insertion of multiple lymphatic trunks; operation completed

Four lymphatic trunks have been inserted into the venous lumen following the technique described above. Two of the lymphatics shown are double channels. This has the advantage of providing drainage of two lymphatic trunks through *one single* lymphatic insertion. When performing multiple anastomosis the surgeon must be extremely careful not to disrupt the already completed insertions. Good planning in the placement of the lymphovenous shunts along an adequate segment of vein is very important to prevent twisting, tension and overcrowding of lymphatics in a small area, which may result in damage to the vein with the consequent risk of thrombosis.

The wound is closed in layers. Fine sutures should be used to approximate the subcutaneous tissue and avoid tension in the lymphovenous shunts. No drainage is necessary.

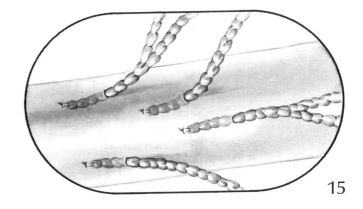

True lymphovenous anastomosis

An alternative to lymphatic insertion is the construction of a true lymphovenous anastomosis. A 5 mm incision is made longitudinally in the lymphatic wall after cannulating the lymphatic with a small grooved needle. A similar incision is made in the vein. A complete anastomosis is then performed with single interrupted sutures of 10/0 monofilament material. This type of lymphovenous anastomosis is time-consuming and more difficult to perform than the technique of lymphatic insertion. We have always used the latter and believe that the results obtained by others[4,7], with the use of the true anastomosis, do not justify the added time and technical difficulties.

OPERATION FOR LYMPHOEDEMA OF THE UPPER EXTREMITY

In cases of secondary lymphoedema of the upper extremity (following mastectomy, radiation or trauma), the same basic principles described for the lower extremity are utilized. The operation is performed as follows.

The skin incision is made along the medial edge of the biceps and approximately in the middle third of the arm.

The subcutaneous tissue is carefully separated with a curved mosquito forceps. We use the Miller-Semb retractors with sharp prongs. The lymphatic channels of the medial group are identified by their blue colour since they collect the patent blue dye injected one hour before.

A 5 cm segment of lymphatics should be dissected free in as many trunks as possible. The lymphatic vessels are not as friable as one might suspect given their small size.

The fascia that covers the medial edge of the biceps muscle is incised and the brachial vein identified and dissected.

Once the lymphatic channels and the vein have been dissected and vessel loops passed around both ends of the vein, the same steps described for the lymphovenous shunts of the lower extremity are performed. If the vein is considered to be too small, instead of using grooved needles or Teflon catheters to facilitate insertion of the lymphatics into the vein, we prefer to perform a small incision in the vein (2–3 mm) and insert the lymphatic directly with fine Adson tissue forceps at the same time that traction is exerted on the lymphatic with the two monofilament sutures previously placed in the edge of the distal end of the lymphatic trunk. The two edges of the small phlebotomy can be kept open by placing a 5/0 stay suture at each side of the incision. As many lymphatics as possible should be inserted into the vein. The operation is completed in the same manner as described for the lower extremity.

Postoperative care

Absolute bedrest is essential for 3–4 days. The Trendelenburg position must be continued for as long as necessary. Active mobilization of joints and muscles is encouraged to facilitate the venous drainage. The use of intermittent pneumatic compression of the lower leg or forearm is recommended for 30–45 minutes 3–4 times a day. On the fourth day the patient is allowed to get out of bed and walk to stimulate the dynamics of the lymphatic circulation.

We recommend the use of elastic bandages in the leg (from foot to knee) when the patient becomes ambulatory. They should be removed whenever the patient is in bed. Sitting for periods of more than 15 minutes should be prohibited during the first 2 weeks of the postoperative period.

Results

The results obtained with this technique in the 293 patients operated on by Cordeiro and Baccarat vary from a partial reduction of the oedema to an almost complete resolution of the problem[7].

The improvement after surgery is gradual and reaches its maximum benefit 6–9 months after operation. We have had patients, however, who have lost 15 cm of circumference during the first month after surgery. The patient should be aware that the improvement will be gradual and that no miraculous cure is to be expected.

In our own experience, we have had marked improvement in 75 per cent of the patients followed from 1 to 6 years. Marked improvement is defined as: mean reduction of the leg or arm circumference of at least 15 per cent from the original measurements; improvement in the patient's ability to move the extremities; greater freedom of movement of the joint areas; less heaviness and overall patient satisfaction with the results. Of the remaining 25 per cent, 16 per cent had less than 15 per cent mean reduction in circumference but reported less heaviness and greater freedom of movements especially around the joint areas. Nine per cent of patients did not benefit from the operation (5 per cent had lymphoedema of the upper and 4 per cent of the lower extremities). Our results revealed that 24 per cent of patients had recurrences at from 1 to 6 years.

There has been both radiological (lymphography) and isotopic evidence that there is passage of lymph through the lymphovenous anastomosis[4] and postoperative lymphography has revealed a clear improvement of the lymphatic circulation

At the present time, there is evidence that a considerable number of patients can benefit by this type of procedure and there is minimal morbidity and mortality. No patient in our experience has been made worse by the operation.

References

1. Kinmonth, J. B. Lymphangiography in man: a method of outlining lymphatic trunks at operation. Clinical Science 1952; 11:13–20

2. Kinmonth, J. B., Taylor, G. W., Harper, R. K. Lymphangiography. A technique for its clinical use in the lower limb. British Medical Journal 1955; 1:940–942

3. Kinmonth, J. B. Lymphatics: diseases, lymphography and surgery. London: Edward Arnold, 1972

4. Cordeiro, J. A., Sanchez-Fabela C. Sindrome de linfedema y fibredema. In: Diaz, B. F., Paramo, D. M., eds. Los grandes sindromes vasculares. Mexico: Institute Mexicano del Seguro Social, 1984: 595

5. Hewson, W. Experimental inquiries: Part the second. Containing a description of the lymphatic system in the human subject and other animals. London: J. Johnson, 1774

6. Foster, M. Harvey and the circulation of the blood: the lacteals and lymphatics. Lectures on the history of physiology. Cambridge: Cambridge University Press, 1901: 25–53

7. Cordeiro, K. A., Bacarat, F. F. Linfologia. Edit. Fundo Editor. BYK-PROCIENX. Sao Paolo, Brazil, 1984

8. Degni, M. New technique of drainage of the subcutaneous tissue of the limbs with nylon net for the treatment of lymphedema. VASA 1974; 3: 329–341

Illustrations by Anita Matthews

Operative management of lymphoedema

Elethea H. Caldwell MD
Associate Professor of Plastic Surgery, University of Rochester
School of Medicine and Dentistry, Rochester, New York, USA

Introduction

Lymphoedema, the excessive accumulation of pro-teinaceous extracellular fluid, may appear in numerous pathological states. Two general types are recognized: congenital and acquired lymphoedema. Unfortunately little is known about the basic aetiology and pathophysiology of either type. Congenital lymphoedema is represented by various states of hypoplasia, dilatation or aplasia of lymphatic vessels with dermal backflow of lymph. Acquired lymphoedema is an obstructive phenomenon secondary to mechanical blockage by parasites, tumour, scarring following infection, surgery or radiation.

Congenital and acquired lymphoedema may involve the upper or lower extremities. They are different clinical entities, yet they are managed in a similar fashion. The types most frequently subjected to (and most amenable to) surgery are idiopathic lymphoedema of the leg and postoperative lymphoedema of the arm.

The arm lesion is an obstructive one due to damage to the lymphatic trunks, either by the operation for clearance of axillary lymph nodes or by subsequent irradiation. Venous obstruction may complicate the condition, in which case the oedema will appear within a few hours of surgery. Pure lymphatic obstruction may take a long time to become evident. Swelling begins in the arm and spreads distally to involve the hand. Function is limited by the weight, bulk and tension on the tissue. The aesthetic impact may be appreciable. Recurrent cellulitis and lymphangitis following the most minor trauma is common, and this in turn leads to further fibrosis and lymphatic obstruction.

Lymphoedema of the lower extremity is usually congenital, with typical onset at the age of puberty. It may be unilateral and is more common in the female. Similar to what occurs in the upper extremity, the disability consists of impaired function, aesthetic deformity and recurrent cellulitis usually secondary to β-haemolytic streptococcus causing increased fibrosis and further disability. When the process is uncontrolled the skin becomes hyperkeratotic, with a loss of skin appendages, thinning of the epidermis and increase in dermal collagen.

Gratifying response and long-term control may be attained in early cases, before skin changes occur, by continuous external compression, scrupulous hygiene and prompt, adequate antibiotic treatment for even the most minor infection. This approach should be tried initially in all early and moderate cases. Surgical intervention should be considered when conservative means fail to control the progression of oedema, when recurrent bouts of cellulitis occur, when advanced vegetative dermatitis appears, and when the bulk of the limb undermines function.

It must be realized that lymphoedema cannot be cured by surgical means. The large number of procedures proposed stands as a testimony to the fact that normal lymphatic function is not restored by any procedure and that surgical intervention is aimed at symptomatic control of the lymphoedema.

Two general types of surgical approaches have been suggested in the past: either an attempt to reconstruct or substitute an adequate lymphatic system, or excision of the diseased lymphatics and their host tissue and fascia.

Five procedures are currently employed: omental transposition[1]; buried dermal flap[2]; microsurgical lymphatic anastomosis[3]; staged skin and subcutaneous excision beneath flaps[4]; and the Charles procedure[5]. Physiologically designed procedures attempt to improve intrinsic lymphatic drainage. Handley[6] used silk threads buried in the subcutaneous tissue to improve lymphatic drainage in postmastectomy oedema of the arm. Kondoléon attempted to establish communication between the diseased lymphatics and the deep muscle compartment. This concept was based on the observation that the deep muscle compartment was not involved in the oedematous process.

Thompson[2] extended Kondoléon's plan and incorporated principles of Sistrunk's[7] flap operation to produce the buried dermis flap procedure. This involves denuding a posteriorly based skin flap of its epithelium, a generous excision of diseased subcutaneous tissue, and insertion of the resulting dermis flap through the incised fascia into the muscle compartment. The bulk of the leg is reduced by the excision and the egress of lymph is felt to be improved as evidenced by improved clearance of tagged albumin. However, a significant amount of current clinical and laboratory information indicates that new lymphatic drainage is not provided and improvement is heavily dependent upon the amount of subcutaneous tissue excised[8].

Advances in microsurgical techniques hold substantial promise for the future, particularly in the management of acquired lymphoedema[3].

Excisional techniques have provided the most consistent success in the treatment of lymphoedema of the extremities. These procedures represent the antithesis of attempts to improve intrinsic lymphatic drainage. The most extensive procedure of this type was introduced by Charles in 1912[9]. He advocated excision of the diseased skin and subcutaneous tissue down to fascia with resurfacing by split-thickness skin grafts.

Grafts may be obtained from excised skin if it is of good quality. It has been learned that the use of split-thickness skin grafts often leads to weeping of lymph through the grafts and subsequent development of vegetative dermatitis. This condition may be more deforming than the original lymphoedema. It has been emphasized that full thickness or very thick split-thickness grafts should be used. The thicker grafts provide superior and more durable coverage. This procedure is very effective in reducing the bulk of the limb and is the procedure of choice in advanced cases[10].

A more moderate form of excisional therapy is the staged subcutaneous excision of diseased tissue under intact skin flaps[11]. The majority of the subcutaneous tissue can be removed by staged excision beneath skin flaps without producing the postoperative deformity of the Charles procedure.

Preoperative preparation

Preoperative preparation includes 3–4 days of preliminary hospitalization for optimum control of oedema by strict bedrest and elevation. Reduction in size is substantial. Antibiotic coverage should be established during this period. Selection of the drug is based on control of the flora of any open wound, plus β-haemolytic streptococcus which is frequently present in the lymphatic lakes and blind channels. Skin hygiene is attended to by frequent washes with Betadine soap. Although a tourniquet is used during the procedure, blood must be available for transfusion.

Anaesthesia

General anaesthesia is most appropriate because of the length of the procedure and probable extent of blood loss.

The operations

STAGED SUBCUTANEOUS EXCISION BENEATH INTACT SKIN FLAPS

1

The incision

Excision is performed in stages at 3-month intervals through curvilinear incisions on the volar and dorsal aspects of the arm. Skin flaps are approximately 1.5 cm thick.

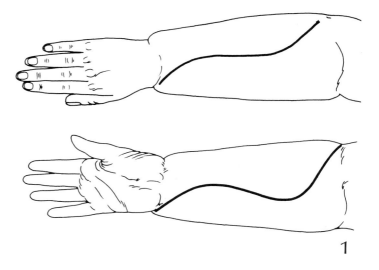

1

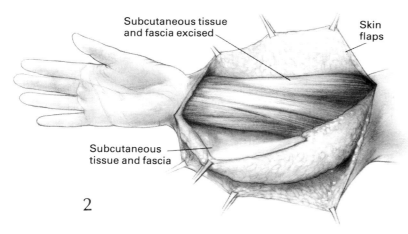

Subcutaneous tissue and fascia excised

Skin flaps

Subcutaneous tissue and fascia

2

2

Excision of subcutaneous tissue

All underlying fibroadipose tissue is removed, including the muscle fascia. Excess skin is excised to allow accurate approximation.

3

Closure

Closure is carried out using interrupted 5/0 Vicryl in the subcutaneous tissue and the skin is closed with a continuous 3/0 Dermalene suture. Two drainage catheters are inserted and connected to constant suction.

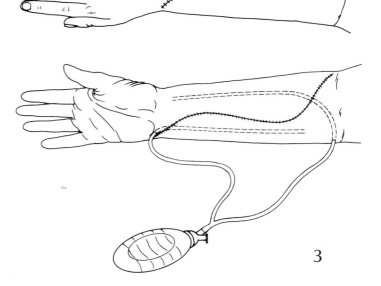

3

EXCISION AND SKIN GRAFT (CHARLES PROCEDURE)

4

The incision

The limb may be suspended by a calcaneal pin. Incisions are made as noted to remove the skin in one piece.

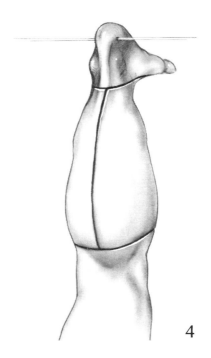

4

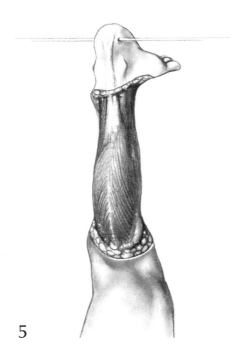

5

5

Removal of subcutaneous tissue

All subcutaneous tissue and fascia are removed. Margins of the subcutaneous tissue are tapered. Some subcutaneous tissue is left over the Achilles tendon and over the fibular head.

6

Replacement of skin

If disease changes in the skin are not marked, the skin is returned as a free graft. The specimen is pinned to a board or glued to a firm surface such as a dermatome drum. The tissue is thinned to 15–18 μm. If local skin has significant change, split skin grafts are obtained from a distant source.

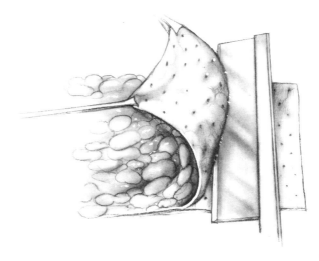

6

7

Closure

The skin graft is returned in one piece using a posterior or medial suture line. If haemostasis is not satisfactory, the wound may be dressed snugly and the skin stored in a moist saline sponge at 4°C for application in 2–3 days.

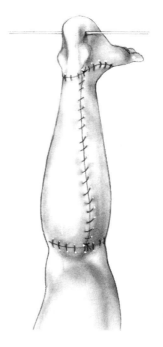

7

Postoperative care

The extremity is immobilized in a large, bulky dressing. Drainage catheters are connected to constant suction. Bedrest with elevation of the extremity is necessary for a period of 10–14 days. Intravenous antibiotics are continued for 72 hours postoperatively. After 2 weeks the extremity is measured for an elastic stocking. An Ace bandage may be used for support during ambulation until the stocking is available.

Results

The extent of improvement following any procedure for the treatment of lymphoedema of the extremities is directly related to the magnitude of excision of subcutaneous tissue. The Charles procedure provides the most radical excision of subcutaneous tissue and fascia, but the severe cutaneous defect produced at times is more disfiguring than the original lymphoedema. Staged subcutaneous excision beneath intact skin flaps provides a significant improvement in the lymphoedematous extremity without the deformity and possible development of vegetative dermatitis which is associated with free skin graft techniques.

References

1. Goldsmith, H. D., De Los Santos, R., Beattie, E. J. Relief of chronic lymphedema by omental transposition. Annals of Surgery 1967; 166: 573–585

2. Thompson, N. The surgical treatment of chronic lymphoedema of the extremities. Surgical Clinics of North America 1967; 47: 445–503

3. O'Brien, B. M., Sykes, P., Threlfall, G. N., Browning, F. S. C. Microlymphaticovenous anastomoses for obstructive lymphedema. Plastic and Reconstructive Surgery 1977; 60: 197–211

4. Miller, T. A. Surgical management of lymphedema of the extremity. Plastic and Reconstructive Surgery 1975; 56: 933–941

5. Dellon, A. L., Hoopes, J. E. The Charles procedure for primary lymphedema. Long-term clinical results. Plastic and Reconstructive Surgery 1977; 60: 589–595

6. Handley, W. S. A prospective cure for elephantiasis. Lancet 1909; 1: 31–33

7. Sistrunk, W. E. Further experiences with the Kondoléon operation for elephantiasis. Journal of the American Medical Association 1918; 71: 800–806

8. Danese, C. A., Papaioannou, A. N., Morales, L. E., Mitsuda, S. Surgical approaches to lymphatic blocks. Surgery 1968; 64: 821–826

9. Charles, H. Elephantiasis screti In: Latham, A., English, T. C., eds. A System of Treatment, Vol. 3. London: Churchill, 1912: 504–516

10. Miller, T. A. Charles procedure for lymphedema: a warning. American Journal of Surgery 1980; 139: 290–292

11. Miller, T. A., Harper, J., Longmire, W. P., Jr. The management of lymphedema by staged subcutaneous excision. Surgery, Gynecology and Obstetrics 1973; 136: 586–592

Illustrations by J. Akister and Robert N. Lane

Sympathetic ganglion block

Alastair J. Gillies MB, ChB
Professor, Department of Anesthesiology, and Professor of Pharmacology,
University of Rochester School of Medicine and Dentistry, Rochester, New York, USA

Introduction

The sympathetic ganglia may be temporarily blocked by the injection of a local anaesthetic agent. The injection may be made at a number of sites, of which the most usual are the stellate (inferior cervical) ganglion, the upper thoracic ganglia, the splanchnic nerves and adjacent ganglia, and the lumbar ganglia. Semipermanent interruption of the lumbar ganglia may be obtained with the injection of phenol. Complications have followed the injection of alcohol and phenol at other sites and their use is not recommended, except in the lumbar chain.

Preoperative

Indications

These are similar to those listed for the appropriate sympathectomy. Sympathetic block is done to estimate the benefit which is likely to result from a surgical sympathectomy and to differentiate the varieties of vasospastic diseases. In addition, sympathetic ganglion block is useful in the treatment of post-traumatic dystrophies and acute arterial dysfunction, secondary to emboli, thromboses and crush injuries. Relief of pain, due to carcinoma of the pancreas, acute pancreatitis and various causalgias may be obtained from appropriate sympathetic block. Phenol block has also been employed as an alternative to lumbar sympathectomy[1] in poor-risk patients.

Premedication

None is required, yet the occasional apprehensive patient may benefit from intramuscular diazepam 10 mg as a sedative 1 hour before block.

Apparatus

Thin lumbar puncture needles or long 22 gauge needles, preferably graduated in centimetres, are satisfactory for the main injection.

The operations

STELLATE OR INFERIOR CERVICAL GANGLION BLOCK

Position of patient

The route may be anterior, lateral or posterior; the anterior is preferred. The patient lies flat on his back with his arms by his sides and the head in line with the trunk. The neck and head are extended.

1

Lateral approach

The midpoint of the clavicle is marked and the skin and deeper structures above and medial to this point anaesthetized with 0.5 per cent lignocaine. A lumbar puncture needle or a 22 gauge needle at least 8 cm long is then introduced at an angle of 45° to the sagittal plane towards the body of the 7th cervical vertebra and advanced until the point strikes this bone.

A syringe is applied and aspirated to ensure that the needle is not in either the subarachnoid space or a blood vessel; 10 ml of 0.5 per cent lignocaine are injected. It is unwise to attempt the injection of this ganglion with alcohol or phenol. A successful injection produces a temporary Horner's syndrome as well as the desired diagnostic or therapeutic response.

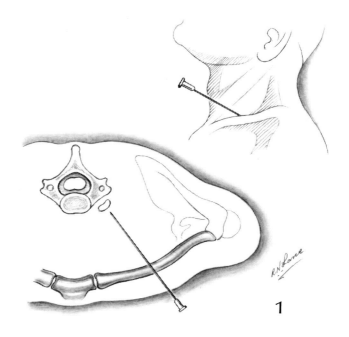

1

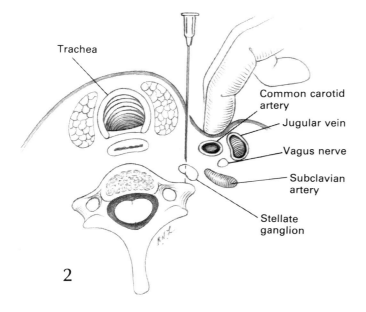

Trachea

Common carotid artery

Jugular vein

Vagus nerve

Subclavian artery

Stellate ganglion

2

2

Anterior approach

A skin weal is raised approximately 1.5 cm lateral and 1.5 cm superior to the suprasternal notch. A 6 cm needle is directed posteriorly between the trachea and the carotid sheath to the lateral aspect of the vertebral body. The needle is redirected to miss the vertebral body and contact the transverse process. At this point the needle is withdrawn 0.5 cm to place the tip in the correct fascial plane; 10 ml of 0.5 per cent lignocaine are injected. As above, succesful injection produces a temporary Horner's syndrome.

UPPER THORACIC GANGLION BLOCK

Position of patient

The patient is placed on his side, with the head, hips and knees flexed as for a lumbar puncture, the head being supported on a pillow so that the spine is in a straight line.

3

The spines of the upper four thoracic vertebrae are located and the injections made in line with these 4 cm from the midline. After infiltration of the skin and deeper structures with 0.5 per cent lignocaine, 10 cm lumbar puncture needles are introduced at right-angles to the skin until the point strikes the transverse process. Each needle is manipulated until it lies at the lower edge of this bone. It is now angled to about 20° to the saggital plane and advanced until the point strikes the body of the vertebra.

The sympathetic chain lies at an average depth of 3 cm from the transverse process against the side of the vertebral body. If possible the needle should be marked in centimetres so that it can be placed in this position after these two bony points have been located by the needle point. If aspiration produces neither blood, cerebrospinal fluid nor air, then the injection can be made for a diagnostic block; 5 ml of 0.5 per cent lignocaine are injected into each of the upper four thoracic ganglia.

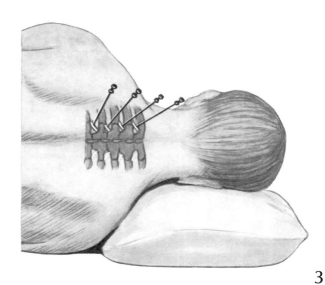

3

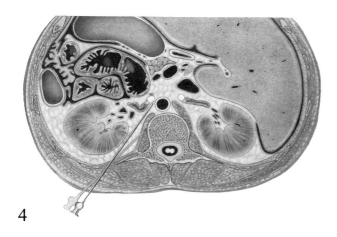

4

LUMBAR GANGLION BLOCK

Position of patient

The patient lies face downwards with a pillow beneath the abdomen to reduce the lumbar lordosis. The patient can be positioned on his side as for a lumbar puncture.

4

The injection is made 3 cm from the midline at the level halfway between the 2nd and 3rd spinous processes. After infiltration of the skin and deeper structures with 0.5 per cent lignocaine, a 10 cm lumbar puncture needle is inserted and advanced until it strikes the transverse process of the appropriate lumbar vertebra. It is then manipulated until it passes just above or below this bone.

The needle is now angled so that the point is directed medially towards the body of the vertebra. As soon as it strikes this bone it is carefully aspirated and, if neither blood nor cerebrospinal fluid is withdrawn, the injection is made – 30 ml of 0.5 per cent lignocaine for a temporary block, 10 ml of 6 per cent phenol in water for a semipermanent denervation. A rise in the skin temperature of the appropriate foot and toes indicates a satisfactory nerve block.

POSTERIOR SPLANCHNIC BLOCK

Position of patient

The patient is placed in a semiprone position with the side to be injected turned upwards.

5

This procedure will induce a block of the coeliac plexus in front of the first lumbar vertebra which in turn will affect the visceral autonomic nerve fibres in the coeliac ganglia. The injection is made four finger breadths from the midline at the level of the first lumbar spine, or four finger breadths from the midline immediately below the 12th rib.

A 12 cm short bevelled needle is inserted at an angle of 70° through the erector spinae to strike the body of the first lumbar vertebra. The needle is withdrawn for 3 cm and redirected forwards – at about 80° – passing the vertebra and into the retroperitoneal space. Aspiration will confirm that the needle is not in a blood vessel or the subarachnoid space. About 40 ml of a 0.5 per cent lignocaine solution are injected, producing anaesthesia on both sides from one injection.

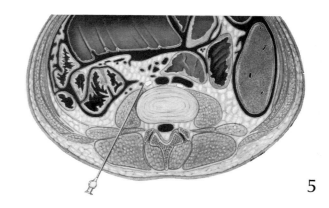

5

Reference

1. Haxton, H. A. Chemical sympathectomy British Medical Journal 1949; 1: 1026–1028

Sympathectomy of the upper extremity

Richard M. Green MD, FACS
Clinical Assistant Professor of Surgery, University of Rochester Medical Center, Rochester, New York, USA

Charles G. Rob MC, MChir, MD, FRCS, FACS
Professor of Surgery, Department of Surgery, Uniformed Services University of the Health Sciences,
F. Edward Hébert School of Medicine, Bethesda, Maryland, USA

Introduction

Sympathetic denervation of the upper extremity and most of the axilla can be achieved by removal of the lower portion of the stellate or inferior cervical ganglion and the second and third thoracic ganglia. This portion of the sympathetic chain may be approached by one of five routes: cervical; transaxillary through the bed of the first rib; transaxillary via the third interspace; anterior thoracic; or posterior. The cervical is the preferred approach and is most commonly used because it causes the patient less inconvenience than any of the others. The transaxillary and axillary via the third interspace may be preferred when the ganglionectomy should be taken below the level of the third thoracic ganglion as in hyperhidrosis. The anterior thoracic approach provides excellent exposure but means a thoracotomy and the posterior approach has been largely abandoned.

Indications

Upper extremity sympathectomy has been recommended for a number of diseases when the disability has been sufficiently severe and non-operative methods have failed. Results have not been uniformly good, often because of poor patient selection, and the operation has a bad reputation amongst some surgeons. It is essential, therefore, that patients are properly selected for sympathectomy. When there is doubt as to the value of the procedure in a particular patient one or more diagnostic stellate ganglion blocks may be performed.

The best long-term results with upper extremity sympathectomy are obtained in patients with true causalgia and other autonomic nerve dystrophies. These must be demonstrated by objective criteria such as digital plethysmography or an element of vasospasm. Patients with hyperhidrosis should also do well although they may develop excessive body sweating after operation. Results in patients with digital artery occlusion from embolus, thrombosis or frostbite and with thrombo-angiitis obliterans depend on the degree of occlusion and the amount of tissue destruction. If vasospasm is a significant

aspect of the problem a satisfactory result can be achieved.

The greatest controversy in terms of operative indications comes in the group of patients with Raynaud's phenomena. Since this is a broad diagnostic grouping of a great many diseases patients must be carefully screened prior to recommending operation and even then patients must be made aware that symptoms are likely to recur. Patients with primary Raynaud's Disease and with symptoms of pure vasospasm should get relief of their symptoms for a prolonged period. The problem lies in defining these patients as many develop collagen vascular diseases later in life and have recurrent symptoms of vasospasm. Many patients with collagen vascular disease develop obliterative digital artery occlusive disease which when severe may not respond to sympathetic ablation. In the latter group sympathectomy may be useful in the short term to heal digital ulcerations that are refractory to non-operative therapy.

Anatomy of the sympathetic chain

The cervical sympathetic outflow is composed of a superior cervical ganglion from the fused C1 through C4 ganglia, a middle cervical ganglion from C5 and C6, and an inferior cervical ganglion from C7 and C8. The inferior cervical ganglion and the first thoracic ganglia fuse to form the stellate ganglion. In man, sympathetic outflow to the upper extremities is usually from spinal segments T2–T9 but in 10 per cent of cases fibres from T1 contribute to arm innervation. There may also be a direct connection between the second and third thoracic ganglia and the brachial plexus, the nerve of Kuntz.

Regeneration

Return of preoperative symptoms has led some to implicate regeneration of ganglion cells as an explanation of disappointing results. We do not believe that this occurs. A more frequent cause of recurrence is an incomplete primary operation or progression of the basic disease.

The operations

CERVICAL APPROACH

The patient is placed in the supine position with the head of the operating table elevated to prevent venous engorgement. The head is rotated to the opposite side and the arms are placed by the side of the body.

1

The incision

The incision is made in a skin crease a fingerbreadth above the clavicle. It begins medially at the anterior border of the sternomastoid muscle and extends laterally about 7.5 cm to the external jugular vein. The incision is then carried down through the platysma muscle with the electrocautery knife.

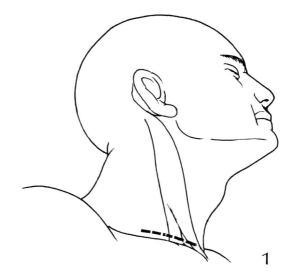

2

Partial division of sternomastoid muscle

The external jugular vein is divided between suture ligatures and the supraclavicular nerves are spared when possible. The sternomastoid muscle is exposed and its lateral border identified. The clavicular head is divided with electrocautery. Care must be taken to avoid injury to the internal jugular vein which lies under the muscle. We use forceps to elevate pieces of the muscle before dividing it.

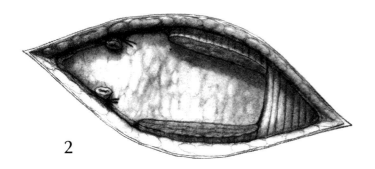

3

Exposure of anterior scalene muscle

The dissection is now carried down through the scalene fat pad. The omohyoid muscle and a number of small vessels are divided. The lateral margin of the internal jugular vein is mobilized and the medial border of the anterior scalene muscle is identified. The phrenic nerve lies deep to the investing fascia of the muscle and should be isolated and retracted medially with the internal jugular vein. During this and other parts of the dissection it is important not to retract laterally as this might inadvertently injure the upper trunks of the brachial plexus.

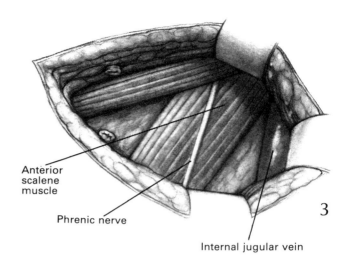

Anterior scalene muscle

Phrenic nerve

Internal jugular vein

3

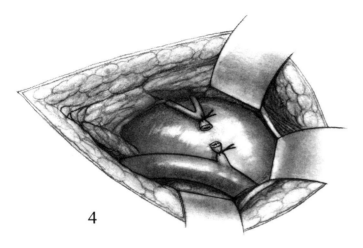

4

4

Exposure of subclavian artery

The muscle is isolated over a distance of 2.5 cm and is then carefully divided, a few fibres at a time. This protects the subclavian artery which may lie directly under the muscle although it usually is somewhat caudad. The medial aspect of the brachial plexus should be identified but not dissected. It is usually found directly beneath the already divided external jugular vein. The subclavian artery can be easily identified and controlled once the anterior scalene muscle is divided. The artery must be moved downwards and it is usually necessary to divided one or two small branches which leave the superior aspect of the artery.

5

Mobilization of pleura

Once the artery is retracted downwards the suprapleural membrane (Sibson's fascia) is encountered. Division of this membrane is the key to the operation and is best done with the operator's finger. The suprapleural membrane is divided on the inner side of the triangle bounded by the brachial plexus, subclavian artery and internal jugular vein by pushing downward against the vertebral column with the finger. When Sibson's fascia is penetrated the operator's finger falls into the retropleural space and the pleura can be stripped from the side of the vertebral column. Small malleable retractors are useful here to keep the pleura and the subclavian artery out of the way. At this point in the operation lighting can best be achieved with a headlight worn by the operator.

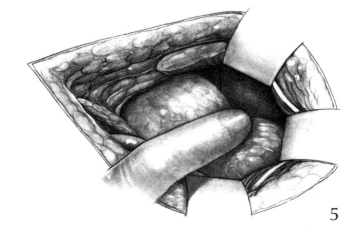

5

6

Identification of sympathetic chain

The sympathetic chain is most easily identified by palpation against the vertebral column at the neck of the first rib. Once the chain has been localized in this manner a dissecting swab can be used to expose the stellate ganglion fully and its identity can be confirmed visually. A nerve hook or a right-angled clamp is passed around the chain and with a swab the remainder of the chain down to the third ganglion is exposed. Several intercostal veins will be seen crossing the trunk; these should be avoided if possible or controlled with small hemoclips if necessary. Bleeding from these veins can be troublesome if appropriate care is not exercised.

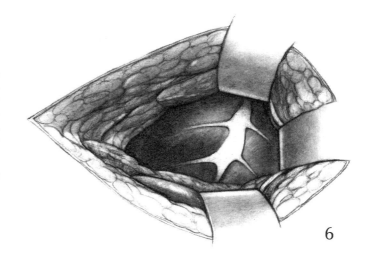

6

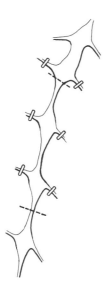

7

7

The sympathectomy

Removal of the stellate ganglion will cause sympathetic denervation of the face and eye, resulting in a permanent Horner's syndrome, and should be avoided. It is necessary to remove only fibres from the T1 segment and to leave the cervical segments intact. Our preference is to divide the ganglion in its lower aspect where the rami communicantes from the first thoracic nerve enter. Once divided the distal end is clamped and traction is applied to facilitate the remainder of the dissection. Hemoclips are used prior to dividing each ramus and the chain is divided below the third ganglion and removed.

Closure

The lung should be inflated prior to closure and if a pneumothorax is present a small catheter should be inserted which can be removed after the incision is completely closed. The divided sternomastoid muscle is repaired, the platysma layer is closed and the skin sealed with skin clips. No drains are employed.

TRANSAXILLARY APPROACH (FIRST RIB RESECTION)

8

The patient is positioned on the operating table by the surgeon prior to scrubbing. A standard thoracotomy position is used with padding between the knees and under the contralateral axilla. Wide adhesive tape placed across the uppermost hip and sandbags placed parallel to the trunk help to secure the patient in the proper position. The ipsilateral arm, chest, back and shoulder are prepared and the arm is placed in a sterile stockinette. We wrap an elastic bandage around the elbow to keep the stockinette in place during retraction of the arm.

The incision

The incision is made just beneath the axillary hairline between the latissimus dorsi and the pectoralis major muscle.

9

Resection of first rib

The incision is carried down to the chest wall and then with finger dissection carried up to the first rib. The intercostobrachial nerve may need division and there is often an arterial branch from the axillary artery which needs division between Hemoclips. The superior surface of the first rib is exposed after division of the anterior scalene muscle. A periosteal elevator is used to strip the intercostal muscles off the inferior surface of the rib and the pleura is gently pushed off the inside of the rib with the operator's finger. The rib is then removed and the ends are smoothed off with rongeurs.

10

Exposure of sympathetic chain

Once the rib is removed the dome of the pleura is exposed and this must be gently dissected away from the lateral mediastinum with the operator's finger. The sympathetic chain is identified by palpation between the T1 nerve root and the subclavian artery. A nerve hook is then passed around it and a sympathectomy can be accomplished in the same manner as described above. As the dissection is carried downwards the pleura can be retracted by a narrow malleable retractor. Lighting can best be achieved with a headlight as the dissection approaches the fourth ganglion.

Closure

The wound is filled with saline, the lung inflated and if there is no pneumothorax, closure can be started. If the pleura has been injured a fenestrated catheter is inserted into the pleural space, brought out through the wound and connected to a water seal. A postoperative chest X-ray is obtained in the recovery room and if the lung is completely inflated the tube is withdrawn. If not, the tube can be connected to suction.

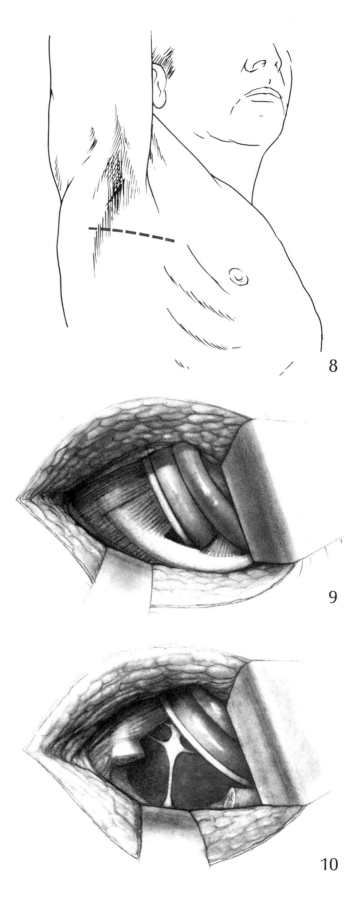

8

9

10

TRANSAXILLARY APPROACH (THIRD INTERSPACE)

This is a transpleural operation and is therefore contraindicated if there is evidence that the patient has many adhesions between the visceral and parietal pleura in the region of the apex of the lung. The patient is positioned as for a first rib resection but the arm need not be in the operative field.

The incision

The incision is made in the axilla and follows the line of the third rib. It passes downwards and forwards across the thoracic wall of the axilla from the posterior to the anterior axillary fold and is usually about 15 cm long. In women the incision should stop at least 2.5 cm before the anterior axillary fold is reached because a major reason for using this approach is the production of a less obvious scar.

11

Exposure of third rib

After the attachment of skin towels the incision is carried down to the periosteum of the third rib. The pectoral muscles and breast are retracted well forwards and the latissimus dorsi, teres major and subscapularis muscles backwards. The long thoracic nerve is identified and placed under the posterior retractor. The lateral thoracic artery usually appears in the posterior portion of the wound and requires division. The third rib is exposed by incising the overlying fibrofatty tissue of the axilla and removing the serratus anterior from its attachment to this bone. The periosteum on the rib is incised with a diathermy knife throughout the full length of the wound and then separated from the upper surface of the rib and from the back of the rib on its upper part. In large patients the incision can be purely intercostal; for others it is necessary to remove a variable length of the third rib to produce sufficient exposure.

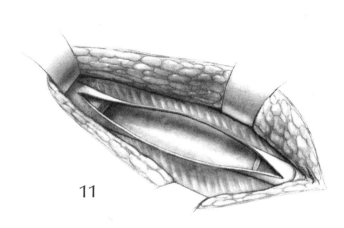

12

Exposure of sympathetic chain

The pleura is opened through the periosteum in the upper part of the bed of the third rib. This avoids damage to the intercostal vessels and nerve and this zone is relatively avascular. A rib spreader is now inserted and the thorax opened to a width of about 10 cm. This usually provides sufficient exposure but if it does not the rib above may be divided subperiosteally and about 2.5 cm resected. A large gauze pack is placed in the chest and the lung retracted downwards. This exposes the dome of the pleura and the upper part of the mediastinal pleura covering the bodies of the upper five thoracic vertebrae and the posterior portions of the corresponding ribs. The sympathetic chain can easily be seen beneath the pleura as it lies on the heads and necks of these ribs.

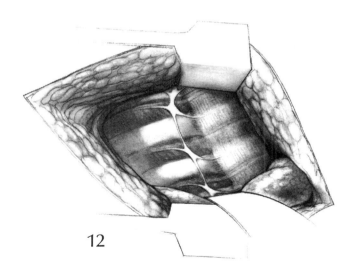

13

Mobilization of sympathetic chain

The parietal pleura is opened with scissors as it lies over the sympathetic chain and swept back for a short distance on each side with a gauze swab on a longer holder. The chain is then lifted up with a nerve hook below the fourth or fifth thoracic ganglion and divided. Traction is now applied to the chain and the rami communicantes divided. The chain is then divided above the second ganglion and removed. It is not possible to remove the whole of the stellate ganglion with safety through this axillary incision, but the inferior portion can often be excised.

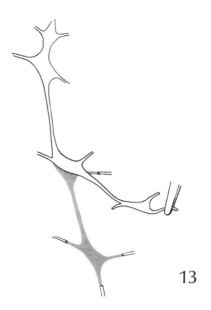

13

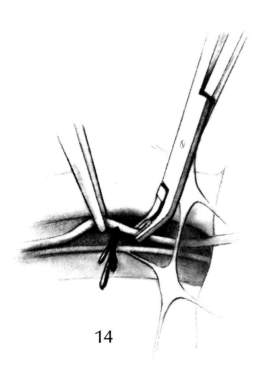

14

14

Control of haemorrhage

Great care should be used in dissection to prevent bleeding, as this may be difficult to control. A small gauze swab on a long holder, preferably a dental roll held in a long straight artery forceps, should be pressed firmly on the bleeding point for 5 min; the artery can then be picked up with a long artery forceps and coagulated with diathermy or controlled with a haemostatic clip. As the bleeding usually comes from an intercostal artery or vein, a meticulous technique should be employed, otherwise the accompanying nerve may be damaged and painful neuralgia may follow.

Wound closure

Once a dry field has been obtained the lung can be inflated and the wound closed. The pleura overlying the bed of the sympathetic chain is not sutured. A chest tube is inserted and attached to low pressure suction. The ribs are approximated and the periosteum and pleura bed in the rib bed closed with a continuous catgut suture. The fascia is then sutured and the skin closed. It is unwise to perform the axillary operation on both sides at the same operation.

Special postoperative complications

A Horner's syndrome follows division of the rami from the first thoracic nerve to the stellate ganglion and may be unavoidable in as many as 10 per cent of cases. The syndrome consists of ptosis of the lid, enophthalmos and miosis, dryness of the nasal mucosa and loss of facial sweating. It may be avoided by not dividing the stellate ganglion but this risks inadequate sympathetic arm denervation in 10 per cent of cases. The problem of a Horner's syndrome should be completely discussed with the patient pre-operatively but when the operative indication is strong the patient usually can accept the risk. Excessive dryness of the hands may be noticed. This can be treated with daily applications of a moisturizer.

Cervical approach

Gentle retraction, particularly in the region of the brachial plexus, is essential to avoid a temporary nerve palsy.

On the left side the thoracic duct may be injured. This is recognized by an escape of lymph. The treatment is careful ligation of the duct with transfixion sutures. The advantage of this route is that both the hospital stay and period of disability are shorter than with the other procedures.

Further reading

Atkins, H. J. B. Sympathectomy by the axillary approach. Lancet 1954; 1: 538–539

Goetz, R. H. Sympathectomy for the upper extremities. In: Dale, W. A., ed. Management of arterial occlusive disease. Chicago: Year Book Medical Publishers, 1971: 437

Kirtley, J. A., Riddell, D. H., Stoney, W. S., Wright, J. K. Cervicothoracic sympathectomy in neurovascular abnormalities of the upper extremities: experiences in 76 patients with 104 sympathectomies. Annals of Surgery 1967; 165: 869–879

Kuntz, A. Distribution of the sympathetique rami to the branchial plexus. Archives of Surgery 1927; 15: 871

Roos, D. B. Experience with first rib resection for thoracic outlet syndrome. Annals of Surgery 1971; 173: 429

Telford, E. D. The technic of sympathectomy. British Journal of Surgery 1935; 23: 448

Illustrations by Anita Matthews

Lumbar sympathectomy

John J. Ricotta MD
Assistant Professor of Surgery, University of Rochester
School of Medicine and Dentistry, Rochester, New York, USA

Preoperative

Indications

Lumbar sympathectomy for arterial occlusive disease was first performed in 1924. In the era prior to arterial reconstruction, this was the most commonly performed procedure for arterial ischaemia. Results with sympathectomy were erratic and with the advent of direct vascular reconstruction, the operation fell into disrepute, and its role in arterial disease has remained controversial. However, this has in large part been due to the lack of consistent selection criteria. While it has been generally accepted that lumbar sympathectomy is not indicated for treatment of uncomplicated claudication, many authors have reported gratifying results when sympathectomy is employed in patients with rest pain or localized tissue loss[1,2]. Removal of the sympathetic chain is most effective in patients with evidence of adequate collateral circulation of the extremities. This may be demonstrated by: good clinical response of the extremities to warming (increase in distal skin temperature); adequate perfusion of the distal thigh and calf reflected in segmental pressure gradients on plethysmographic tracings; or collateral circulation evident on angiography[3]. In general, lumbar sympathetic block has been an inconsistent predictor of the efficacy of sympathectomy. Diabetes mellitus may cause neuritis and autonomic nerve destruction, resulting in 'autosympathectomy'. Such patients clinically have warm, dry feet which do not sweat, and in these instances surgical sympathectomy is not indicated. Sympathectomy may give good results in selected patients with diabetes, however.

The effects of sympathectomy are limited by underlying arterial occlusive disease and it should not be used as a substitute for arterial reconstruction when the latter is feasible. However, there is evidence that sympathectomy will further augment bloodflow increases seen after arterial reconstructive surgery and, as such, it may be a valuable adjunct to aortoiliac or femoropopliteal reconstruction[4].

Other less common indications for lumbar sympathectomy include hyperhydrosis, causalgia and vasospastic conditions such as acrocyanosis, erythrocyanosis and Raynaud's phenomenon with evidence of tissue ulceration. Although these problems are rare, the role of lumbar sympathectomy is less controversial in these diseases than in occlusive arterial disease of the lower extremity.

When undertaken, sympathectomy must be technically adequate and the level of denervation must be appropriately selected. In general, removal of ganglia L2–L4 denervates the limb from the lower third of the thigh distally; inclusion of the first lumbar ganglion raises the level of denervation to the groin; and the lower two thoracic ganglia need to be removed if the buttock is to be included. Bilateral removal of the first lumbar ganglion may interfere with ejaculation in males and this ganglion should be preserved on one side in males whenever possible[5].

Anaesthesia

General anaesthesia is usually employed.

The operation

In general, an anterior retroperitoneal approach is adequate for the removal of the L2–L4 sympathetic ganglia.

1

Position of patient and incision

The patient is placed supine. A small sandbag or rolled towel may be used to elevate the operative side 15°–30°. The incision is slightly curvilinear and begins medially at the lateral border of the rectus abdominis extending laterally to the tip of the 12th rib. The incision may be extended medially for additional exposure.

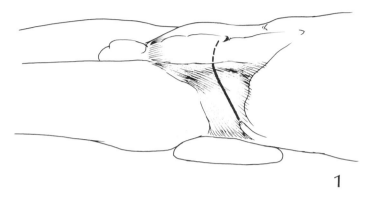

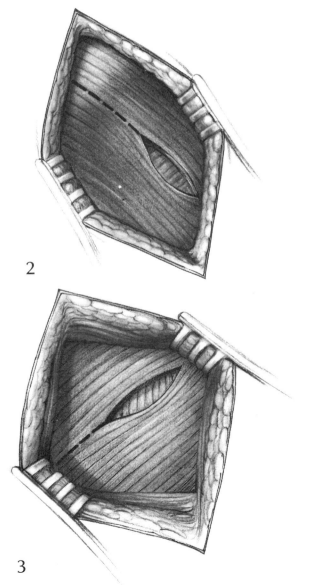

2, 3 & 4

Incision of the muscles

The external and internal oblique muscles are incised along the lines of their fibres. The transversus abdominis is then incised parallel to and between the intercostal nerves which are protected. If additional exposure is necessary, the lateral portion of the anterior and posterior rectus sheath may be incised and the rectus muscle retracted.

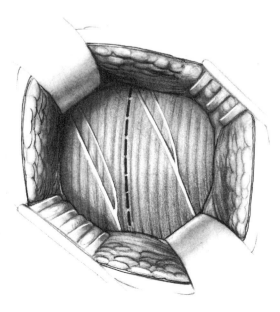

5

Extraperitoneal dissection

The retroperitoneal fat and peritoneal contents are displaced towards the midline using blunt dissection. Retroperitoneal fat should be left posteriorly. Dissection should begin laterally to minimize the possibility of entering the peritoneal cavity. If the peritoneum is inadvertently entered, it may be closed with a running absorbable suture or the peritoneal contents may be packed out of the operative field with a tagged gauge pack. It is important at this point to identify the psoas major muscle and to maintain the plane of dissection anterior to it. This muscle is often more anteriorly located than one might anticipate. As dissection proceeds the genitofemoral nerve is identified on the anterior border of the psoas major and the ureter is identified and retracted medially with the intraperitoneal contents.

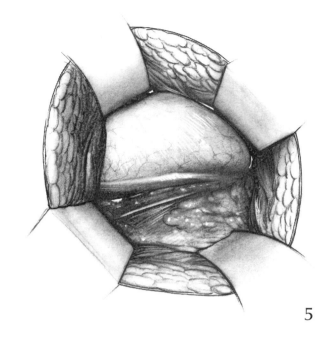

5

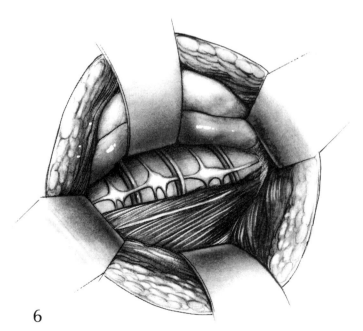

6

6

Exposure of the sympathetic chain

The sympathetic chain is identified on the anterolateral aspect of the vertebral column. On the left, the ganglia lie close to the lateral wall of the aorta, while on the right they are covered by the inferior vena cava. The sympathetic chain is most readily identified by palpation. It is a firm structure, fixed to the vertebral column by the rami communicantes, and the ganglia are readily palpated. The L4 ganglion may be most readily palpable at the sacral promontory. Occasionally two or more of the sympathetic ganglia may be fused but distal dissection should always proceed to the level of the sacral promontory. Occasionally, the sympathetic ganglion may be confused with retroperitoneal lymph nodes or, more rarely, the genitofemoral nerve.

7

The sympathectomy

Once exposed, the sympathetic chain is mobilized with a long nerve hook. The rami communicantes are divided between silver clips and the sympathetic ganglia freed up. Dissection should proceed cephalad as far as possible and caudad to the pelvic brim. At this point, the dissection will be stopped by the iliac vessels. During mobilization of the sympathetic chain, caution must be exercised to avoid damaging the lumbar veins. Most commonly these pass behind the sympathetic chain, but occasionally, especially on the right, one or more veins may pass anterior to it. When this occurs, the veins should be divided between clips or the chain threaded out from behind them. Occasionally the sympathetic chain may be divided in the middle between clamps to facilitate dissection cephalad or caudad. When doubt arises about the identification of the sympathetic trunk, its identity should be confirmed by frozen section prior to wound closure.

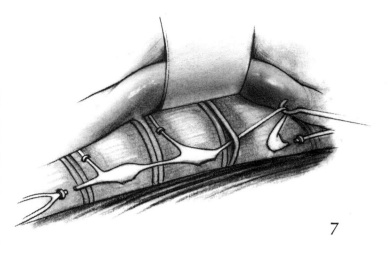

7

Closure

Haemostasis is established with particular attention to the lumbar vessels. The wound is then closed in layers using absorbable suture (polyglycolic acid 2/0). If the rectus sheath has been opened, its anterior and posterior aspects are closed separately with interrupted sutures. The transversus abdominis and obliques are closed separately with a simple running suture. Once again, it is important to protect the intercostal nerves.

Postoperative care

Usually no special measures are required in the convalescent period. If the pleura has been entered, a chest X-ray should be obtained in the recovery room. Paralytic ileus, although usually mild, may occur and require gastric decompression. Pain may develop 1–3 weeks after sympathectomy over the lateral thigh and buttock. Often quite discomforting, this pain is best treated with analgesics and will resolve within 2–3 months[6].

References

1. Haimovici, H., Steinman, C., Karson, I. H. Evaluation of lumbar sympathectomy: advanced occlusive arterial disease. Archives of Surgery 1964; 89: 1089–1095

2. Szilagyi, D. E., Smith, R. F., Scerpella, J. R., Hoffman, K. Lumbar sympathectomy: current role in treatment of arteriosclerotic occlusive disease. Archives of Surgery 1967; 95: 753–761

3. Yao, J. S. T., Bergan, J. J. Predictability of vascular reactivity relative to sympathetic ablation. Archives of Surgery 1973; 107: 676–680

4. Collins, G. J., Rich, N. M., Anderson, C. A., Hobson, R. W., McDonald, P. T., Kozloff, L. Acute hemodynamic effects of lumbar sympathectomy. American Journal of Surgery 1978; 136: 714–718

5. May, A. G., DeWeese, J. A., Rob, C. G. Changes in sexual function following operation on the abdominal aorta. Surgery 1969; 65: 41–47

6. Raskin, N. H., Levinson, S. A., Hoffmann, P. M., Pickett, J. B. E., Fields, H. L. Post sympathectomy neuralgia: Amelioration with diphenylhydantoin and carbamazepine. American Journal of Surgery 1974; 128: 75–78

Illustrations by Robert Wabnitz

Amputations

Richard M. Green MD, FACS
Clinical Assistant Professor of Surgery, University of Rochester Medical Center, Rochester, New York, USA

Charles G. Rob MC, MChir, MD, FRCS, FACS
Professor of Surgery, Department of Surgery, Uniformed Services University of the Health Sciences,
F. Edward Hébert School of Medicine, Bethesda, Maryland, USA

Introduction

There are four levels of amputations of the lower extremity for complications of peripheral vascular disease; above-knee; below-knee; transmetatarsal; and local removal of toes and metatarsals. In the upper limb, only amputations of the digits will be considered in this chapter. Other amputations, through the forearm or arm, resemble above- or below-knee amputations in the lower limb and are therefore not discussed separately.

Preoperative

Indications

The usual indications for amputation are gangrene, severe rest pain, and spreading or intractable infection associated with diabetes or ischaemia. Amputation may also be performed for acute irreversible arterial occlusion, to preserve the patient's life and renal functions by removing a large mass or necrotic muscle. When an amputation becomes inevitable the procedure must achieve a definitive result. The correct selection of the level is crucial for both medical and psychological reasons.

Selection of amputation level

Clinical judgement, arteriography and non-invasive testing have been used to guide the surgeon in selecting an appropriate level of amputation[1-5]. Clinical signs are subjective, and experience which is often gained only by trial and error is necessary to predict accurately the lowest amputation level which will heal. Arteriography, while essential in making a decision regarding arterial reconstruction, is imprecise and often misleading in determining the proper level of amputation. Non-invasive testing can be helpful especially when used in conjunction with the clinical findings.

We have established certain clinical guidelines concerning amputation level. The presence of at least one palpable ankle pulse should ensure healing after local excision of tissue, a transmetatarsal amputation or the amputation of a toe and metatarsal head. These patients are often diabetic with infection and neuropathy; ischaemia plays a lessor role. Diabetics with palpable ankle pulses and gangrene of the great toe present a difficult clinical problem and we feel it is often wise to amputate all the toes at the first operation. This produces a foot which can easily fit into a slightly modified shoe and the smaller toes do not present a threat of future gangrene. On the other hand if only one of the four smaller toes is gangrenous and the great toe is normal, only the gangrenous small toes need to be removed.

In patients with peripheral arterial disease the transmetatarsal amputation is in our opinion rarely indicated. It is usually better to amputate all the toes and the metatarsal heads separately. This leaves a series of natural skin bridges between the digits which hold the skin together and assist healing. In some patients the dorsal skin over the distal foot is necrotic and then a transmetatarsal amputation with a plantar flap is preferred. It is usually a mistake to do a transmetatarsal amputation unless at least one ankle pulse is palpable.

When gangrene or severe ischaemia extends proximal to the mid-foot, amputation at the level of the leg or thigh becomes indicated. Deciding on an above- or below-knee amputation can be difficult. We feel that primary wound healing can be achieved below the knee when the skin of the proximal calf is free of trophic changes. The presence or absence of palpable pulses may be misleading but we believe a patent profunda femoris artery is essential for healing below the knee, and therefore we would not perform a below the knee amputation when the femoral pulse is absent. A palpable popliteal pulse is not required for healing below the knee. The presence or absence of bleeding and the status of the muscles at the time of operation are the final clinical factors and one should not hesitate to move to a higher level if these are not satisfactory.

Non-invasive measurements of arterial pressures are not an absolute guide to choosing a below-knee amputation[4]. A very helpful finding, however, is the absence of an audible Doppler arterial signal in the popliteal space. This is uniformly associated with failure of a below-knee amputation. Several laboratories have established segmental pressure criteria to predict the level of healing. Most feel that a below-knee pressure of 70 mmHg or greater is predictive of healing but admit that healing can occur at lower arterial pressures.

The circulation of the foot and toes can be evaluated with digital plethysmography[5]. In non-diabetics a digit blood pressure above 10 mmHG is predictive of foot amputation healing. In diabetics, 25 mmHg is predictive of healing.

Technical considerations

1. A modern amputation in no way resembles the classic procedures of the past. The surgeon should operate gently and carefully and should not hurry.
2. The skin must not be traumatized. The only instruments which should touch the skin are the knife and the needle.
3. Haemostasis should be complete.
4. The skin flaps must not be under tension.
5. If the wound is to be sutured, a two-layer closure is essential.
6. Closed suction drainage should be employed.
7. A proper adhesive dressing should be applied.

An open or closed wound

Amputations of the toes and the local excision of tissue for ischaemia are best left open while other amputations are best closed. This means that most amputations for infected or neuropathic gangrene in diabetic patients should not be sutured. An alternative to primary closure of a transmetatarsal amputation when a satisfactory plantar flap is not available is the delayed application of a split-thickness skin graft.

Immediate casting and early ambulation

In the absence of severe infection, diabetic patients undergoing below the knee amputations should be fitted with a cast dressing in the operating room by a trained prosthetist[6]. The next morning a pylon device is put on the cast and physical therapy begins. Ambulation training continues for 7–10 days when the cast is changed and the wound inspected. A new cast is applied and the patient discharged. Another cast is applied 10 days later. A temporary prosthesis can be used 30 days after the amputation.

The benefits of the immediate fit prosthesis are a result of the rigidity of the dressing and prevention of oedema[7-10]. Wound immobilization may also limit postoperative pain and prevent knee flexion contracture. Early ambulation reduces pulmonary complications, facilitates nursing care and increases the psychological well-being of the patient. Some surgeons feel that a plaster cast prevents access to the wound and recommend a Jobst air splint.

The operations

AMPUTATION OF ONE TOE FOR GANGRENE

The incision

The incision is circular and is made around the proximal phalanx. It is important to remember that the skin will not be sutured unless the blood supply is excellent and this is rarely the case. The skin incision is made about 1 cm distal to the base of the proximal phalanx so that the skin will be loose and fall together over the defect. The tendons are then divided as high as possible and the digit removed through the metatarsophalangeal joint. Any bleeding points are now secured and the head of the metatarsal bone removed with rongeurs. A formal resection of the metatarsal head requires an extension of the circular incision and because this may compromise the blood supply of the skin, it should be avoided.

1 & 2

Removal of the distal metatarsal

A small pair of rongeur forceps are now introduced into the wound, and the head of the metatarsal bone together with the distal 2 or 3 cm of the shaft is removed piece by piece. Multiple small bites are taken until this portion of the bone has been removed and the cut end of the shaft of the metatarsal is smooth. Loose fragments of tendon or fascia are then trimmed with scissors. The wound is irrigated with saline and dressed by placing a light absorbent dressing across the surface and securing it loosely with an elastic bandage. It is important not to pack the wound. This will lead to skin necrosis and delay or prevent healing.

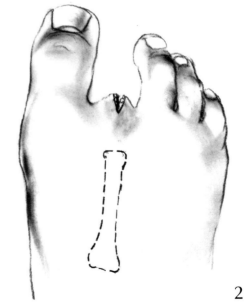

1

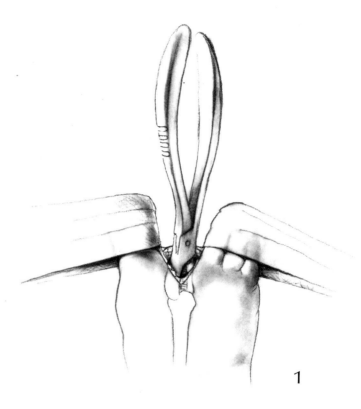

2

AMPUTATION OF A TOE AND THE METATARSAL BONE

In some patients with infective or neuropathic gangrene it may be possible to excise the toe and metatarsal bone, leaving the rest of the foot. As a good blood supply is essential for healing, this procedure is not indicated if the foot is ischaemic. In addition the infected tendons and fascia are excised.

3

The incision

An incision is made around the base of the toe and extended along the plantar surface of the foot. It is deepened to expose the flexor tendons of the involved toe and the metatarsal bone.

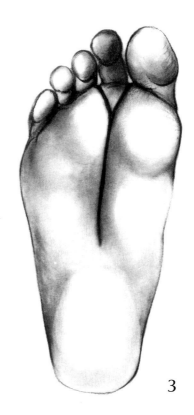

3

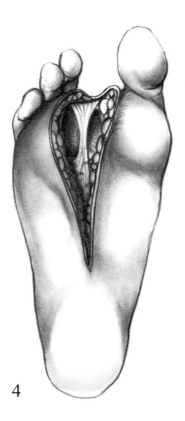

4

4

Removal of the toe and metatarsal

The infected flexor tendons and fascia are divided as far proximal as possible and the base of the metatarsal bone is disarticulated. The metatarsal bone and extensor tendon are then freed from the dorsal skin. The wound is now irrigated with saline and any additional necrotic tissue removed with scissors. The wound is not sutured. An elastic bandage is applied to approximate the remaining toes.

AMPUTATIONS OF ALL THE TOES

5

We believe that this procedure is superior to a transmetatarsal amputation and should be used when the condition of the skin permits. It should also be used in most diabetic patients with ischaemic, neuropathic or infective gangrene of the great toe even though the other four toes are still viable. Once the great toe has been removed in a patient with this type of gangrene, there is considerable risk that the other toes will soon become gangrenous. The procedure is the same as that described for the amputation of one toe. Again it is stressed that the skin incision is circular and about 1 cm distal to the base of the proximal phalanx. The toe is removed through the metatarsophalangeal joint and then the head and distal shaft of each metatarsal are removed piece by piece with a small pair of rongeurs; the skin incisions are neither sutured nor packed. The skin is dressed with a light absorbent dressing so that the edges are approximated and the bridges of skin between the toes are carefully preserved. These skin bridges hold together the dorsal and plantar skin.

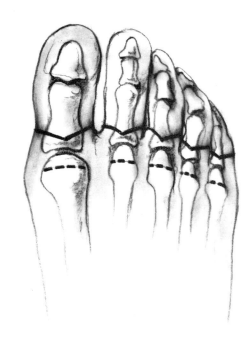

5

Postoperative care

The wounds should be dressed as infrequently as possible. They should never be packed. If there was preoperative infection, the appropriate antibiotic drugs should be administered systemically for 5 days beginning 12 hours before the operation.

In general these patients should rest in bed for the first week, and after that when possible keep the leg horizontal but not elevated above the heart until healing is well advanced. During the period of bedrest, ankle, knee and hip exercises should be encouraged.

Associated diabetes mellitus, cardiac and other abnormalities must also be actively treated.

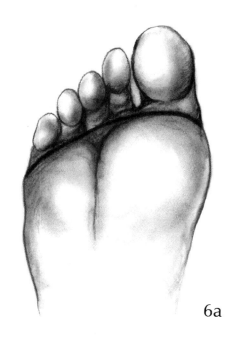

6a

THE TRANSMETATARSAL AMPUTATION

6a & b

The incision

We prefer to amputate the toes and distal metatarsals individually so that the skin bridges between the toes aid healing. However, if the skin of the distal part of the dorsum of the foot between the toes is gangrenous, a transmetatarsal amputation is indicated.

The plantar skin incision is made as close to the digits as possible and the dorsal incision crosses the foot about 3 cm from the base of the toes. The plantar flap is fashioned by cutting as close as possible to the metatarsals and the plantar tendons. The flexor tendons are then divided individually.

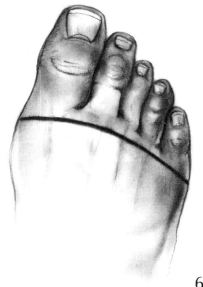

6b

7

Division of the metatarsals

Each metatarsal is now identified from the plantar surface and the shaft divided with bone-cutting forceps or a wire saw about 2 cm from its base. After all five metatarsals have been transected the tendons and other soft tissues are divided with scissors or a knife and the amputated specimen is removed. All bleeding points are now secured. Any redundant portions of fascia or tendon are removed and the whole area is irrigated with saline.

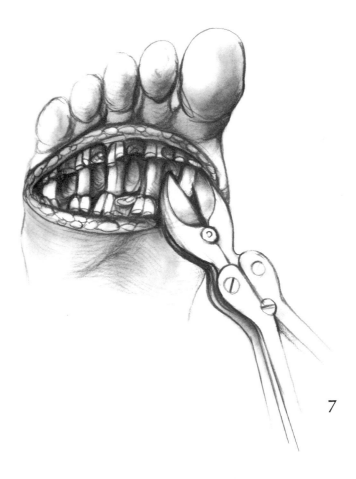

7

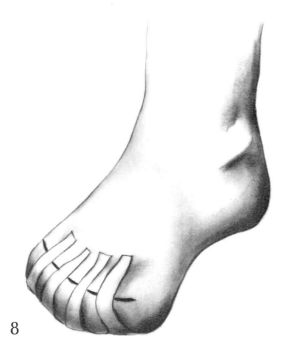

8

8

Skin closure

The skin flaps should be loose and under no tension. The skin must be treated very gently. It should not be picked up with forceps. When possible the deep fascia is closed with interrupted absorbable sutures. Drainage through a small stab incision in the plantar flap is usually recommended. Sometimes it is possible to close the skin with Steri-Strips, but otherwise interrupted skin sutures are required. The wound is now dressed with a light absorbent dressing.

Postoperative care

If the toes were infected, the patient should be treated with the appropriate antibiotics. The drain is removed on the fifth postoperative day.

After a transmetatarsal amputation, bedrest is recommended for 5–7 days. Full hip, knee and ankle exercises are encouraged but early ambulation or early weight-bearing may delay healing and should be avoided.

The advantage of a transmetatarsal amputation is that, when ambulation begins, the patient can soon wear an ordinary boot or shoe with the space in the front filled with a soft sponge pad. A prosthesis is not required.

THE BELOW-KNEE AMPUTATION

Patients with lower-limb ischaemia often have serious cardiorespiratory problems. For this reason we prefer to perform this procedure with the patient lying on his back rather than in the face-down position.

9

The incision

Equal anterior-posterior flaps may be cut, but a long posterior flap containing part of the calf muscles is preferred. The best level of bone sections is 10–12 cm distal to the medial join line. The anterior skin incision should be placed about 2 cm distal to the level of the bone section and is taken directly through the deep fascia except over the tibia where it is taken through the periosteum. The posterior flap is cut about 14 cm distal to the level of bone section and the incision goes through the deep fascia into the calf muscles. It is useful to cut the posterior flap longer than necessary to ensure that there is no suture line tension.

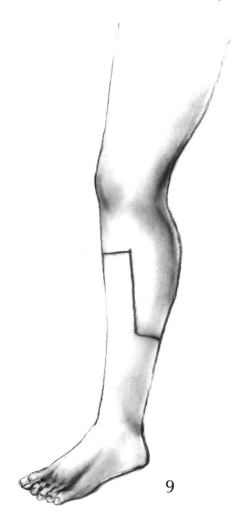

9

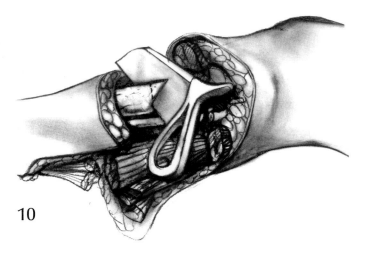

10

10

Division of muscles and other soft tissues

The fibrous attachments to the periosteum are raised with an elevator from the anteromedial surface of the tibia for a distance of 1 cm. The deep fascia is also retracted upwards at this time. The surgeon now divides the calf muscles obliquely so that a thick muscular cutaneous posterior flap is fashioned. The other muscles are divided transversely. In amputations for ischaemia, tourniquet should not be used so all bleeding points must be secured at this time. The nerves should be tied with fine catgut and allowed to retract.

11

Division of the bones

The fibula is freed with a periosteal elevator and divided with heavy bone forceps about 1 cm proximal to the proposed level of section of the tibia. The skin flaps and soft tissues are now gently retracted and the tibia divided so that the anterior surface or tibial crest is bevelled. Distally and posteriorly the first saw cut is angled obliquely so that it will meet the next vertical cut at an angle of 45°. The initial cut is then made and the anterior fragment removed to provide a smooth anterior surface to the tibial stump. Any irregularities of the bone end should now be removed with a bone file or rongeurs. A Gigli saw may also be used.

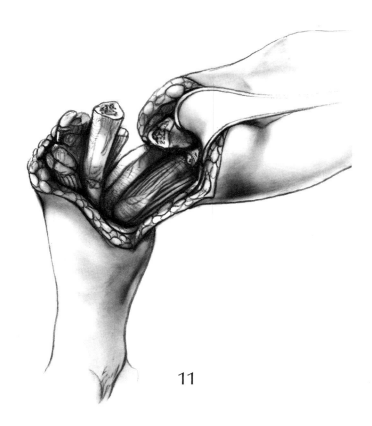

11

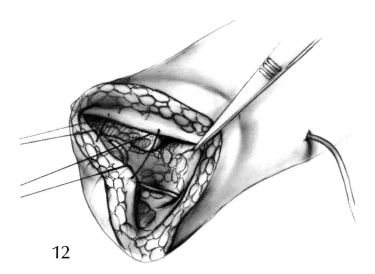

12

12

Drainage and closure of the deep fascia and periosteum

The wound is thoroughly irrigated with saline, loose fragments of tendon muscle or fascia are excised and a final check is made to confirm that haemostasis is complete. A Haemovac suction drain is introduced through the skin above the level of the knee joint and usually on the lateral side of the limb, the suction tube being passed into the wound beneath the deep fascia. This fascia is now closed with a series of interrupted synthetic absorbable sutures. This is an important step and must be performed gently so that the fascia, subcutaneous tissues and skin are not contused or otherwise damaged. The central part of the anterior layer of this closure consists of the periosteum of the tibia which has previously been freed for this purpose.

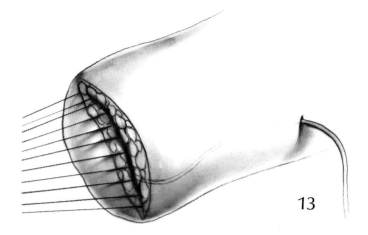

13

13, 14 & 15

Skin closure

Gentleness is essential whenever the skin is touched. Skin healing is important and in patients with vascular disease, a simple step such as picking up the skin edge with forceps may cause sufficient injury to delay or prevent healing. We believe that only two instruments should touch the skin in these patients: the knife when the incision is made, and the needle when it is closed. The skin should not be touched with dissecting or other forceps. When the skin closure is complete, a dressing is applied and the Haemovac drain or suction adjusted to its final postion.

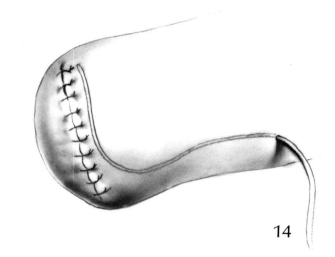

14

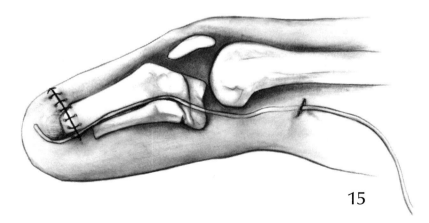

15

16

The plaster cast

The plaster cast dressing controls oedema, protects the stump from trauma and reduces patient discomfort. In our opinion a dressing of this type should be applied to most below-knee amputations.

The cast can be applied as shown here or according to the method described by Burgess, Romano and Zettl[7]. We have not advised early weight-bearing but there is increasing evidence that early partial weight-bearing on a properly applied postoperative prosthesis is not harmful[6,9]. In this system of management full weight-bearing on the amputation stump is not allowed until the permanent prosthesis has been applied. Early ambulation as contrasted with early weight-bearing is recommended in every patient.

Postoperative care

The patient is encouraged to stand by the bed on the evening of the operation or, at the latest, 24 hours later. This is coupled with physiotherapy in the physiotherapy department as soon as possible including limb exercises and walking between parallel bars on the first day if possible and then with a walker.

Antibiotics and analgesic drugs are given if necessary and associated conditions such as diabetes mellitus and cardiac problems are treated. The Haemovac drain is removed on the third postoperative day. The plaster cast is removed on the seventh day and the sutures removed from the wound. If confusion, increased wound pain or unexplained fever occurs the cast should be removed and the wound inspected. The plaster-of-Paris cast is then immediately reapplied and the prosthesis fitted so that the patient can begin weight-bearing as soon as the plaster has dried. Even if healing is not complete, the cast must be reapplied. The rigid protection aids healing even if the

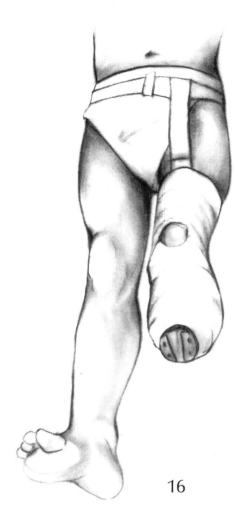

16

wound is partially open and infected. In such patients weight-bearing may await the more complete healing of the wound.

It is important to stress the role of rehabilitation in patients who have a below-knee amputation. The aim is to rehabilitate these patients so that they can walk at least with a cane and hopefully without one. This is often possible in patients aged 75 years or over.

THE ABOVE-KNEE AMPUTATION

17

The skin incision

The skin flaps must be loose and under no tension when closed. A common error is for them to be too short. To avoid this the skin flaps are equal, that is, the amputation is almost circular and the anterior incision is placed at the level of the proximal or superior border of the patella. The skin incision should pass through deep fascia. At this time the long saphenous vein may need ligating. It is stressed that the skin must not be traumatized during the operation. The skin and deep fascia are then dissected proximally for a distance of about 4 cm in the plane just below the deep fascia.

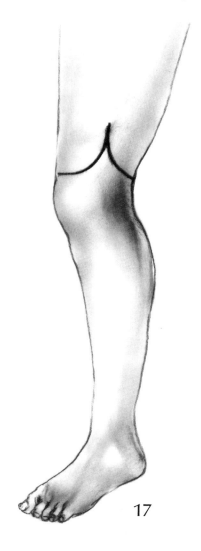

17

18

Division of the soft tissues

The muscles are divided circumferentially at a level 2–3 cm proximal to the level of the skin and fascial section. The femoral artery and veins are clamped and divided. The artery is usually occluded and the vein is usually open. The sciatic nerve is gently pulled down and divided. Frequently it is accompanied by a small vessel which requires a ligature. Posteriorly and laterally there may be several small terminal branches of the profunda femoris artery which require ligature.

18

19

Division of the bone

The periosteum is now divided circumferentially and elevated proximally with a periosteal elevator. Along the linea aspera of the femur there may be some difficulty in elevating the periosteum but the surgeon should persist until the optimum level of bone section 22–28 cm distal to the tip of the great trochanter is reached. The muscles are then protected with a gauze pack or preferably a stump retractor, the bone is divided with a saw and the limb removed.

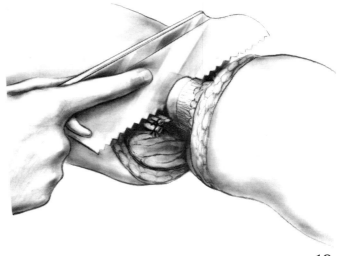

19

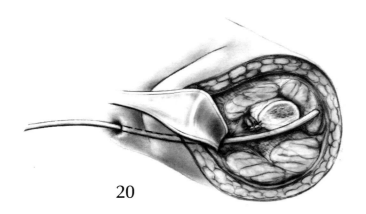

20

20

Checking for haemostasis and drainage

The wound is now thoroughly irrigated with saline to remove all debris. It is carefully inspected and all residual bleeding points are secured. At the same time any loose tags of muscle or fascia are removed. When haemostasis is complete a Haemovac drain is placed across the wound. This is introduced high on the outside of the thigh so that it can be removed without disturbing the dressing.

21 & 22

Closure of wound

The deep fascia is now closed with interrupted synthetic absorbable sutures. It is not necessary to suture the muscles. This fascial closure is important and should be performed with care. As with the below-knee amputation, the skin should only be touched with the needle and the knife. It should not be picked up with dissecting forceps. When the closure is complete, the wound is dressed with a light absorbent dressing and elastic gauze bandage is applied. We recommend that unless complications develop, this dressing should not be changed for 2 weeks, when the sutures are removed. In our opinion healing is best achieved by applying a plaster-of-Paris cast shaped as a cap over the stump. This adds protection as well as rigidity.

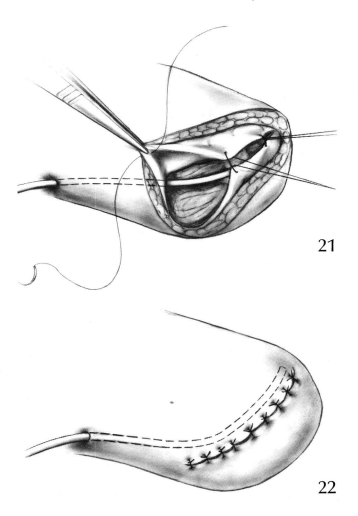

21

22

Postoperative care

The aim is early ambulation and this applies especially to older patients. Within 24 hours of the conclusion of the operation, the patient should be standing by his bed on his sound limb. The rehabilitation will include early walking between parallel bars, with a walker, and with crutches. Stump exercises are begun immediately and a temporary prosthesis is fitted as soon as possible. This makes it easier for the patient to balance and adds a feeling of security. We do not recommend full weight-bearing until after the sutures are removed, usually on the 14th day. Before this, protected weight-bearing between parallel bars can be initiated in favourable cases.

If there is excessive stump pain or evidence of a wound infection, the dressing must be removed and the stump examined. The Haemovac drain is removed on the third day without disturbing the cast or dressings.

After the sutures are removed and a temporary limb fitted, exercises and ambulation should be supervised by the physiotherapists. The patient must be taught to bandage his stump. As soon as this has shrunk sufficiently, the permanent prosthesis is fitted.

Patients with an above-knee amputation often gain weight. The patient should be kept on a diet so that he does not exceed his preoperative weight. This important point will require active control and supervision for the rest of the patient's life.

AMPUTATION OF A FINGER, PART OF A FINGER OR THE THUMB

Ischaemia in the hand differs from ischaemia in the foot. Vasospastic diseases such as Raynaud's phenomenon may lead to thrombosis of the digital arteries and gangrene of a digit. Embolization of the digital arteries may also be secondary to a cervical rib. In lesions of these types the wrist pulses may be normal and the ischaemic problem confined to the digits. This means that most of these amputations can be closed with sutures in contrast to amputation of the toes which are usually left open.

In the hand, preservation of tissue is especially important. This applies particularly to the thumb.

For ischaemia of the fingers, regional or general anaesthesia is preferred; local digital nerve block may be harmful. It is stressed that healing rather than the cosmetic result is the essential element in amputations of ischaemic digits.

Amputation through the middle phalanx

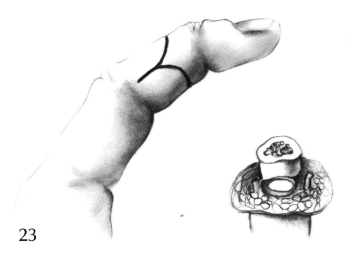

23

The incision

Almost equal flaps are fashioned, the palmar being slightly longer than the dorsal. The superficial tissues and extensor tendons are divided. The palmar flap is then fashioned and the flexor digitorum profundus tendon is divided. The middle phalanx is divided just distal to the attachment of the flexor digitorum sublimis tendon.

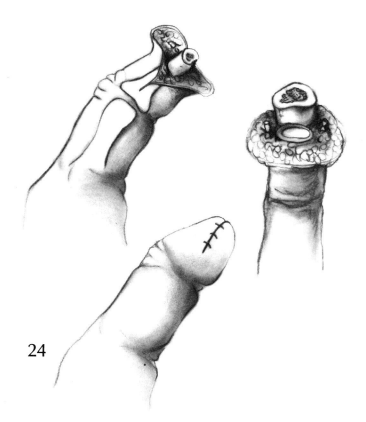

24

Haemostasis and closure

Bleeding points are secured, and the incision is closed with a series of interrupted skin sutures. A dressing is then applied.

Amputation distal to the metacarpophalangeal joint

25

The incision

A circular incision is made at the level of the skin web between the fingers. This is carried down to the bone circumferentially. Bleeding points are secured and the divided tendons are allowed to retract. The shaft of the proximal phalanx is divided with bone forceps and the finger is removed. The proximal portion of the phalanx is then removed with rongeur forceps.

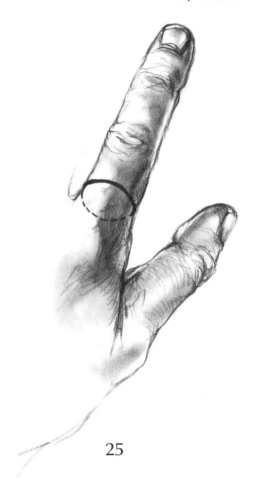

25

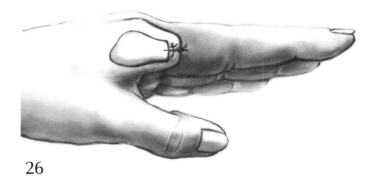

26

26

Closure

The wound is irrigated with saline and any loose tags of tendon or fascia are excised. The wound is then closed with interrupted skin sutures.

Postoperative care

The problem is wound healing when the reason for amputation was ischaemia. This means that the hand should be kept at rest for the first 3 or 4 days. It is wise to inspect the wound daily and to remove the sutures if the blood supply is in doubt.

References

1. Moore, W. S. Determination of amputational level: measurement of skin blood flow with xenon Xe 133. Archives of Surgery 1973; 107: 798–802

2. Murdoch, G. Level of amputation and limiting factors. Annals of the Royal College of Surgeons of England 1967; 40: 204–216

3. Cranley, J. J., Krause, R. J., Strasser, E. S., Hafner, C. D. Below the knee amputation for arteriosclerosis obliterans: with or without diabetes mellitus. Archives of Surgery 1969; 98: 77–80

4. Barnes, R. W., Shanik, G. D., Slaymaker, E. E. An index of healing in below-knee amputation: leg blood pressure by Doppler ultrasound. Surgery 1976; 79: 13–20

5. Barnes, R. W., Thornhill, B., Nix, L., Rittgers, S. E., Turley, G. Prediction of amputation wound healing: roles of Doppler ultrasound and digit photoplethysmography. Archives of Surgery 1981; 116: 80–83

6. Condon, R. E., Jordan, P.H., Jr. Immediate postoperative prosthesis in vascular amputations. Annals of Surgery 1969; 170: 435–447

7. Burgess, E. M., Romano, R. L., Zettl, J. H. The management of lower extremity amputations, 1969 (TRIO-6 available for $7.50 from Superintendent of Documents, US Government Printing Office, Washington, DC 20402)

8. Burgess, E. M., Romano, R. L., Zettl, J. H., Schrock, R. D. Amputations of the leg for peripheral vascular insufficiency. Journal of Bone and Joint Surgery 1971; 53A: 874–890

9. Committee on Rehabilitation of the amputee. Hospital resources for a quality amputation program: peripheral vascular disease. Circulation 1972; 46: A-293–A-304

10. Kendrick, R. R. Below knee amputation in arteriosclerotic gangrene. British Journal of Surgery 1957; 44: 13–17

Illustrations by Diane Elliott and Anita Matthews

Fasciotomy

Richard M. Green MD, FACS
Clinical Assistant Professor of Surgery, University of Rochester Medical Center, Rochester, New York, USA

James A. DeWeese MD, FACS
Professor and Chairman, Division of Cardiothoracic Surgery,
University of Rochester Medical Center, Rochester, New York, USA

Preoperative

Indications

Painful swelling of the muscles in the compartments of the lower leg may occur following active exercise, fractures, crush injuries, revascularization of an ischaemic limb and acute deep venous thrombosis or ligation of a major deep vein. The diagnosis should be considered whenever severe pain occurs in the above circumstances. It can be confirmed by redness and glossiness of the skin over the involved compartment and tender swelling. If untreated at this stage, distal hypaesthesia, loss of arterial pulses and muscle necrosis occur. Fasciotomy is most beneficial when used early and will be of no benefit when irreversible ischaemia has occurred. Therefore, the need for fasciotomy must be recognized early and appropriate decompression performed.

A single operative approach for all cases cannot be recommended. One must decide whether all four leg compartments need decompression or whether single compartment decompression will suffice. Attempts at measuring tissue pressures in the various compartments have been helpful but not uniformly reliable. The actual pressure at which neuromuscular degeneration occurs has not been defined but pressures of 45 mmHg are thought to be harmful[1-2].

The operations

Limited fasciotomy

ANTERIOR COMPARTMENT

In most cases an adequate fasciotomy can be accomplished through limited skin incisions[3]. In these cases the fascia and not the skin is the restricting structure. There is very little morbidity associated with this procedure. This approach is clearly the treatment of choice in the anterior compartment syndrome. The anterior compartment contains the extensor digitorum longus, extensor hallucis longus and peroneus tertius muscles, the peroneal nerve and the anterior tibial artery. Compression of this compartment causes anaesthesia of the first web space, loss of dorsiflexion initially of the great toe and then of the ankle and loss of the dorsalis pedis pulse[4]. Fasciotomy through limited skin incisions should be curative and is recommended as the initial procedure in most cases except for specific situations requiring extensive decompression[5].

1

The incision

A 5 cm longitudinal incision is made two fingers' breadths lateral to the tibia beginning two fingers' breadths distal to the tibial head. Occasionally, a second incision is necessary above the ankle.

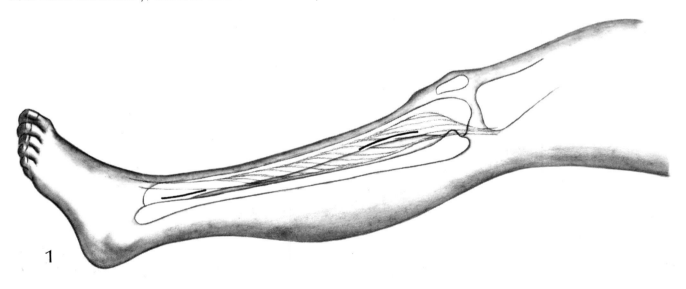

1

2

Fascial incision

The investing fascia is identified, a short incision is made in the deep fascia and the muscle inspected. Bulging of the muscle through the fascia further confirms the diagnosis. Grey or brown muscle may be found late but should not be excised.

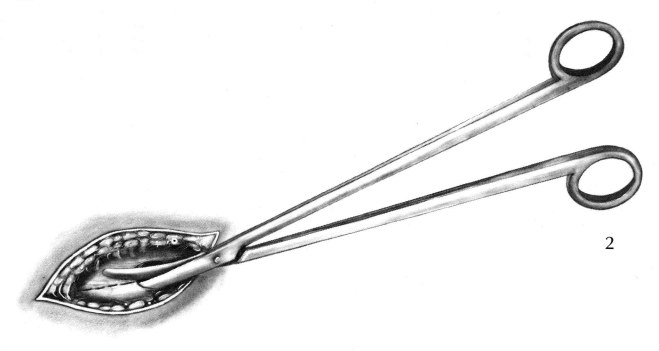

2

3

Splitting of fascia

Using long scissors the muscle is split to ankle level. Fasciotomy knives are available but long scissors inserted subcutaneously are just as satisfactory. The subcutaneous tissue is not approximated. The skin may be closed with interrupted sutures or delayed primary closure can be performed in 5 or 6 days when the swelling has subsided. If undue tension persists, split-thickness skin grafts can be applied for coverage.

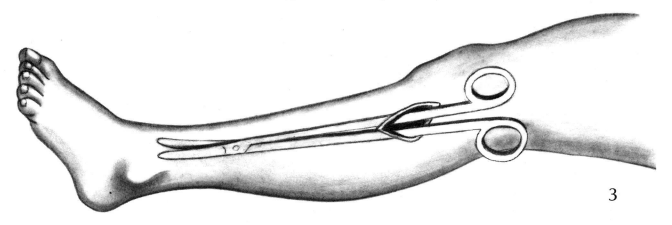

3

LATERAL COMPARTMENT

4

Exposure

Involvement of the lateral compartment may be confused with involvement of the anterior compartment because of their close proximity. Therefore, this compartment should be decompressed whenever primary involvement is suspected or whenever exploration of the anterior compartment reveals normal muscle. The lateral compartment can be reached by lateral retraction of the incision made for the anterior compartment fasciotomy until the fascia over the peroneus muscle is identified[6].

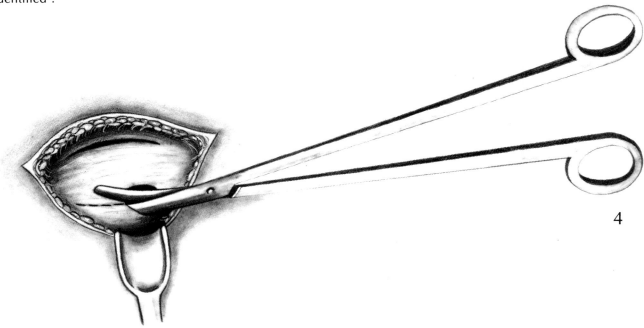

4

POSTERIOR COMPARTMENT

5

The incisions

Decompression of the posterior compartment is rarely necessary. Usually two incisions are necessary. They are made of 5 cm longitudinal incisions over the bulging gastrocnemius muscles on the medial and lateral posterior aspect of the leg. Scissors are used to divide the fascia proximally and distally.

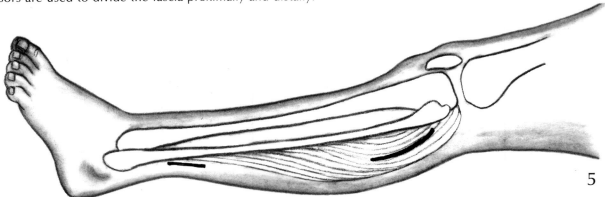

5

Complete four-compartment fasciotomy

Severe vascular impairment can occur after massive soft tissue injury in the absence of a major vascular injury[7]. These patients may have sustained a severe crush injury and have a major long bone fracture. They usually present with massive swelling, absent arterial pulses, paralysis and anaesthesia. In these situations, the skin itself may play an important role in the compartmental compression and long skin incisions are necessary as well as decompression of all four compartments. In some cases fasciotomy should be carried out *before* the start of the operative procedure. This should be considered when there has been a long delay between injury and operation, when significant muscle dysfunction is clearly present and when there is an associated major vessel injury. Four-compartment fasciotomy can be accomplished through multiple incisions or through a long lateral incision with or without resection of the fibula. The lateral incision is more efficient and has replaced the multiple incision approach.

6a & b

Four-compartment fasciotomy via lateral leg incision

The anterior, lateral and both posterior compartments can be decompressed by an incision made over the fibula from its neck to just above the lateral malleolus. This incision exposes the fascia of the lateral compartment. A long incision in this fascia decompresses the peroneal muscles.

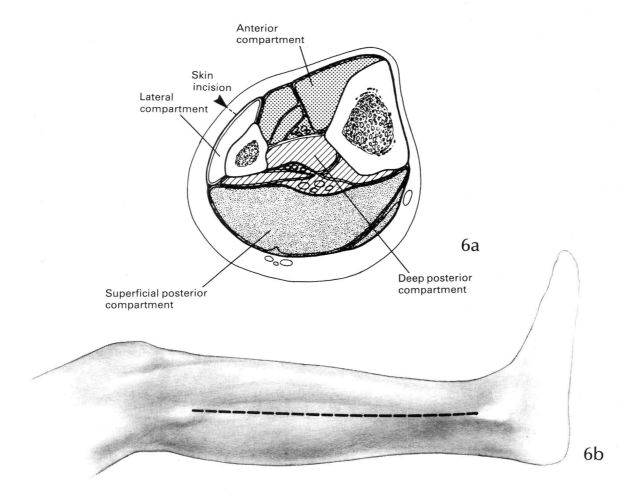

Anterior compartment

Skin incision

Lateral compartment

Deep posterior compartment

Superficial posterior compartment

6a

6b

7a & b

Decompression of anterior compartment

The anterior skin flap is retracted, exposing the anterior compartment. A long fascial incision is then made to decompress the long extensors of the foot. The superficial peroneal nerve should be identified and avoided.

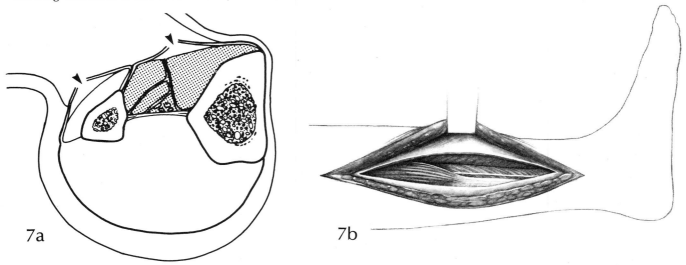

7a

7b

8a & b

Decompression of posterior compartments

The fascia of the superficial posterior compartment is incised to decompress the gastrocnemius and soleus muscles. The deep posterior compartment is approached by detaching the soleus from the fibula and incising the fascial investment overlying the peroneal vessels.

Partial fibulectomy can be accomplished through this lateral incision and will also decompress all four compartments. This approach has not been widely accepted because of concern over subsequent ankle deformity and impaired function[8].

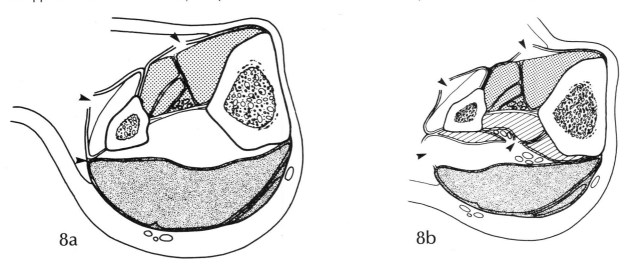

8a

8b

Skin closure

The wounds are left open after four-compartment fasciotomy and sterile antiseptic-soaked dressings are applied. When the swelling has subsided delayed primary closure can be performed or split-thickness skin grafts applied.

Postoperative care

The leg is elevated. If a foot drop has already occurred, a posterior splint is applied to maintain dorsiflexion of the foot. Active and passive exercises are begun early but bed-rest is maintained until the swelling has disappeared.

References

1. Rollins, D. L., Bernhard, V. M., Towne, J. B. Fasciotomy: An appraisal of controversial issues. Archives of Surgery 1981; 116:1474–1481

2. Matsen, F. A., Winquist, R. A., Krugmire, R. B. Diagnosis and management of compartmental syndromes. *Journal of Bone and Joint Surgery* 1980; 62A:286–291

3. Rosato, F. E., Barker, C. F., Roberts, B., Danielson, G. K. Subcutaneous fasciotomy – description of a new technique and instrument. Surgery 1966; 59:383–386

4. Moretz, W. H. The anterior compartment (anterior tibial) ischaemia syndrome. American Surgeon 1953; 19:728–749

5. Leach, R. E., Zohn, D. A., Stryker, W. S. Anterior tibial compartment syndrome. Archives of Surgery 1964; 88:187–192

6. Reszel, P. A., Janes, J. M., Spittel, J. A. Jr Ischemic necrosis of the peroneal musculature, a lateral compartment syndrome: report of case. Proceedings of Staff Meetings of the Mayo Clinic 1963; 38:130–136

7. Patman, D. R., Thompson, J. E. Fasciotomy in peripheral vascular surgery: report of 164 patients. Archives of Surgery 1970; 101:663–672

8. Kelly, R. P., Whitesides, T. E. Jr Transfibular route for fasciotomy of the leg. Journal of Bone and Joint Surgery 1967; 49A: Pt 2:1022–1023

Illustrations by Robert Wabnitz

Meralgia paraesthetica

Charles G. Rob MC, MChir, MD, FRCS, FACS
Professor of Surgery, Department of Surgery, Uniformed Services University of the Health Sciences,
F. Edward Hébert School of Medicine, Bethesda, Maryland, USA

James A. DeWeese MD, FACS
Professor and Chairman, Division of Cardiothoracic Surgery,
University of Rochester Medical Center, Rochester, New York, USA

Preoperative

Meralgia paraesthetica is an irritative neuritis of the lateral cutaneous nerve of the thigh. The symptoms are worse after hard exercise and when lying in bed and consist of numbness, paraesthesia or pain in the distribution of the lateral cutaneous nerve of the thigh. It is characteristic that flexion of the hip relieves the symptoms and so the patient may soon learn that they are relieved by sitting on the side of the bed or in an upright chair.

These symptoms are caused by compression of the lateral cutaneous nerve of the thigh as it passes through the inguinal ligament. The normal situation is for this nerve to pass behind the inguinal ligament. In patients with meralgia paraesthetica it passes through the inguinal ligament and is compressed and stretched over the deep fasciculus of this ligament.

It is important to stress that these symptoms are not relieved by division of the nerve. They are relieved, however, by removal of the compression of the nerve. The responsible agent is the deep fasciculus of the inguinal ligament which lies behind the nerve. Division of this band frees and preserves the nerve and cures the patient. Division of the superficial fasciculus of the inguinal ligament which lies in front of the nerve does not free the nerve from compression and does not relieve the symptoms.

Anaesthesia

General anaesthesia is preferred, but local anaesthesia is satisfactory.

The operation

Exposure of nerve

The lateral cutaneous nerve of the thigh normally passes behind the inguinal ligament, but in patients with meralgia paraesthetica it passes through this ligament, so that in these patients a portion of the ligament lies posterior to the nerve. The incision commences 0.5 cm below the anterior superior spine of the ileum. It then follows the line of the inguinal ligament for a distance of 4–6 cm. It is carried down so that the lateral portion of this ligament is exposed. The lateral cutaneous nerve of the thigh is then identified just below the inguinal ligament.

1

Division of posterior fasciculus of inguinal ligament

The surgeon now follows the lateral cutaneous nerve of the thigh to the inguinal ligament. If the nerve passes through this ligament the diagnosis is confirmed. If it passes behind the inguinal ligament the diagnosis probably has been mistaken. The surgeon mobilizes and divides all of the inguinal ligament which lies behind the nerve, after which the deep fascia and skin are closed in the usual manner.

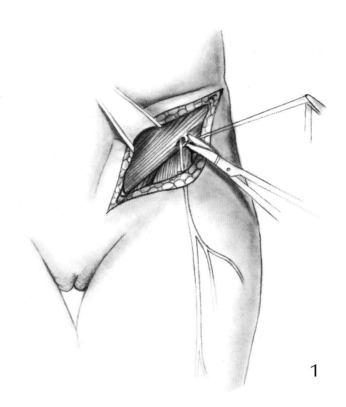

1

Postoperative care

The patient may get up from bed as soon as he has recovered from the anaesthetic. He may leave the hospital the next day and 1 week later the sutures are removed.

Further reading

Ecker, A. D., Woltman, H. W. Meralgia paraesthetica: a report of 150 cases. Journal of the American Medical Association 1938; 110: 1650–1652

Stevens, H. Meralgia paraesthetica. Archives of Neurology and Psychiatry 1957; 77: 557–574

Illustrations by Lou Sadler

Thoracic outlet syndrome

Harold C. Urschel, Jr MD
Clinical Professor of Thoracic and Cardiovascular Surgery, University of Texas Health Science Center,
Baylor University Medical Center, Dallas, Texas, USA

The syndrome

Rob coined the term thoracic outlet syndrome to describe compression of the subclavian vessels and brachial plexus at the superior aperture of the thorax[1]. It was previously designated according to presumed aetiologies, such as scalenus anticus, costoclavicular, hyperabduction, cervical rib, and first thoracic outlet rib syndrome. The various syndromes are similar and the specific compression mechanism is often difficult to identify. However, the first rib seems to be a common denominator against which most compressive factors operate[2-4]. The symptoms are either neurological, vascular, or mixed, depending upon which component is compressed. Occasionally, the pain is atypical in distribution and severity, experienced predominantly in the chest wall and parascapular area, and simulating angina pectoris[5].

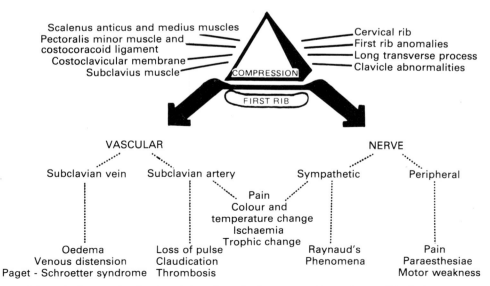

Schematic diagram showing the relation of muscle, ligament and bone abnormalities in the thoracic outlet that may compress neurovascular structures against the first rib

Diagnosis

1

Diagnosis in the nerve compression group can be objectively substantiated by determination of the ulnar nerve conduction velocity (UNCV)[6,7]. The ulnar nerve is electrically stimulated in the supraclavicular fossa, the mid-upper arm, below the elbow and the wrist. Action potentials which are generated in the muscles of the hypothenar eminence are recorded and the conduction velocity from the point of stimulation to the muscles of the hypothenar eminence is determined. Normal average conduction velocity values of 59.1 m/s in the forearm, 55.8 m/s around the elbow and 72.2 m/s through the thoracic outlet have been obtained by this method. An average UNCV value of 58.7 m/s across the outlet has been observed in patients with thoracic outlet compression. The ulnar nerve conduction test has widened the clinical recognition of this syndrome and has improved diagnosis, selection of treatment and assessment of therapeutic results[6,8].

In the vascular compression group, diagnosis can be established clinically, rarely requiring the use of angiography. Arteriograms are indicated for supraclavicular bruit, aneurysms, emboli or chronic obstructive occlusive disease. Venograms are indicated in patients with the Paget-Schroetter syndrome or chronic swelling of the arm[4,9].

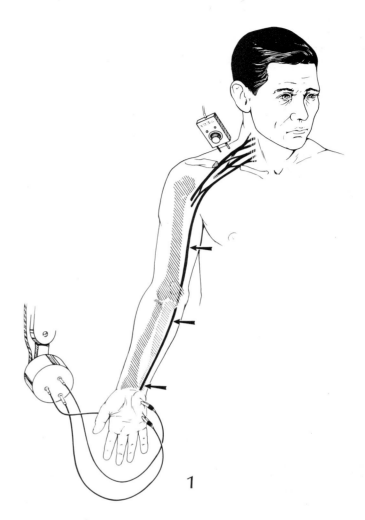

1

Preoperative

To improve posture and strengthen the shoulder girdle muscles, physiotherapy is employed initially in most cases and is successful in cases of mild compression. Surgical therapy involves extirpation of the first rib, usually through the transaxillary approach as introduced by Ross in 1966, and is reserved for cases of severe nerve compression (UNCV 60 m/s) which have not responded to medical therapy[10]. First rib resection without thrombectomy is employed for patients with demonstrated venous obstruction and arterial aneurysm. Occlusive disease is treated by subclavian to axillary artery bypass and subsequent first rib resection.

The operation: transaxillary resection of first rib

Position of patient

Under general, endotracheal anaesthesia the patient is placed in the lateral position with the involved extremity abducted to 90° by traction straps wrapped carefully around the forearm and attached to an overhead pulley. An appropriate amount of weight, usually 1.4–2.3 kg (3–5 lb), depending on the build of the patient, is used to maintain this position without undue traction. Traction can be increased intermittently for exposure by an assistant. Hyperabduction or hyperextension greater than 90° or severe or prolonged traction are common causes for brachial plexus injuries, or 'stretch', and should be assiduously avoided. The axilla and forearm are prepared and draped.

2a & b

Exposure of rib

A transverse incision is made below the hairline between the pectoralis major and latissimus dorsi muscles and deepened to the external intercostal fascia. Care should be taken to prevent injury to the intercostobrachial cutaneous nerve, which passes from between the first and second ribs of the chest wall to the subcutaneous tissue in the centre of the operative field. The dissection is extended cephalad along the external intercostal fascia to the first rib. With gentle dissection the neurovascular bundle is identified and its relation to the first rib and both scalene muscles clearly outlined to avoid injury to these structures.

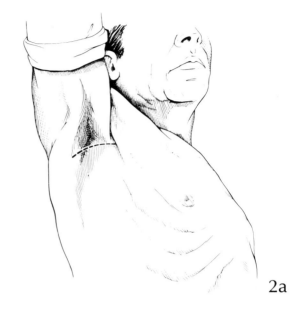

2a

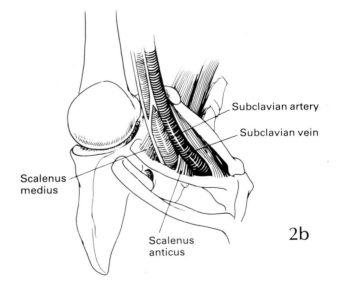

Subclavian artery

Subclavian vein

Scalenus medius

Scalenus anticus

2b

3

Division of rib

The insertion of the scalenus anticus muscle on the first rib is dissected and the muscle divided. The first rib is dissected subperiosteally with a periosteal elevator and carefully separated from the underlying pleura to avoid pneumothorax. The rib is divided at its middle portion.

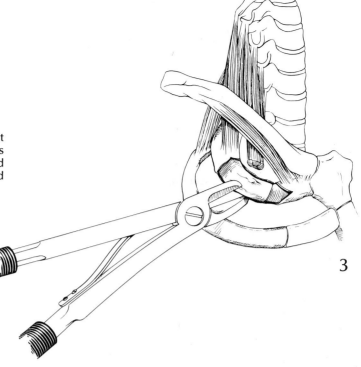

4

Removal of anterior rib

Using an alligator forceps, the anterior portion of the rib is pulled away from the vein; the costoclavicular ligament is cut and the rib is divided at its sternal attachment. The anterior venous compartment is thus decompressed.

5

Dissection of posterior rib

The posterior segment of the rib is grasped with alligator forceps and retracted from its bed to facilitate its dissection and separation from the subclavian artery and brachial plexus posteriorly. It should be emphasized that the scalenus medius muscle should not be cut from the rib but rather stripped with the subperiosteal dissection to avoid injury to the long thoracic nerve which lies on its posterior margin. The dissection of this rib segment is carried to its articulation with the transverse process of the vertebra and divided. If the dissection is kept in the subperiosteal plane, no damage occurs to the first thoracic nerve root which lies immediately under the rib. An attempt is also made to fragment and destroy the integrity of the periosteum to prevent callus formation and 'regeneration' of the rib, but only after the rib has been removed subperiosteally.

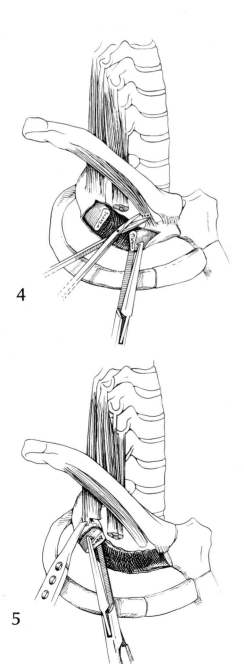

6

Excision of posterior rib

Complete removal of the neck and head of the first rib is achieved by means of a special long, reinforced double-action pituitary rongeur. The eighth cervical and first thoracic nerve roots can be visualized clearly at this point. If a cervical rib is present, it is removed at this time, and the seventh cervical nerve root identified. Although partial rib resection will alleviate symptoms in most patients, most of the recurrent symptoms result from regrowth of bone and scar from the ends of the remaining rib. Therefore, complete rib resection is recommended during the initial surgery in all patients[11].

Closure of incision

A round Jackson-Pratt drainage catheter is placed to avoid haematoma, which is often responsible for recurrent symptoms. Only the subcutaneous tissues and skin require closure, since no large muscles have been divided. Intermittent firm traction is rarely required for exposure, and the shoulder should never be hyper abducted or hyperextended to 90°. No evidence of brachial plexus stretching or neuritis has been observed.

Postoperative care

Exercises

The patient is encouraged to use the arm normally with mostly a passive range of shoulder motion for 3 weeks, after which there can be a gradual return to normal activity. Patients are discharged from the hospital 2–3 days following surgery. The patient is treated by gentle range of motion exercises and graduated to active exercises only after 6 weeks to allow a smooth healing process. Conduction velocity studies are performed at 3 months postoperatively as a baseline, and thereafter only if symptoms recur.

Results of therapy

The clinical results of first rib resections in properly selected patients are good in 85 per cent, fair in 10 per cent and poor in 5 per cent. A good result is indicated by complete relief of symptoms, a fair result by improvement with some mild residual or recurrent symptoms, and a poor result by no change from the preoperative status.

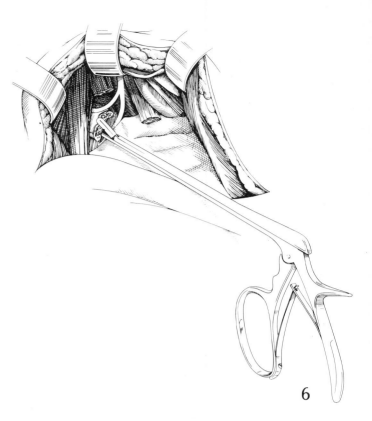

6

Uniform improvement of symptoms is usually obtained in patients with primarily vascular compression. However, in patients with predominantly nerve compression, two general groups with different rates of improvement are observed. The first group includes patients with the classic manifestation of ulnar neuralgia and elicitation of pulse diminution, in whom an average preoperative UNCV is reduced to 53 m/s. Ninety-five per cent of this group are improved by first rib resection. In the second group are patients with atypical pain distribution who may or may not have shown pulse changes by compression tests, and in whom the average preoperative UNCV was only reduced to 60 m/s. Surgery is performed in such cases as a therapeutic trial after prolonged conservative therapy has failed. Although many patients in the second group are improved, others do not fare as well[6].

A high correlation between UNCV and the clinical status has been observed. Patients with good postoperative results have a preoperative average of 51 m/s and an average of 72 m/s after operation. In those who have fair results, the preoperative UNCV averages 60 m/s and increases to an average of 63 m/s after operation. In the poor result group there is no appreciable change from the preoperative values[6,7].

Table 1 Correlation of UNCV and clinical status in patients with thoracic outlet syndrome

Clinical result	Average UNCV (m/s)	
	Preoperative	Postoperative
Good	51	72
Fair	60	63
Poor	61	58

No hospital mortality has been directly related to this procedure. Postoperative morbidity after the transaxillary approach includes clinically inconsequential pneumothorax in 15 per cent of cases, haematoma in 1 per cent and infection in less than 1 per cent[7]. The average hospital stay is reduced from 6 days for patients operated by the posterior approach to 3 days for those treated through the transaxillary approach. Less pain and a more rapid return to full range of motion of the shoulder are apparent in the transaxillary group.

In patients with recurrent symptoms and a decreased UNCV the posterior approach is recommended for removal of residual or regenerated rib, neurolysis of the nerve roots and brachial plexus and decompression of the vessels[11].

References

1. Rob, C. G., Standeven, A. Arterial occlusion complicating thoracic outlet compression syndrome. British Medical Journal 1958; 2: 709–712

2. Clagett, O. T. Presidential address: research and prosearch. Journal of Thoracic and Cardiovascular Surgery 1962; 44: 153–166

3. Rosati, L. M., Lord, J. W. Neurovascular compression syndromes of the shoulder girdle. p. 168. New York: Grune & Stratton, 1961

4. Urschel, H. C. Jr., Paulson, D. L., McNamara, J. J. Thoracic outlet syndrome. Annals of Thoracic Surgery 1968; 6: 1–10

5. Urschel, H. C. Jr., Razzuk, M. A., Hyland, J. W. et al. Thoracic outlet syndrome masquerading as coronary artery disease (pseudoangina). Annals of Thoracic Surgery 1973; 16: 239–248

6. Urschel, H. C. Jr., Razzuk, M. A., Wood, R. E., Parekh, M., Paulson, D. L. Objective diagnosis (ulnar nerve conduction velocity) and current therapy of the thoracic outlet syndrome. Annals of Thoracic Surgery 1971; 12: 608–620

7. Urschel, H. C. Jr., Razzuk, M. A. Management of the thoracic outlet syndrome. New England Journal of Medicine. 1972; 286: 1140–1143

8. Caldwell, J. R., Crane, C. R., Krusen, U. L. Nerve conduction studies: an aid in the diagnosis of the thoracic outlet syndrome. Southern Medical Journal 1971; 64: 210–212

9. Adams, J. T., DeWeese, J. A., Mahoney, E. B., Rob, C. G. Intermittent subclavian vein obstruction without thrombosis. Surgery 1968; 63: 147–165

10. Roos, D. B. Transaxillary approach for first rib resection to relieve thoracic outlet syndrome. Annals of Surgery 1966; 163: 354–358

11. Urschel, H. C. Jr., Razzuk, M. A., Albers, J. E., Wood, R. E., Paulson, D. L. Reoperation for recurrent thoracic outlet syndrome. Annals of Thoracic Surgery 1976; 21: 19–25

Illustrations by Anita Matthews

Excision of carotid body tumours

John J. Ricotta MD
Assistant Professor of Surgery, University of Rochester
School of Medicine and Dentistry, Rochester, New York, USA

Introduction

Carotid body tumours are one type of a larger group of tumours known as 'chemodectomas'. These tumours arise from paraganglionic tissue of neural crest origin and as such may be present at multiple sites throughout the body including the glomus jugulare, middle ear, aortic arch, mediastinum and retroperitoneum. Paraganglionic cells may function as chemoreceptors and are sensitive to changes in blood pH, Po_2 and Pco_2. These tumours may rarely produce catecholamines. Chemodectomas may be multicentric and a familial distribution has been reported by several investigators.

Carotid body tumours are slow growing and rarely metastasize. Differentiation of 'benign' and 'malignant' tumours on histological grounds alone is difficult. Despite their relatively indolent course, progression is inexorable in most instances and the tumours are generally not responsive to radiotherapy. While most lesions present as an asymptomatic mass at the angle of the jaw, if neglected, they may grow and produce symptoms by local extension and compression of adjacent structures and organs. Avoiding the latter constitutes the main rationale for treating these lesions. Current treatment of these lesions is surgical in most instances, especially in patients with an otherwise long life expectancy[1].

Preoperative angiography characteristically demonstrates widening of the carotid bifurcation and neovascularity pathognomonic of the tumour. Angiography may also be useful in predicting the difficulty of dissection and the necessity for concomitant arterial resection. Early surgical series reported significant mortality, most often associated with hemiplegia following ligation of the internal carotid artery. Modern vascular techniques using shunting and interposition vein graft have significantly reduced this complication rate and make surgical resection the treatment of choice for this lesion. Special difficulties may be encountered with extensive or distally located tumours. These will be discussed at the end of this chapter.

The operation

Preparation of the patient

Resection of carotid body tumours may require partial or total resection of the carotid bifurcation. In these cases reconstruction may require a saphenous vein patch or a venous interposition graft. Since this cannot be predicted preoperatively, one leg should always be prepared for harvesting the saphenous vein. Vein may be taken from the groin or at the ankle. When the distal vein is of adequate calibre, this should be removed preferentially so that the proximal saphenous can remain available if needed at some later date.

1

The incision

This is the same as that for carotid endarterectomy. When possible, a curvilinear incision following the skin folds in the neck is preferred for cosmetic reasons. In large tumours, an incision along the anterior border of the sternocleidomastoid may be necessary. The superior portion of the incision should proceed upward along the anterior border of the sternocleidomastoid muscle with care being taken to preserve the greater auricular nerve.

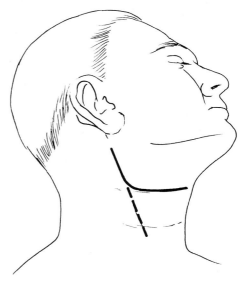

1

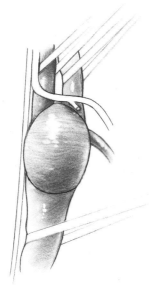

2

2

Isolation of the carotid vessels

The platysma is divided along the skin incision and the sternocleidomastoid is retracted laterally. The common, external and internal carotid arteries are isolated close to the margin of the tumour and encircled with tapes. The hypoglossal nerve is isolated at this point and protected. It may be necessary to divide the ansa hypoglossi to allow superior retraction of the hypoglossal nerve.

3

Mobilization of the tumour

The tumour is circumferentially mobilized from the periphery toward the carotid vessels. These tumours are quite vascular and meticulous haemostasis with fine 4/0 silk ties is essential. Any obviously enlarged lymph nodes are removed. As dissection approaches the artery, the tumour becomes increasingly adherent. A subadventitial plane is established in the common carotid artery and dissection proceeds cephalad toward the bifurcation. Haemorrhage from the tumour itself can most often be controlled by compression. Often the tumour can be totally or nearly totally removed without clamping the carotid or its branches. As much dissection as possible should be done with the arteries looped but not clamped. Dissection proceeds from the common to the external carotid artery.

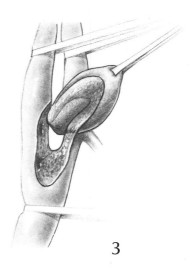

3

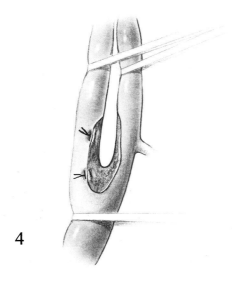

4

4

Control of bleeding

Dissection may at times result in small tears through the arterial wall. In some instances these may be controlled by pressure. Superficial horizontal mattress sutures may be required for other more significant tears. If the bleeding is from the external carotid artery this branch can be ligated.

5

Carotid resection

Resection of the carotid bifurcation or a portion of the internal carotid artery may be necessary because of tumour adherence. This is not necessarily a sign of malignancy. When this occurs, the external carotid artery is ligated and after the patient has been systemically heparinized, the common and internal carotid arteries are clamped and divided.

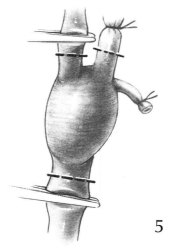

5

6

Insertion of shunt

After the tumour and adherent vessels have been resected, the defect is bridged by a saphenous vein interposition graft. A suitable segment of vein is harvested and placed over an Argyle shunt[2]. The shunt is then inserted temporarily to reestablish blood flow during vascular repair. The shunt is first inserted distally into the internal carotid artery and then the proximal end is placed in the common carotid artery. The shunt may be secured by Rommel tourniquets or Javid clamps. This is usually done without difficulty although stay sutures may be helpful to control the cut ends of the artery.

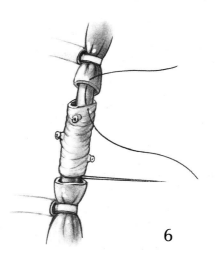

6

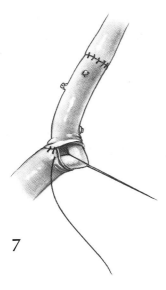

7

7

Vein graft interposition

Once the shunt is in place, a leisurely end-to-end anastomosis between the transected artery and saphenous vein is possible. This is performed using the triangulation technique with three stay sutures. The stay sutures are connected by continuous 6/0 Prolene suture to complete the anastomosis. The shunt is removed just before the last few sutures are placed.

Extensive tumours

Carotid body tumours, if discovered late, may grow from the bifurcation toward the jugular foramen. These lesions have been deemed inoperable in the past because of inability to achieve distal control. Schick[3] has reported preoperative embolization of a large chemodectoma followed by resection in a young man. Several operative techniques have been developed recently to facilitate exposure of the distal internal carotid artery. The first approach, described by Fry[4], involves anterior subluxation of the jaw while the patient is under general anaesthesia. This allows an additional 2–3 cm of distal exposure. Subluxation is maintained during surgery by wiring the jaw with arch bars.

8

The second approach, described by Purdue[5], is more complex. The approach was initially described by Arena[6] for resection of tumours of the temporal bone and glomus jugulare. An incision is made along the anterior border of the sternocleidomastoid muscle and curved up along either side of the ear. The auricle can be retracted superiorly and with the mastoid process resected, the distal internal carotid can be exposed up to the base of the skull. This technique requires a cooperative approach, with both the vascular surgeon and otolaryngologist participating. The details of exposure will not be given here but the interested reader should consult the references listed at the end of this chapter.

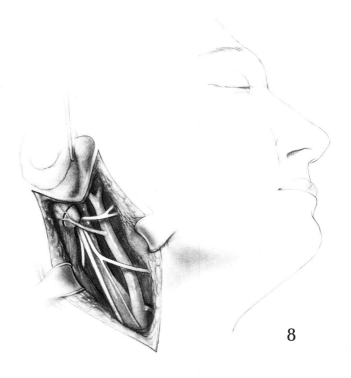

8

Closure

Following removal of the tumour, haemostasis is secured. As mentioned, the external carotid may need to be ligated. The carotid bifurcation may require partial resection and repair. After haemostasis has been achieved, a closed suction drain is placed alongside the carotid artery. If heparin was given for carotid clamping, this is reversed with protamine. The drain is brought out through a stab incision and the platysma is reapproximated followed by subcuticular closure of the skin.

Postoperative care

Major complications are bleeding and carotid artery occlusion. Early occlusion may be diagnosed with oculopneumoplethysmography (OPG-GEE) which is easily done in the recovery room. If occlusion occurs, prompt reoperation may avoid permanent neurological deficit.

References

1. Javid, H., Chawlan, S., Dye, W. *et al*. Carotid body tumor: resection or reflection. Archives of Surgery 1976; 111: 344–347

2. Dent, T. L., Thompson, N. W., Fry, W. J. Carotid body tumors. Surgery 1976; 80: 365–372

3. Schick, P. M., Hieshima, G. B., White, R. A. *et al*. Arterial catheter embolization followed by surgery for large chemodectoma. Surgery 1980; 87: 459–464

4. Fry, R. E., Fry, W. J. Extracranial carotid artery injuries. Surgery 1980; 88: 581–587

5. Purdue, G. F., Pellegrini, R. V., Arena, S. Aneurysms of the high internal carotid artery: a new approach. Surgery 1981; 89: 268–270

6. Arena, S. Tumor surgery of the temporal bone. Laryngoscope 1974; 84: 645–670

Vascular access

Allyn G. May MD
Professor of Surgery, University of Rochester Medical Center, Rochester, New York, USA

Carl H. Andrus MD
Clinical Associate Professor of Surgery, University of Rochester Medical Center, Rochester, New York, USA

Introduction

Vascular access may be defined as the means by which to take from and deliver fluids into the circulatory system at a rate of 200 ml or more per minute for lengthy intervals of time.

The demonstration by Wilhelm Kolff[1] that chronic intermittent haemodialysis could save lives gave impetus to the development of useful techniques and materials for vascular access. At first, segments of artery and vein needed to be sacrificed for each treatment. Then Quinton, Dillar and Scribner[2], using biologically compatible Teflon cannulae and Silastic tubing, found that one operation could establish useful vascular access often for months and, sometimes, for years. The arterial and venous tubes were connected while the shunt was not in use so that the constant flow of blood prevented clotting in the device. Thus, it could be used repeatedly for haemodialysis. In 1966, Brescia et al.[3] reported their experience with the radiocephalic arteriovenous fistula constructed subcutaneously at the wrist. This procedure ensured that the cephalic vein would be kept distended even though blood was continuously and rapidly withdrawn from the vein. The blood was then passed through the dialyser and returned to the proximal segment of the same arterialized vein or to another vein. The advantages of the 'Brescia-Cimino fistula' over the 'Scribner shunt' were the absence of perpetual defects in the skin through which infection could more easily enter and the absence of implanted prosthetic materials. The disadvantage was its need frequently for time to mature before use and, therefore, its unsuitability for emergencies.

Because the Scribner shunt could be used immediately, it became the device of choice for emergency vascular access. However, venous catheters designed for percutaneous insertion have made the Scribner shunt obsolete. These catheters are usually inserted through a subclavian vein into the superior vena cava or right atrium. With proper care a catheter may be used safely for weeks or months before requiring removal and introduction of a new catheter in the contralateral vein. They do not interfere at all with the patient's activity. The catheters may be biluminal or uniluminal. The latter require special equipment which allows for alternate aspiration and infusion of small volumes of blood, which are passed through the dialysis cartridge and then back to the patient through the same needle. There is more 'recirculation' inefficiency with this device than with biluminal catheters. Percutaneous catheterization of the femoral vein is less satisfactory because it is more difficult to maintain cleanliness and sterility in the groin, because of the more severe consequences of iliofemoral venous thrombosis, and because of the limitations the device imposes upon walking and sitting.

There are many choices of device or technique for achieving vascular access. The simplest one which offers reasonable success should be used. For example, the radiocephalic arteriovenous fistula should always be chosen before a brachiocephalic fistula, a basilic vein interposition fistula or a saphenous vein transplant fistula. The latter three techniques should be considered successive back-up procedures to be used in case construction of a simpler fistula is not possible.

In order to select the best location for construction of an arteriovenous fistula for vascular access, the surgeon must be sure that the vein to be used is adequate to promote success of the fistula and that the arterial supply remaining is adequate to ensure satisfactory perfusion of the limb. Often patients who need vascular access have had chronic illness and have required repeated phlebotomies and intravenous infusions which may have caused thrombosis of many superficial veins. The venous lumen must be patent at the anastomosis and proximally. This can be determined by application of a tourniquet high on the arm and inspection and palpation of the vein. To ensure an adequate arterial supply to the limb after construction of a fistula the surgeon makes sure the following conditions are fulfilled: (1) an alternative arterial supply is available, i.e. in the upper extremity the Allen test should be negative; (2) the artery is not interrupted, i.e. a side-to-side or, preferably, a side-to-end arteriovenous anastomosis is constructed, and (3) the anastomosis should be made as peripheral as possible, or, if necessity requires a more central location between larger vessels such as the brachial artery and cephalic vein, the anastomosis should be made small enough to avoid a steal syndrome.

Procedures

PERCUTANEOUS CATHETERIZATION OF THE SUBCLAVIAN VEIN

1

Position of patient

The patient is positioned supine in bed with a folded towel along the thoracic spine in order to allow the shoulders to fall back.

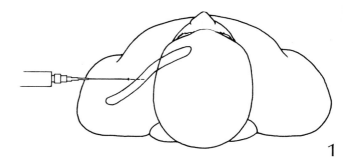

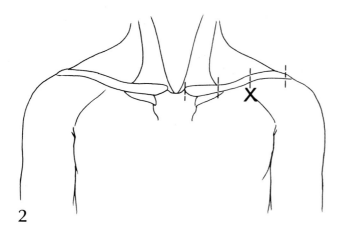

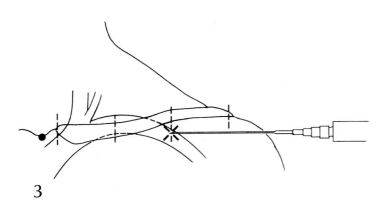

2

Preparation

The shoulder and adjacent parts of the neck, chest and arm are prepared antiseptically and draped to expose the clavicular region. An area of skin just below the junction of the middle and distal thirds of the clavicle is anaesthetized.

3

Catheter insertion

The long hypodermic needle with syringe attached (3.43 mm external diameter or 11 Fr as supplied in commercial kits) is passed through this skin, then placed horizontally and inserted toward the suprasternal notch while suction is applied. This should result in the needle's tip entering the subclavian vein at which point venous blood will flow easily into the syringe.

Without moving the needle further, the syringe is removed and the wire is inserted into the needle flexible end first. The wire is advanced until it is well into the superior vena cava. It should advance easily and should never be forced.

The needle is next withdrawn over the wire which is held stationary. The catheter is then passed over the wire into the superior vena cava and finally the wire is removed leaving the catheter in the desired position. Fluoroscopy often is helpful and occasionally is necessary for the success of this procedure.

The catheter should be filled with heparin (1000 u/ml) but not overfilled to avoid a systemic effect and the attendant increased risk of bleeding. A chest X-ray film should be obtained as soon as the catheterization is completed so as to detect any air or fluid in the pleural space and to define the position of the catheter.

The catheter should be securely sutured to the skin and a sterile dressing applied to the puncture site.

RADIOCEPHALIC FISTULA

4

The incision

A transverse incision is made and proximal and distal skin flaps are developed to allow exposure of adequate lengths of vessels.

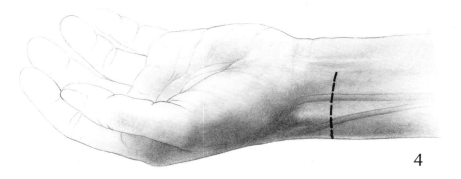

4

5

Exposure

To expose the artery the deep fascia is incised longitudinally along the palpable radial pulse. Branches are tied with silk and divided so that the artery can be lifted from its bed.

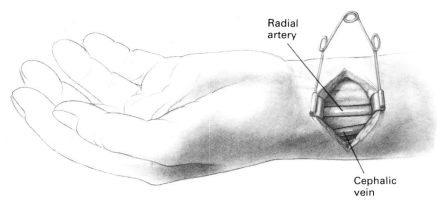

Radial artery

Cephalic vein

5

6

Isolation of vessels

The vein is tied distally, controlled proximally with a vascular clamp and divided just proximal to the ligature. The isolated segment is dilated gently with a clamp and irrigated with heparinized saline.

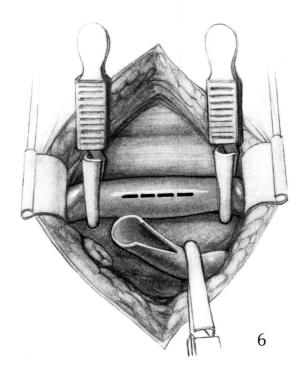

6

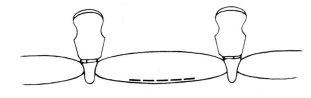

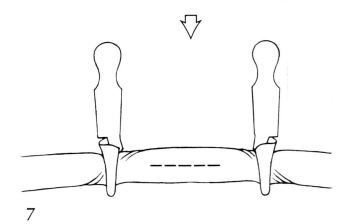

7

7

Arteriotomy

The artery is controlled with vascular clamps applied perpendicularly and is rotated medially to present the lateral aspect of the vessel for anastomosis. A longitudinal arteriotomy two to three times the width of the lumen is made and flushed free of blood or clot with heparinized saline.

Anastomosis

8

The cephalic vein end is spatulated to fit the arteriotomy. The anastomosis is constructed with two running 6/0 or 7/0 monofilament Prolene sutures inserted at the proximal and distal vertices, with the help of lateral and medial stay sutures.

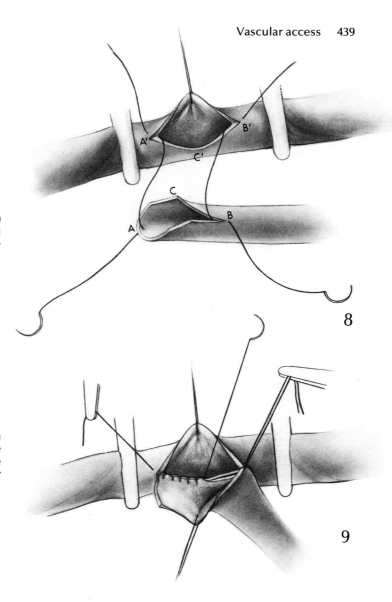

8

9

The 'back wall' of the anastomosis is constructed through the open anastomosis with the knots tied outside. The vein should describe a gentle curve as it passes from the anastomosis to its native bed and should not be kinked or twisted.

9

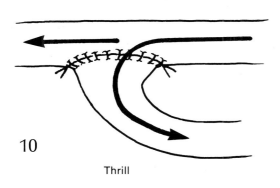

10

Thrill

10

Evaluation

When the vascular clamps are removed, the vein is checked for filling and for a palpable thrill. Haemostasis is ascertained.

Finally, the wound is closed with a single row of continuous vertical mattress sutures of 4/0 monofilament nylon. A loose dressing which is not circumferential is applied to the incision. The patient is advised to make ordinary use of the extremity, to avoid placing it in a dependent position and not to modify the dressing (except to remove it, if wetted).

In men with large veins, this sort of fistula can be used for dialysis in a week or two. In women and children, who tend to have small vessels, a period of maturation of several weeks or months may be desirable before easy use without risk of loss of the fistula.

BRACHIOCEPHALIC FISTULA

11

The incision

A curved incision is made in the antecubital fossa for exposure of the cephalic or medial cubital vein and the brachial artery.

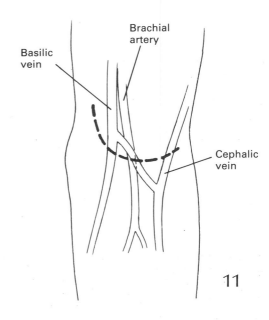

11

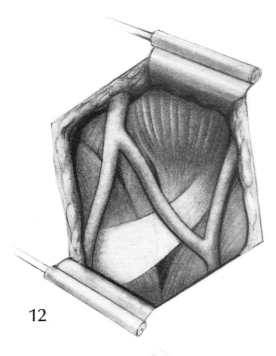

12

12

Exposure

Either vein can be used for the anastomosis, but it is important that only the cephalic vein be arterialized and not the basilic vein which is too deep in its native position to be useful.

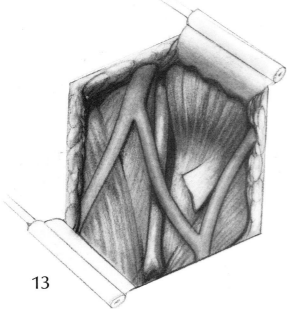

13

13

Mobilization

The lacertus fibrosus is incised parallel to the course of the brachial artery as it can be felt entering the antecubital fossa. Small branches are divided after ligation in continuity with silk to free 2–2.25 cm of artery. The vein is controlled by ligation at one end and placement of a vascular clamp at the other.

14

The brachial artery is controlled proximally and distally with atraumatic clamps as in construction of the radiocephalic fistula. An arteriotomy is made on its anteriolateral surface. To minimize the risk of a steal syndrome and ischaemia of the hand, the length of the arteriotomy should not exceed the diameter of the artery. Both vessels are irrigated with heparinized saline.

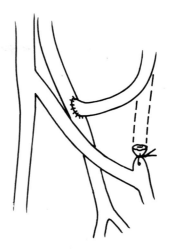

14

15

If the median antecubital vein is used it should be flushed with heparinized saline without a clamp in order to detect valves which might interfere with blood flow. It is occasionally possible to poke out the valves in the forearm portion of the cephalic vein by means of a probe inserted through the median cubital vein. This will allow arterialization of a longer segment of the cephalic vein.

The vein may be dilated gently and spatulated if necessary. A side-to-end anastomosis is performed with a running suture of 6/0 monofilament Prolene. The venous clamp is removed. Then the distal arterial clamp is released to evacuate any clot into the vein in order to minimize the risk of distal embolization. Last, the proximal arterial clamp is removed. The wound is closed with absorbable suture in the subcutaneous layer and a running monofilament suture in the skin, or by means of a single row of skin sutures. Again, a loose, non-circumferential dressing is applied to the wound with advice to the patient as before.

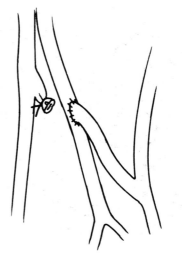

15

BASILIC VEIN TRANSPOSITION FISTULA

16

The incision

The basilic vein is exposed through a curvilinear incision passing from the antecubital fossa medially 2 cm anterior to the medial epicondyle of the humerus.

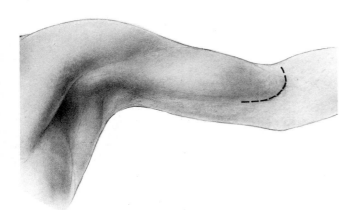

16

17

Exposure

Care should be taken to avoid injury to the medial cutaneous nerve of the forearm, which runs alongside the vein, and the median nerve which is deep in the antecubital fossa.

18

Mobilization

The vein is followed proximally by extension of the incision high into the axilla. Branches are ligated with silk ties and microhaemoclips, and then divided. The basilic vein is freed to its junction with the axillary vein. Occasionally there are large branches connecting the basilic and brachial veins. These must be divided and oversewn.

The brachial artery is exposed in the groove medial to the distal belly of the biceps. Small branches are divided after ligation in continuity and 3 cm of vessel is freed and encircled with vessel loops. A subcuticular tunnel is made from the antecubital portion of the incision passing along the anteromedial aspect of the biceps muscle and emerging in the axillary portion of the incision. The tunnel should be made wide at the proximal and distal ends.

The distal end of the basilic vein is ligated and divided. A vascular clamp controls the most proximal end of the vein in the axilla. The vein is gently dilated and irrigated with heparinized saline.

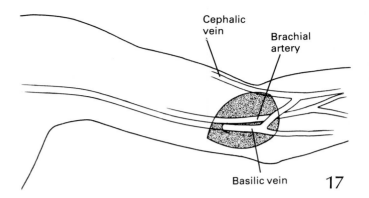

Cephalic vein

Brachial artery

Basilic vein

17

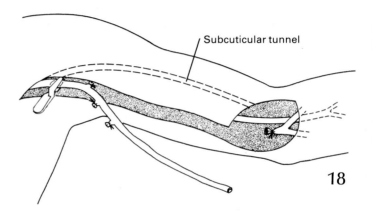

Subcuticular tunnel

18

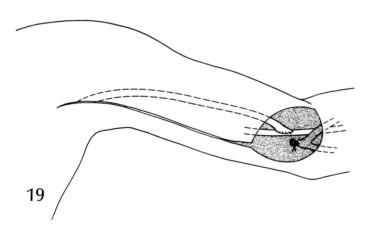

19

19

Anastomosis

The distal end is then drawn through the tunnel, carefully avoiding kinks and twists. It is helpful to close the upper part of the incision temporarily with towel clips to be sure the course of the tunnel is correct.

The artery is controlled with vascular clamps, and an arteriotomy, the length of which should not exceed the diameter of the artery, is made on its anteromedial surface. A side-to-end anastomosis is performed with running suture of 6/0 monofilament Prolene with the help of appropriate stay sutures. After completion of the anastomosis the vascular clamps are removed in the order described above.

When haemostasis is ascertained, the wound is closed with a running absorbable suture for the fascia, and non-absorbable sutures or staples for the skin. The dressing should not be circumferential in order to avoid compression of the fistula. The fistula should not be used for at least 2 weeks. Earlier use, before there is obliteration of the tunnel space by healing, will risk a perivenous haematoma.

SAPHENOUS VEIN TRANSPLANT FISTULA

20

Radial artery fistula

The key element in this procedure is the transplantation, usually of an autologous segment of saphenous vein, to a subcuticular tunnel in the upper extremity. Ideally, the configuration of the vein should be straight from, for example, the radial artery at the wrist to the median cubital or brachial vein.

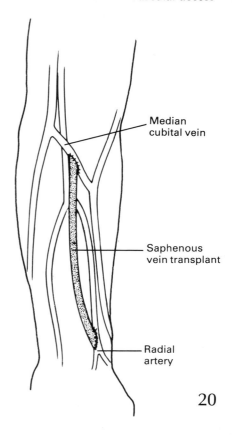

Median cubital vein

Saphenous vein transplant

Radial artery

20

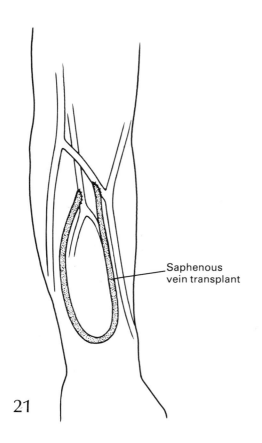

Saphenous vein transplant

21

21

Loop fistula

However, if a distal artery is not available, then a 'loop fistula' can be constructed by making a curved subcuticular tunnel from the brachial artery down the lateral aspect of the forearm, across and up the medial aspect of the forearm to the venous anastomosis at the median cubital or brachial vein.

Attention to certain details of these procedures is important for a successful result. The vein should be inserted so that its valves do not interfere with blood flow. If a 'loop fistula' is constructed, a counter-incision across the course of the tunnel at its distal extremity must be used to allow passage of the vein through the tunnel without a twist. If the vein transplant crosses the elbow joint, it should do so on the medial or lateral aspects of the joint so that flexion does not cause kinking of the vein. This type of fistula should not be used for at least 2 weeks for the reasons given above.

Complications

PERCUTANEOUS CATHETERS

Most percutaneous catheters for vascular access are introduced into the subclavian vein. Because of the proximity of the parietal pleura to the subclavian vein, pneumothorax, haemothorax, or haemopneumothorax can occur. Consequently it is mandatory to obtain chest films after catheterization and before the catheter is used. If there is evidence of such a complication, the catheter should be withdrawn, and, if necessary, a chest tube inserted for control of the pleural space. Because bilateral complications of this kind are extremely hazardous, the contralateral subclavian vein should not be catheterized immediately. If immediate access is necessary after having induced a pneumo- or haemothorax, then the femoral vein may be catheterized.

If infection of a percutaneous catheter is suspected, it should be used to obtain blood cultures, then removed. If signs of infection persist after its removal, the patient should be treated with specific antibiotics for endothelial infection. During antibiotic therapy a new venous catheter may be placed at another site and the sites of catheterization should be changed frequently. As an alternative approach peritoneal dialysis may be used.

ARTERIOVENOUS FISTULAE

Early complications

Most early complications of arteriovenous fistulae can be avoided by attention to the detail of the surgical procedure. Haemostasis must be satisfactory in order to avoid a perivenous haematoma which will compress the vein and therefore obstruct blood flow and result in failure of the fistula by clotting. The arteriovenous anastomosis must be done without a twist or kink in the vein because these interfere with blood flow and result in failure. After the anastomosis has been completed and the wound closed, it is necessary to be sure that blood flow is adequate in order to minimize the chance of an unexpected venous obstruction. The best physical signs of good blood flow are a palpable thrill throughout the vein and an audible bruit. In contrast a venous pulse is *not* a reliable sign of good blood flow, e.g. an exaggerated venous pulse may be present briefly distal to a complete venous obstruction.

Failure of fistula

Failure of a fistula may occur after it has been used successfully for months or years. This often happens as the result of contraction of the patient's blood volume such as may occur by inadequately replaced surgical blood loss or by excessive haemoconcentration during dialysis. The first sign of this is a lessened turgidity of the arterialized vein. Then the thrill and bruit disappear. The fistula can sometimes be salvaged non-operatively in these circumstances, if the problem is detected promptly, i.e. before extensive clotting has developed. If palpation of the vein does not reveal a large thrombus, then restoration of the blood volume should be begun and the offending thrombus, which is usually confined initially to the venous side of the anastomosis, can be dislodged by vigorous massage through the skin. Lubrication of the skin is of assistance. This manoeuvre has never been followed by symptoms or signs of pulmonary embolus in our experience. The technique should *not* be used when the thrombus is palpable (i.e. large) and it should not be used if the patient is known to have a cardiac septal defect.

Heart failure and distal ischaemia

Heart failure and distal ischaemia may rarely and correctly be attributed to arteriovenous fistulae for vascular access. These complications always occur in patients who have a particular susceptibility to them. They usually can be successfully treated and, preferably, may be prevented by attention to simple technical details during the construction of the fistula.

Severe myocardial or valvular disease predisposes the patient to development of 'high output' heart failure after construction of an arteriovenous fistula, and diabetes mellitus predisposes to development of distal ischaemia. The incidence of both complications can be minimized by using the most distal site for construction of the fistula. This results in a smaller fistulous blood flow, less burden on the heart, and less 'steal' from the distal arterial circulation. If larger, proximal vessels must be used, then the anastomosis should be kept small. Furthermore, no more than the vein to be used for dialysis should be arterialized. For example, in the case of brachiocephalic fistula, it is possible inadvertently to arterialize both the basilic vein and the cephalic vein, if the cephalic vein distal to the median cubital is connected to the brachial artery. This can result in unnecessarily large blood flow through the fistula and congestive failure or distal 'steal' ischaemia.

Banding of vein

22

If the anastomosis is determined to have been made too large and to be the cause of congestive failure or distal ischaemia, then the vein can be 'banded' to limit its blood flow.

To do this, the venous segment adjacent to the anastomosis is exposed surgically and encircled with a piece of Dacron about 5 mm in width. A mandril of a diameter equal to the desired narrower lumen is laid beside the vein and within the Dacron strip.

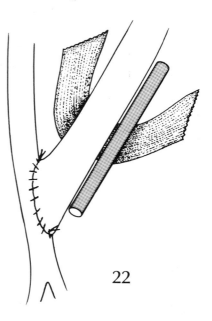

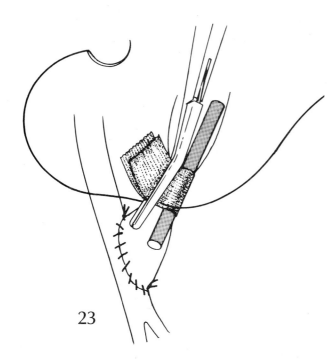

23

The patient is heparinized. The Dacron strip is then tightened about the vein and mandril so as to occlude completely the venous lumen. The Dacron is then clamped with a haemostat and sewn into a closed cuff beneath the haemostat.

24

The haemostat is removed and the excess Dacron resected. Finally the mandril is removed to allow the vein to open to the size of the mandril. The heparin is reversed with protamine and the wound closed.

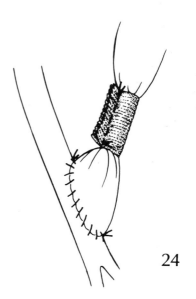

Stenosis at venous outflow

25

Excessive 'recirculation' and inefficient haemodialysis can occur when a venous stenosis develops in the vein beyond that part used for access. This may happen with simple arteriovenous fistulae, with a saphenous vein transplant fistula or fistulae constructed with prosthetic materials. With the latter two techniques the stenosis usually develops at the venous anastomosis.

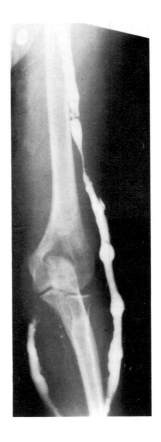

25

26

Physiological effects

The stenosis slows blood flow to such an extent that blood, already having passed through the dialysis machine, is recycled through the dialyser several times before it leaves the arterialized vein through the stenosis. The percentage recirculation can be calculated by means of the formula:

$$\text{Percentage recirculation} = \frac{BUN_P - BUN_A}{BUN_P - BUN_V} \times 100$$

where BUN = blood urea nitrogen concentration
        A = arterial line
        V = venous line
        P = peripheral venous

Arteriovenous fistulae for haemodialysis should not have more than 10 per cent recirculation. Correction of the problem may be achieved surgically by application of a vein or prosthetic patch to widen the stenosis, by reimplantation of the vein or prosthesis, or by use of a 'jump' graft. Vein is the preferred material.

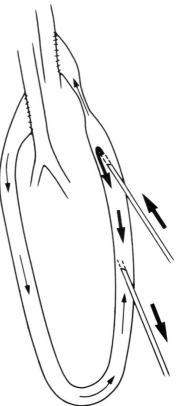

26

Venous hypertension of hand

Venous hypertension of the hand may develop after construction of a radiocephalic fistula. The hand becomes oedematous, uncomfortable and susceptible to infections after minor injuries. The incidence of this problem can be minimized by the use of a side-to-end arteriovenous anastomosis. However, if large enough collateral veins with incompetent valves develop, then symptomatic venous hypertension can occur even with a side-to-end anastomosis. The proper treatment is ligation of the collateral veins.

Conclusion

This consideration of vascular access has not been exhaustive. There are many devices which have been promoted for the purpose. Some are occasionally useful, many are costly, and all are composed of prosthetic or other foreign material. The Allen-Brown and Thomas shunts are Silastic tubes bonded to Dacron prostheses which can be used to construct a shunt without ligation of a vessel. The Hemasite device and others like it are prostheses with a chronic percutaneous extension through which vascular access can be 'atraumatically' achieved. Expanded polytetrafluoroethylene, bovine arterial, fetal umbilical venous, and Dardik grafts have been used in place of autogenous vein for construction of arteriovenous fistulae, but the authors believe that autogenous vein remains by far the best tissue for construction of long-term vascular access.

References

1. Kolff, W. J. First clinical experience with the artificial kidney. Annals of Internal Medicine 1965; 62: 608–619

2. Quinton, W. E., Dillar, D., Scribner, B. H. Cannulation of blood vessels for prolonged hemodialysis. Transactions of the American Society of Artificial Internal Organs 1960; 6: 104–113

3. Brescia, M. J., Cimino, J. E., Appel, K., Hurwich, B. J. Chronic hemodialysis using venipuncture and a surgically created arteriovenous fistula. New England Journal of Medicine 1966; 275: 1089–1092

Index

Abdominal aorta
  anastomosis to common femoral artery, 131, 132
  anastomosis to iliac artery, 130
  aneurysms
    anaesthesia for, 124
    anastomoses in, 129, 130
    infrarenal, 125
    operative procedures, 123, 125
    postoperative care, 134
    preoperative considerations, 124
    removal of content, 128
    suprarenal, 133
    symptoms, 123
    treatment of, 123–135
  arteriovenous fistula with common iliac vein, 234
  arteriovenous fistula with inferior vena cava, 234
  exposure of, 143
    below renal vessels, 52, 53
    extraperitoneal, 53
    transperitoneal, 52
  high proximal control of, 126
  infrarenal control of, 127
  operations on
    causing injury to iliac vein, 233
    causing injury to inferior vena cava, 233
    suprarenal, endarterectomy of, 150
Abdominal lymphatics, anatomy and pathology, 368
Acrocyanosis, 394
Adams-DeWeese clip, 326, 328
Amaurosis fugax, 73, 92
Ambulatory venous pressures, 260
Amputations, 398–414
  above knee, 409
  arm, 398
  below knee, 405
  finger, 412
  immediate casting in, 399
  indications for, 399
  leg, 398
    levels of, 398

Amputations (cont.)
  risk from arterial ligation, 229
  technical considerations, 399
  thumb, 412
  toes, 400, 401
  transmetatarsal, 403
Anastomoses, 63–72
  Blalock sutures in, 67
  end-to-end by modified Carrel method, 65
  to include plaques, 69
Aneurysms
  abdominal aorta, 125–135
    anaesthesia for, 124
    operative procedures, 125
    postoperative care, 134
    preoperative considerations, 124
    symptoms, 123
  anastomotic, 209
  aortic arch, 111
  atherosclerotic, in femoral artery, 208
  cirsoid, resection of, 248
  coeliac artery, 213
  descending thoracic aorta, 111, 119
  extracranial carotid artery, 211
  false, to femoral artery, 237
  femoral artery, 208–209
  following aortofemoral grafting, 209
  hepatic artery, 212
  infrarenal abdominal aorta, 125
  intrathoracic
    coronary bypass with coronary perfusion in, 112, 116
    postoperative care, 122
    preoperative considerations, 111
    treatment of, 111
  mycotic, causing arteriovenous fistulae, 239
  peripheral arterial, 207–213
  popliteal artery, 210–211
  renal artery, 213
  splenic artery, 212
  superior mesenteric artery, 213

Aneurysms (*cont.*)
  thoracic aortic
    diagnosis, 105
    indication for operation, 105
    postoperative care, 110
    preoperative considerations, 105
    prosthesis, 108, 110
    reapproximation of aorta, 107
    types I and II, 106
    type III, 109
    valve replacement, 106
  thoracoabdominal, 122
    postoperative care, 122
    preoperative considerations, 111
    treatment of, 111
  vertebral artery, 212
  visceral artery, 212
Angiography
  operative, 70–72
  postreconstruction completion, 72
  prereconstruction, 71
Angioplasty
  complications of, 35
  dilatation and balloon size, 25
  femoral, 29
  iliac, 25
  pathophysiology of, 25
  patient selection, 25
  percutaneous, in treatment of peripheral vascular disease, 24
  results of, 34
  run-off vessels, 34
  technique, 25, 26
Ankle
  blood vessels, arteriography of, 16
  venous drainage of, 310
Ankle flare, 311
  in varicose veins, 271
Ankle-brachial index, 6, 7
Ankle-perforating veins
  anatomy of, 313
  incompetence of, 311
  involvement in deep vein thrombosis, 312
  ligation of, 310–317
    extrafascial operation, 314
    indications for, 311
    postoperative care, 316
    preoperative preparation, 312
    subfascial operation, 315
    technique, 313
    wound closure, 316
  location of, 313
Anterior compartment syndrome, 416
Aorta
  abdominal (*see* Abdominal aorta)
  anastomosis, in renal artery construction, 170
  aneurysms, associated with aortic valve insufficiency, 113
  approach to, 137
    thoracoabdominal retroperitoneal, 163
  direct puncture of, 21
  embolectomy, 203
  embolus, 203
  exposure of, 113, 138
    above renal vessels, 49
  extended retroperitoneal approach, 149
  hypoplasia, 137
  innominate bypass, 93, 94
  insertion of grafts in, 107, 109
  occlusive disease
    reconstruction in, 136
    thromboendarterectomy, 137
  reapproximation of, 107
  to superior mesenteric and coeliac artery bypass, 161

Aorta, ascending, aneurysms, 111, 112
Aorta, descending, exposure of, 37, 40, 109
Aorta, infra-abdominal, aneurysms, 125
Aorta, suprarenal, approach to, 149
Aorta, thoracic
  aneurysms, 104, 112
    diagnosis of, 105
    indications for operation, 105
    postoperative care, 110
    treatment, 104
  exposure of, 40
  suturing, 111
Aortic arch
  aneurysm, 111, 116
  exposure of, 40
  occlusion of
    operations for, 93, 103
    preoperative considerations, 92
    treatment of, 92–103
Aortic bifurcation, 53
Aortic bypass grafts
  for aortoiliac reconstruction, 136
  reimplantation of visceral vessels to, 165
Aortic valve
  insufficiency, 113
  replacement of, 106
Aortocarotid bypass, for carotid artery occlusion, 101
Aortofemoral bypass grafts
  anastomosis, 145, 146, 147
  in aortoiliac reconstruction, 143
  clotting graft, 144
  flushing graft, 148
Aortofemoral grafting, aneurysm following, 209
Aortography, 21
Aortoiliac bypass graft
  in aortoiliac reconstruction, technique, 143
  clotting graft, 144
  flushing graft, 148
Aortoiliac obstruction, 179
Aortoiliac reconstruction, 136–151
  aortofemoral bypass graft in, 143
  aortoiliac bypass graft in, 143
  bypass grafts in
    anastomosis, 145, 146, 147
    closure, 148
    flushing graft, 148
    by renal vein in, 144
  complications, 151
  eversion endarterectomy in, 141
  mortality rate, 136
  postoperative care, 151
  reimplantation of inferior mesenteric artery in, 149
  results of, 136
  semi-closed endarterectomy in, 141, 142
  thromboendarterectomy and bypass graft in, 136
  vasculogenic impotence after, 151
Aortoinnominate bypass operation, 93, 94
Aortorenal artery graft, in renal artery reconstruction, 169
Arm
  amputations, 398
  chronic swelling of, 425
  intermittent compression symptoms, 263
  intermittent venous obstruction, 269
  lymphatic channels, 366
  lymphoedema, 377
    surgical procedures, 375
  oedema of, 318, 378
Arterial circulation, peripheral, evaluation of, 2
Arterial disease, in small vessels, 4
Arterial pulse volume recording, 4
Arterial embolectomy, 201–206
  intraoperative evaluation, 206

Arterial embolectomy (*cont.*)
   postoperative care, 205
   preoperative considerations, 201
   preparation for, 202
Arterial reconstruction, below the inguinal ligament, 183–200
   anastomoses, 189
   autogenous venous bypass procedures, 185
   choice of procedure, 184
   completion angiogram, 190
   distal bypass, 197
   exposure of arteries, 187
   femoropopliteal thromboendarterectomy with patch graft, 192
   indications for, 184
   in situ saphenous vein technique, 197
   peroneal artery grafting, 199
   postoperative care, 200
   preoperative considerations, 184
   preparation of saphenous vein, 185, 189
   profundoplasty, 195
   tunnelling the vein, 188
   umbilical vein as graft, 191
   use of prosthetic bypass grafts, 191
Arteries
   anastomosis, 63–72
     end-to-end by modified Carrel method, 65
   clamping, release of, 69
   embolism, symptoms of, 201
   end-to-end suture, including plaques, 68, 69
   exposure of, 36–62
     indications and contraindications, 36
     in injury, 220
     postoperative care, 62
     for vertebral artery surgery, 86
   fixation of plaques, 68, 69
   grafts, invagination of, 69
   iatrogenic injuries, 229
   injuries to (*see also specific arteries*), 219–228
     anastomoses in, 220, 221
     clinical evaluation, 219
     principles of repair, 220
   lateral suture, 64
   ligation of, risks in, 229
   occlusion
     diagnosis, 2
     localizing site of, 7
   recanalization, 32
   spasm, in percutaneous catheterization, 23
   stenosis
     localizing site of, 7
     ultrasonic diagnosis, 2, 3
   suturing, 63–72
     Blalock, 67
     diseases tissue, 68
     everting mattress, 66
     indications and contraindications, 63
     interrupted, 66
     lateral, 64
     materials, 63
Arteriography, 15–23
   carotid, 22
   catheters, needles and cannulae for, 16
     insertion, 18, 19
   contrast materials for, 16
     complications from, 23
   equipment for, 15
   false aneurysm of femoral artery following, 237
   femoral artery, 17
   percutaneous catheterization, 17
   preoperative preparation, 17
   pressure injectors for, 15
Arteriosclerosis, peripheral, arteriography for, 16

Arteriovenous fistulae
   acquired, 239–245
     complications of, 245
     exploring fistula, 242
     indications and contraindications for operation, 239
     postoperative care, 245
     preoperative considerations, 239
     quadruple ligation in, 242
     repair by excision and anastomosis, 244
     repair by excision and grafting, 244
     simple repair, 243
     technique of repair, 240
     transvenous repair, 243
   caused by lumbar disc operation, 234
   complications of, 444
   congenital, 246–252
     inoperable lesions, 252
     ligation of afferent arteries, 250
     postoperative care, 252
     preoperative considerations, 247
     symptoms, 246
     therapeutic alternatives, 247
     transcatheter vessel embolization in, 251
     types, 246
   construction of, 435
   dilated veins with, 271
   for haemodialysis, 61, 435
     complications, 444
     distal ischaemia from, 444
     failure of, 444
     heart failure from, 444
     procedures, 436
     radial artery exposure for, 46
     stenosis at venous outflow, 446
   iatrogenic, 229
   in venous reconstruction, 340
Ascending thoracic aorta, aneurysms of, 112
Ascites, in portal hypertension, 343
Atherosclerosis, surgery for, 62
Athlete's hypertrophic veins, 271
Autosympathectomy, 394
Axillary artery
   catheterization of, 20
   exposure of, 42, 43, 180
Axilloaxillary bypass operations, 93, 96
   technique, 100
Axillofemoral bypass, 42, 179

Basilic vein transposition fistula, 441
Blalock suture, 67
Bleeding oesophageal varices, 342
Blood flow
   diagnosis of, 15
   measurement of, 2
   speed of, 3
   turbulence, 3
Blood vessels
   exposure of (*see also specific vessels*), 36–62
     contraindications, 36
     indications for, 36
     postoperative care, 62
   injuries of (*see also specific vessels*), 219–228
     iatrogenic, 229–238
     mechanism of, 219
     principles of repair, 220
Bowel gangrene, 153
Brachial artery
   approach to, 230
   damage from fracture, 45
   exposure of, 44
     at elbow, 45

Brachial artery (*cont.*)
   high bifurcation of, 44
   thrombosis, after coronary angiography, 230–231
Brachial plexus injury, from catheterization, 20
Brachiocephalic fistula, 440
Brain, protection in carotid endarterectomy, 74
Brain stem ischaemia, symptoms of, 82
Brescia-Cimino shunts, 435
Budd-Chiari syndrome, 342, 343

Calf veins
   incompetence of, 312
   phlebography, in thrombosis, 266
Cardiopulmonary bypass
   excision of aortic valve, 114
   with coronary perfusion, 112
Carotid arteries, common
   embolization, 92
   exposure of, 47
   injuries to, 222
   operations for occlusion, 101
Carotid artery
   anastomosis
      to innominate artery, 95
      to subclavian artery, 98, 102
      to vertebral artery, 90
   arteriography, 22
   bifurcation, 48
   bypass to subclavian artery, 97
   Doppler examination, 9, 10, 11
   endarterectomy (*see* Carotid endarterectomy)
   evaluation of, 12
   extracranial aneurysms, 211
   imaging, 13
   injuries to, 222–223
   mobilization in endarterectomy, 75
   occlusion, 434
   percutaneous catheterization, 20, 22
   stenosis, 12
      restenosis following surgery, 13
      strokes and, 13
   trial occlusion, 75
Carotid artery, internal
   blood flow, 12
   Doppler examination, 9
   endarterectomy, 77
   exposure of, 48
   injuries to, 223
   occlusions of, 11
   stenosis, 9, 73
Carotid bifurcation
   arteriography of, 17
   atherosclerotic disease of, 73
   bruits over, 73
   carotid body tumours and, 430
   disease at, 12
   Doppler examination, 10
   exposure of, 74
Carotid body tumours, excision of, 430–434
   insertion of shunt, 433
   postoperative care, 434
   technique, 431
   vein graft interposition, 433
Carotid bruits, 13, 73
Carotid endarterectomy, 73–81
   cerebral protection, 74
   closure of arteriotomy, 79
   completion of, 77
   complications of, 81
   distal tacking, 78
   exposure of bifurcation, 74

Carotid endarterectomy (*cont.*)
   follow-up, 13
   hypertension following, 81
   incision for, 74, 76
   indications for, 73
   insertion of shunt, 78
   mobilization of arteries, 75
   mobilization of plaque, 76
   patch graft, 80
   peripheral nerve deficits following, 81
   postoperative care, 81
   preoperative care, 73
   removal of arterial shunt, 80
   removal of debris, 79
   restenosis following, 13
   technique, 74
   trial occlusion in, 75
Carotid occlusion, with vertebral artery disease, 83
Carotid plaques, 82
Carotid stenosis, associated with vertebral artery disease, 83
Catheters, arterial, 16
   insertion of, 18, 19
   for pressure monitoring, 19
Causalgia, 386, 394
Cellulitis, in lymphoedema, 377
Cephalic vein, repair of brachial artery with, 231
Cerebral ischaemia, 82
Cerebral perfusion, in operations for aortic arch aneurysm, 116
Cerebrovascular circulation, evaluation of, 9
Cerebrovascular disease, diagnosis, 13
Cervical ganglions, 386
Cervical sympathetic outflow, 386
Charles procedure for lymphoedema, 378, 380, 381
Chemodectomas (*see also* Carotid body tumours), 430
Chylo-ascites, 369
Chyloedema, 365, 369
Cirsoid aneurysm of scalp, resection of, 248
Claudication, 7, 136, 183
Clavicle, excision of, 322
Coeliac artery
   aneurysm, 213
   aortic bypass, 161
   chronic occlusion, 160
   reconstruction of, 152
Colon, ischaemia, 152
Common carotid arteries
   embolization, 92
   exposure of, 47
   injuries to, 222
   occlusion, operations for, 101
Common carotid bifurcation, 48
Common femoral artery
   anastomosis to abdominal aorta, 131, 132
   antegrade puncture of, 28
   embolectomy, 203
   evaluation of, 2, 6
   exposure of, 55, 185, 187
   injury during ligation of saphenous vein, 232
   pulses in, 5
   reconstruction, 71
Common iliac artery, exposure of, 54
Common iliac vein, injury to from operation on abdominal aorta, 233
Coronary angiography, brachial artery thrombosis following, 230
Coronary artery disease, 13

Deep calf veins, incompetence of, 312
Deep vein thrombosis
   acute, 255
   diagnosis, 253, 255
      Doppler ultrasound in, 258

Deep vein thrombosis (*cont.*)
   perforating veins in, 312
   phlebography in, 263
Dermal back flow, 357
Descending aorta, exposure of, 37
Decending thoracic aorta
   aneurysms of, 119
   exposure of, 40
Diabetes mellitus
   amputations in, 399
   arteriography in, 23
   autosympathectomy in, 394
   small vessel disease in, 4
Digital artery occlusion, 386
Digital intravenous technique, 83
Distal pulses, evaluation of, 5
Doppler carotid imaging, 11
Doppler examination frequency analysis, 10
Doppler spectral analysis, 3
Doppler ultrasound in diagnosis, 2–3
   cerebrovascular evaluation by, 9
   supraorbital, 9
   in venous disease, 258
Dotter procedure, 24

Embolectomy, 201–206
   intraoperative evaluation, 205
   postoperative care, 206
   preoperative considerations, 201
   preparation for, 202
   suturing, 64
Endarterectomy
   carotid, 73–81
   eversion, in aortoiliac reconstrustion, 141
   semi-closed, 141, 142
   of suprarenal abdominal aorta, 150
   transaortic, 163
Erythrocyanosis, 394
Esmarch's bandage, in repair of arteriovenous fistulae, 240
Exercise testing, 6
External carotid artery
   endarterectomy, 77
   exposure of, 48
External iliac artery, extraperitoneal exposure of, 54
Extracorporeal circulation, exposure of ascending aorta in, 37
Eye pulsation, 12

Fasciotomy, 415–421
   four-compartment, 419
   indications for, 415
   lateral compartment, 418
   limited, 416
   operations, 416
   posterior compartment, 416
   postoperative care, 421
   preoperative considerations, 415
Femoral angioplasty, 29
Femoral artery
   anastomosis to abdominal aorta, 131, 132
   aneurysms, 208–209
      atherosclerotic, 208
      treatment of, 209
   catheterization of, 17
   exposure of, 180, 192
      in Hunter's canal, 57
   false aneurysm, after arteriography, 237
   gunshot wounds, 227
   identification of, 17
   occlusion
      angioplasty for, 32, 34

Femoral artery (*cont.*)
   occlusion (*cont.*)
      results of treatment, 34
      treatment, 28
   oedema following surgery of, 62
   reconstruction, 71
   stenosis, angioplasty for, 30
Femoral artery, common
   antegrade puncture of, 28
   embolectomy, 203
   exposure of, 55, 185, 187
   injury during ligation of saphenous vein, 232
Femoral veins
   bypassing, 338
   exposure of, 331
   interruption of, 331
      complications, 333
      mortality, 333
      partial, 331
      preoperative preparation, 326
      results, 333
      site of, 326
      types of, 326
   ligation of, preventing pulmonary embolism, 325
   partial interruption, 331
   phlebography, 266, 267
   thrombectomy, 321
   thrombosis, 266
   valves in, 339
Femorofemoral bypass grafts, 179, 181
Femoropopliteal grafting, aneurysms following, 209
Femoropopliteal occlusive disease, 183
Femoropopliteal thromboendarterectomy, in arterial
      reconstruction, 192
^{125}I-Fibrinogen scanning, in venous disease, 259
Fibroedema, 370
Finger, amputation of, 412
Foot
   amputations of, 399
   postoperative oedema, 62
   transmetatarsal amputation, 403
Frontal artery, Doppler examination, 9

Ganglion blocks, 383, 384
Gangrene, 399
   amputation of toe for, 400
   in iliofemoral venous thrombosis, 318
Gonadal dysgenesis-Turner syndrome, 365
Grafts, invagination of, 69

Haemangioma
   of knee, *en bloc* excision, 249
   steriods in, 247
Haematoma, from vascular access procedures, 444
Haemodialysis (*see also* Vascular access)
   arteriovenous fistula for, 61, 435
      complications, 444
   exposure of radial artery, 46
   radiocephalic fistula, 433, 437
Haemorrhage
   following repair of arteriovenous fistulae, 245
   from percutaneous catheterization, 23
   postoperative, 62
Hand
   amputations of, 412
   venous hypertension of, 447
Heart failure, following repair of arteriovenous fistula, 245
Hepatic artery, aneurysms, 212
Hepatorenal graft, in renal artery reconstruction, 173
Horner's syndrome, 393

Hyperhidrosis, 386, 394
Hypertension
    in aortic aneurysm, 105
    following carotid endarterectomy, 81
    following renal artery reconstruction 177
    from renal artery stenosis, 166
    leg ulcers and, 302
    portal (see Portal hypertension)
    in thoracic aortic aneurysm, 119
    venous, 447
Hypoglossal nerve, damage to, 81

Iliac angioplasty, 25
Iliac artery
    anastomosis to aorta, 130
    approach to, 137
    embolectomy, 204
    exposure of, 53, 54, 138
        extraperitoneal, 54
    occlusions of, 181
        angioplasty for, 25
        reconstruction in, 136
        thromboendarterectomy, 137
    stenosis, 34
Iliac vein
    obstruction of, ligation for, 312
    thromboectomy, 320
Iliac vein, common
    arteriovenous fistula with abdominal aorta, 234
    injury during operation on abdominal aorta, 233
Iliac vein, internal, incompetence, 272
Iliofemoral junction, exposure of, 56
Iliofemoral venous thrombosis, 318
    phlebography, 267
    thrombectomy for, 318, 319, 324
Impedance plethysmography, 254
Impotence, 8
Inferior cervical ganglion block, 383
Inferior mesenteric artery
    ligation of, 127
    reimplantation in aortoiliac reconstruction, 149
Inferior vena cava
    approach to, 327
    exposure of, 52, 327
    injuries to, 224–226
        during operation on abdominal aorta, 233
    interruption of, 325, 327–330
        complications, 333
        extraluminal, 327
        indication for, 325
        intraluminal, 329
        mortality rate, 333
        passage of clip, 328
        postoperative care, 332
        preoperative preparation, 326
        results, 333
        site of, 325
        type of, 326
        umbrella technique, 329, 330
Infrarenal abdominal aorta, aneurysms of, 125
Inguinal lymph nodes
    anatomy, 366
    lymphography, 359
Innominate artery
    embolization, 92
    exposure of, 38
    lesions of, operations for, 93
Internal carotid artery
    exposure of, 48
    injuries to, 223
    stenosis of, 73

Internal iliac vein incompetence, 272
Internal jugular vein, exposure of, 47
Intestinal ischaemia, 152
    acute, 153
    chronic, 160
Intestines, lymphatics, 368, 369
Intrathoracic aneurysms
    coronary bypass with coronary perfusion in, 112, 116
    postoperative care, 122
    preoperative considerations, 111
    treatment of, 111
Ischaemia, evaluation of, 7
Ischaemic muscle necrosis, 62

Jugular vein, internal, exposure of, 47

Kidney, protection against ischaemic injury, 166
Klippel-Trenaunay syndrome, 271
Knee, haemangioma of, en bloc excision, 249

Laboratory examinations
    arterial disease, 1–14
    interpretations, 7
    venous disease, 253–262
Lateral cutaneous nerve of thigh, 422
Left subclavian artery
    endarterectomy, 99
    thoracic part, exposure of, 39
Leg
    amputations
        above knee, 409
        below knee, 405
        casts for, 399, 408
        indications for, 399
        postoperative care, 408, 411
        selection of level, 399
        technical amputations, 399
    anterior compartment syndrome, 416
    aplasia of lymphatic channels, 367
    bilateral hyperplasia of lymph vessels, 363
    chronic ulcers of, 301–309
        basic principles of treatment, 302
        cleansing, 303
        debridement, 303
        diagnosis, 301
        dressing, 304, 305
        glycerin and ichthyol in, 307
        hypertension and, 302
        infection and, 302
        injection with treatment, 309
        ischaemic element, 302
        medicated bandages in, 308
        pinch grafts in, 307
        in post-thrombotic syndrome, 309
        povidone-iodine in, 306
        prevention of recurrence, 309
        stasis in, 302
        sulphadiazine cream in, 306
        treatment of, 302
    chyloedema, 369
    decompression of, compartments in fasciotomy, 419
    fasciotomy, 416
        anterior compartment, 416
        four-compartment, 419
        lateral compartment, 416
        postoperative care, 421
        posterior compartment, 416
    lymphatics of, anatomy, 366
    lymph nodes, 367

Leg (*cont.*)
  lymphoedema, 377
    surgical procedures for, 372
  oedema of, 356
    in megalymphatics, 362
    in pelvic obstruction, 361
    postoperative, 62
  soft tissue injury, 419
  ulcers, complicating varicose veins, 302
  venous drainage of, 263
Limb pressures, segmental, 2
Long saphenous vein, incompetence, 277
  ligation for, 311
Lumbar disc operation, causing vascular injury, 234
Lumbar ganglion block, 384
Lumbar sympathectomy, 394–397
  anaesthesia for, 394
  operation, 395
  postoperative care, 397
  preoperative considerations, 394
Lung, postoperative care of, 134
Lymphangiography, 370
Lymphatics
  anatomy and pathology, 366
    abdominal, 368
    thoracic, 368
  demonstration of, 357
  direct operations on, 365–376
  hypoplasia, 367
Lymphatic channels, aplasia of, 367
Lymph nodes, 367
  in primary lymphoedema, 367
Lymphoedema, 365
  aetiology of, 365
  cellulitis in, 377
  classification of, 365
  pneumatic compression in, 371, 377
  primary, 356, 365, 377
    lymph nodes in, 367
    lymphography in, 360
  secondary, 365, 377
    surgical procedures, 370
  surgical procedures, 370–375, 377–381
    anaesthesia for, 371, 378
    buried dermis flap procedure, 378
    excision and skin graft (Charles), 378, 380, 381
    immediate preoperative measures, 371
    instruments for, 371
    lymphovenous shunts, 370
    postoperative care, 375, 381
    preoperative, 370, 378
    results, 375, 381
    selection of patients, 370
    staged subcutaneous excision beneath intact
      skin flaps, 379
    techniques, 372
    true lymphovenous anastomosis, 375
Lymphoedema tarda, 365, 370
Lymphography, 356–363
  anaesthesia for, 357
  cannulation and injection, 358
  complications, 359
  demonstration of lymphatics, 357
  dermal back flow, 357
  equipment, 356
  inguinal node, 359
  megalymphatics, 362
  position of patient, 357
  preparation for, 356
  technique, 357
Lymphovenous shunts, 370
Lymph vessels, bilateral hyperplasia of, 363

Mediastinum, entering, 37
Megalymphatics, 362
Meralgia paraesthetica, 422–423
Mesenteric arteries
  chronic occlusion, 160
  reconstruction of, 152–165
  reimplantation during aortoiliac reconstruction, 28
Mesenteric artery, superior
  acute occlusion, 153
  aneurysm, 213
  aortic bypass, 161
  embolectomy
    distal approach, 158
    proximal approach, 155
    special considerations, 159
  exposure of, 51
Mesenteric lymph nodes, 369
Monckeberg's calcinosis, 2
Muscle
  ischaemic necrosis, 62
  painful swellings of, 415
Mycotic aneurysms, causing arteriovenous fistulae, 239

Occlusion, localizing site of, 7
Ocularplethysmography, 12
Ocularpneumoplethysmography, 12, 13
Oedema
  following interuption of vena cava or femoral vein, 333
  in iliofemoral venous thrombosis, 318
  leg, 356
  in leg ulcers, 302
  postmastectomy, 378
  postoperative, 62
  in subclavian thrombosis, 318
  in venous ulcers, 301
Oesophageal varices, 342

Paget-Schroetter syndrome, 425
Paralytic ileus, postoperative, 134
Pelvic obstruction, lymphography in, 361
Percutaneous catheterization, 17
  complications, 23
  haemorrhage from, 23
  thrombosis following, 23
  in vascular access, 436
Percutaneous transluminal angioplasty, 24–35
  complications of, 35
  results of, 34
Perforating veins, incompetent, 292
  ligation of, 283
Peripheral arterial aneurysms, management of, 207–213
Peripheral arterial disease, amputations in, 399
Peripheral arteriosclerosis, arteriography for, 16
Peripheral circulation
  evaluation of, 2
  occlusive disease, 24
  stenosis of, 24
Peripheral nerve deficits, following carotid endarterectomy, 81
Peripheral vascular disease, 13
  percutaneous transluminal angioplasty in, 24–35
Peritonitis, 179
Peroneal artery
  embolectomy, 205
  exposure of, 199
  grafting to, 199
Phlebography, 263–270
  ascending, 370
  complications of, 270
  indications for, 263
  of lower limb, 264

Phlebography (*cont.*)
  normal, 265, 268
  upper extremity, 268
Phleborheography, 256
Photoplethysmography, with arterial compression, 9
Plantar arch, arterial supply to, 5
Plaque, compression of, 25
Plethysmography, 4, 254
  techniques, 12
Polytetrafluorethylene as bypass graft, 191
Popliteal artery
  anatomy of, 214
  aneurysms, 210–211
  arteriography of, 16
  dilatation of vessels below, 34
  embolectomy, 204
  entrapment syndrome, 214–218
    clinical signs, 215
    diagnosis, 216
    operation for, 217
    results of treatment, 218
    types of, 215
  exposure of, 58, 185, 187, 192
    extension of, 61
    medial approach, 58, 59
    posterior approach, 60
  occlusion, 183
  oedema following surgery of, 62
  stenosis of, 34
Popliteal veins
  bypassing, 338
  valves, 339
Portal hypertension, 342–355
  arterialization of portal vein for, 353
  causes of, 342
  cavamesenteric shunts, 350–352
    end-to-side, 350
    H graft mesocaval shunt, 351
  portacaval shunts, 344–349
    central splenorenal, 348
    end-to-side, 344
    H graft interposition, 347
    side-to-side, 347
  preserving portal flow, 353
  selection of procedure, 343
  selective splenorenal shunts in, 353
  shunting in, 342
    selection of patients for, 343
Portal vein
  arterialization of, 353
  H graft interposition in, 247
Posterior splanchnic block, 386
Posterior tibial artery, exposure of, 185
Postphlebitic disease, venous reconstruction in, 334, 335
Postphlebitic limbs, 292
Postphlebitic syndrome, 292
Postreconstruction completion angiography, 72
Post-thrombotic syndrome, 273, 283
  ulcers in, 301, 302, 309
Pregnancy, varicose veins in, 272, 292
Prereconstruction angiography, 71
Profunda femoris artery, occlusive disease, 195
Profundoplasty, 195–196
Prosthetic bypass grafts, 191
Proximal popliteal artery, exposure of, 192
Pulmonary embolism, 325
  following interruption of vena cava, 333
  ligation of femoral veins preventing, 325
Pulmonary oil embolism, following lymphography, 359
Pulse volume recorder, 4
Pulses, following operations of vessels, 62

Radial artery
  exposure of, at wrist, 46
  fistula, 443
Radiocephalic arteriovenous fistula, 435, 437
  anastomosis, 439
  venous hypertension of hand following, 447
Radiotherapy, in arteriovenous fistulae, 247
Raynaud's phenomenon, 386, 394
  laboratory evaluation, 8
Recanalization of arteries, 32
Renal artery
  anastomosis, in reconstruction, 171, 172
  aneurysm, 213
    reconstruction in, 177
  endarterectomy, 176
  exposure of, 49, 168
  graft from aorta to, 169
  main stenosis, 169
  reconstruction, 166–178
    anastomosis in, 171, 172
    in aneurysm of, 177
    aortic anastomosis in, 170
    aortorenal artery graft in, 169
    bilateral stenosis, 176
    dissection of saphenous vein, 169
    exposure, 168
    hypertension following, 177
    intraoperative care, 166
    in main artery stenosis, 169
    operative techniques, 167
    postoperative care, 177
    preoperative assessment, 166
    reimplantation of renal artery in, 173
    renal endarterectomy in, 176
    results of, 178
    in segmental stenosis, 174
    selection of cases, 166
    splenorenal anastomosis in, 172
    stenosis, 166
    with three or more branches, 175
Renal failure, complicating arteriography in diabetics, 23
Renal transplantation, 55
Renal vein, in aortoiliac and aortofemoral bypass graft operation, 144
Rest pain, 399
Reversible ischaemic neurological deficit, 73
Rheumatoid arthritis, leg ulcers and, 302
Ribs, resection of, in thoracic outlet syndrome, 426
Right subclavian artery, exposure, 38
Road traffic accidents, 219
Run-off vessels, angioplasty of, 34

Saphenofemoral junction
  direction of, 289
  exposure of, 279
  ligation, 279
Saphenopopliteal bypass grafts, 338
Saphenous vein
  dissection for renal artery graft, 169
  incompetence, 277
  in situ technique for grafting, 197
  ligation, injury to common femoral artery during, 232
  preparation for bypass, 185, 189, 197
Saphenous vein, long, incompetence, 277
Saphenous vein, short, incompetence, 286
Saphenous vein transplant fistula, 443
Saphenovariax, 291
Scalp, cirsoid aneurysm of, resection, 248
Sclerotherapy (*see also* Varicose veins, injection treatment), in arteriovenous fistulae, 247

Scribner shunt, 435
Segmental limb pressures, 6
Seldinger percutaneous catheterization, 17
Sensory impairment, postoperative, 62
Skin, numbness of, 62
Skin temperature, after clamping arterial supply, 62
Small meal syndrome, 160
Splenic artery, aneurysms, 212
Splenorenal anastomosis, in renal artery reconstruction, 172
Splenorenal shunts, 353
Stellate ganglion block, 383
Stenosis
    localizing site of, 7
    ultrasonic diagnosis, 2, 3
Strokes, 73
    carotid artery atherosclerosis in, 73
    carotid stenosis and, 13
    from ligation of neck arteries, 229
    unstable, 73
Subarachnoid haemorrhage, 166
Subclavian to carotid bypass, for carotid artery occlusion, 101
Subclavian artery
    anastomosis
        to carotid artery, 98
        with vertebral artery, 89
    atherosclerosis of, 83
    to distal carotid artery bypass, 102
    exposure of, 388
        cervical part, 40
    left
        endarterectomy, 99
        exposure of, 39
    occlusive disease of branches, 92–103
        operations for, 93, 96
        preoperative considerations, 92
    percutaneous catheterization, 20
    right, exposure of, 38
Subclavian steal, 92
Subclavian vein
    exposure of, 323
    occlusion of, 269
    percutaneous catheterization of, 436
    thrombosis, thrombectomy for, 318, 322, 324
Sulphadiazine cream, in leg ulcers, 306
Superficial femoral artery
    exposure of, in Hunter's canal, 57
    occlusions, treatment, 32, 34
    stenosis, angioplasty for, 30, 34
Superior mesenteric artery
    acute occlusion, 153
    aneurysm, 213
    aortic bypass, 161
    embolectomy
        distal approach, 158
        proximal approach, 155
        special considerations, 159
    exposure of, 51
Supracondylar fracture, damaging brachial artery, 45
Supraorbital Doppler examination, 9
Suprarenal abdominal aorta
    aneurysms, 133
    endarterectomy of, 150
Suprarenal cava injuries, 225
Sutures and suturing, 63–72
    Blalock, 67
    diseased arteries, 68
    end-to-end, including plaques, 68, 69
    everting mattress, 66
    interrupted, 66
    materials, 63
Sympathectomy, 382
    lumbar, 394–397

Sympathectomy (cont.)
    lumbar (cont.)
        anaesthesia for, 394
        operation, 395
        postoperative care, 397
        preoperative considerations, 394
    of upper extremity, 386–393
        cervical approach, 387, 393
        control of haemorrhage, 392
        exposure of sympathetic chain, 390, 391
        first rib resection, 390
        identification of sympathetic chain, 389
        indications of, 386
        operations for, 387
        postoperative complications, 393
        regeneration after, 386
        third interspace, 391
        transaxillary approach, 390, 391
Sympathetic ganglion block, 382–385
    apparatus for, 382
    indications for, 382
    operations for, 383
    preoperative considerations, 382
Symptoms, history of, 5

Thigh
    chyloedema, 369
    lateral cutaneous nerve of, neuritis, 422
Thoracic aorta
    aneurysm
        diagnosis, 105
        indication for operation, 105
        postoperative care, 110
        preoperative considerations, 105
        prosthesis, 108, 110
        replacement valve, 106
        treatment, 104
        types I and II, 106
        type III, 109
    ascending
        aneurysms of, 112
    descending
        aneurysm, 111, 119
        exposure of, 40
    suturing, 111
Thoracic duct, 368
Thoracic lymphatics, anatomy and pathology, 368
Thoracic outlet syndrome, 424–429
    definition, 424
    diagnosis, 8, 425
    operations, 426
    postoperative care, 428
    results of treatment, 428
Thoracoabdominal aneurysm, 122
    postoperative care, 122
    preoperative considerations, 111
    treatment of, 111
Thrombectomy, venous, 318–324
thrombo-angiitis obliterans, 386
Thromboendarterectomy
    in aortoiliac reconstruction, 136, 139
    suturing in, 64
Thrombophlebitis, in sclerotherapy of varicose veins, 299, 300
Thumb, amputation, 412
Tibial arteries
    embolectomy, 205
    exposure of, 185, 188
        posterior, 61
Tibial grafts, 71

Toe
    amputations of, 400
        complete, 402
        postoperative care, 402, 404
        with metatarsal bone, 401
Transaortic endarterectomy, 163
Transient blindness, 73
Transient ischaemic attacks, 73, 92
Translumbar aortography, 21
Transmetatarsal amputation, 403

Ulcers, venous (see Venous ulcers)
Ulnar nerve conduction velocity, 425, 428
Ultrasound, B-mode, 13
Ultrasound scans
    of carotid arteries, 13
    in venous disease, 258
Umbilical vein graft, 184, 191
Upper thoracic ganglion block, 384

Varicose veins
    ankle flare in, 271
    classification of, 271
    history taking, 292
    incompetent perforating veins, 292
    indications for operation, 273
    injection treatment, 273, 291–300
        advantages of, 300
        bandaging, 298
        contraindications, 292
        equipment, 293
        injection of sclerosant, 297
        insertion of needle, 297
        inspection and palpation, 294
        intra-arterial injection of sclerosant, 390
        pain following, 300
        post-treatment, 300
        prevention of skin abrasion, 299
        principles, 292
        selection of sites, 296
        thrombophlebitis following, 299, 300
    operations for, 271–290
        anaesthesia, 275
        bandaging, 285
        complications, 289
        equipment, 275
        ligation for incompetent perforating veins, 283
        long saphenous incompetence, 277
        position of patient, 276
        postoperative care, 285
        saphenofemoral junction, 279
        for short saphenous vein incompetence, 286
        stripping saphenous vein, 280, 281
        vein stripping, 287
    phlebography, 263
    in pregnancy, 272, 292
    preoperative preparation, 274
    primary, 272
    recurrence at groin, 289
    sclerotherapy in, 273
    secondary, 273
    treatment, 273
    ulcers complicating, 302
Vascular access, 435–447
    arteriovenous fistula for, 435
        complications, 444
        failure of, 444
    banding of vein in, 445
    basilic vein transposition fistula, 441
    brachiocephalic fistula, 440

Vascular access (cont.)
    complications, 444
    distal ischaemia following, 444
    failure of fistula, 444
    heart failure from, 444
    loop fistula in, 443
    percutaneous catheterization of subclavian vein, 436
    procedures for, 436
    radial artery fistula in, 443
    radiocephalic fistula, 433, 437
        venous hypertension of hand following, 447
    saphenous vein transplant fistula, 443
    stenosis at venous outflow, 446
    venous hypertension of hand in, 447
Vascular injuries, 219–228
    clinical evaluation, 219
    iatrogenic, 229–238
Vascular malformations, 246, 247
Vasculogenic impotence, 8
Vasodilators, in percutaneous transluminal angioplasty, 35
Veins
    banding of, 445
    diseases of (see also Deep vein thrombosis, etc.)
        ambulatory venous pressures in, 260
        Doppler ultrasound in, 258
        ^{125}I-fibrinogen scanning in, 259
        phleborheography in, 256
        plethysmography in, 254
        role of vascular laboratory in, 253–262
    drainage, 291
    flow and pressure changes in, 291
    post-thrombotic changes, 267
    reconstruction, 334–341
        adjuvant arteriovenous fistula, 340
        anastomosis, 335
        basic principles of, 335
        cross-pubis (cross-over) bypass graft, 337
        free grafts, 336
        in situ saphenopopliteal bypass graft, 338
        operations, 336
        postoperative care, 341
        in postphlebotic disease, 334, 335
        preoperative considerations, 334
        selection of patients, 334
        spiral venous conduit construction in, 336
        in trauma, 334
        valve transposition, 339
    turbulent flow in, 291
    valvular incompetence, 291
Vein grafts, invagination of, 69
Vein patch, for vertebral surgery, 88
Vena cava, arteriovenous fistula with aorta, 234
Vena cava, inferior
    approach to, 327
    exposure of, 52, 327
    injuries to, 224–226
        during operation on abdominal aorta, 233
    interruption of, 325, 327–330
        complications, 333
        extraluminal, 327
        indications for, 325
        intraluminal, 329
        mortality rate, 333
        passage of clip, 328
        postoperative care, 332
        preoperative preparation, 326
        site of, 325
        type of, 326
        umbrella technique, 329, 330
Vena cava, suprarenal, injuries to, 225
Venous insufficiency, 260
Venous obstruction, intermittent, 269

Venous pressure, ambulatory, 260
Venous thrombectomy, 318–324
    postoperative care, 324
    preoperative care, 318
Venous thrombosis (*see also* Deep vein thrombosis),
    acute, 269
Venous ulcers, 301–309
    diagnosis, 301
    hypertension and, 302
    infection and, 302
    ischaemic element, 302
    in post-thrombotic syndrome, 301, 302, 309
    prevention of recurrence, 309
    stasis in, 302
    treatment of, 302
        basic principles, 302
        cleansing, 303
        concomitant injections, 309
        debridement, 303
        dressings, 304, 305
        glycerin and ichthyol, 307
        medicated bandage, 308
        pinch grafts in, 307
        providone-iodine in, 306
        sulphadiazine cream in, 306

Vertebral artery
    anastomosis
        with carotid artery, 90
        with subclavian artery, 89
    aneurysms, 212
    exposure of, 86
    herniation, 84, 91
    occlusive disease, 84
        indications for operation, 83
        operations for, 82–91
        postoperative care, 91
        preoperative considerations, 83
        preoperative preparation, 84
        transposition for, 90
    origin of, exposure of, 40
    stenosis, 83
        transposition for, 90
        transposition of, 90
    vein patch for, 88
Vertebrobasilar insufficiency, 13
Visceral artery, aneurysms, 212
Vocal cord paralysis, following carotid endarterectomy, 81